COGNITIVE-BEHAVIORAL TREATMENT
OF PERFECTIONISM

Cognitive-Behavioral Treatment of Perfectionism

SARAH J. EGAN

TRACEY D. WADE

ROZ SHAFRAN

MARTIN M. ANTONY

THE GUILFORD PRESS
New York   London

Library of Congress Cataloging-in-Publication Data

Egan, Sarah, author.
  Cognitive-behavioral treatment of perfectionism / Sarah J. Egan, Tracey D. Wade,
Roz Shafran, Martin M. Antony.
       p. ; cm.
  Includes bibliographical references and index.
  ISBN 978-1-4625-1698-8 (hardcover : alk. paper)
  I. Wade, Tracey, author. II. Shafran, Roz, author. III. Antony, Martin M., author.
IV. Title.
  [DNLM: 1. Obsessive-Compulsive Disorder—psychology. 2. Obsessive-Compulsive
Disorder—therapy. 3. Achievement. 4. Cognitive Therapy—methods. 5. Evidence-
Based Practice. 6. Self Concept. WM 176]
  RC533
  616.85′227—dc23
                                                                    2014020241

About the Authors

Sarah J. Egan, PhD, is a senior research fellow and previous Director of Clinical Psychology in the School of Psychology at Curtin University in Perth, Western Australia. She has worked as a clinician for over 15 years. Her primary research interest is cognitive-behavioral therapy (CBT) for clinical perfectionism; she also publishes in the areas of obsessive–compulsive disorder and eating disorders. The recipient of awards for her teaching and high-impact publications, Dr. Egan serves on the editorial board of *Stress and Health* and is chair of the organizing committee of the World Congress of Behavioral and Cognitive Therapies. She has presented numerous workshops and papers on CBT for clinical perfectionism and has over 40 publications in peer-reviewed journals.

Tracey D. Wade, PhD, is Professor and Dean of the School of Psychology at Flinders University in Adelaide, South Australia. She has worked as a clinician in the area of eating disorders for over 20 years. Her research interests are in the etiology, prevention, and treatment of eating disorders. Dr. Wade is Editor-in-Chief of the Australian Psychological Society (APS) journal *Clinical Psychologist* and is a member of the Steering Committee of the National Eating Disorder Collaboration in Australia. She is a recipient of the Ian M. Campbell Memorial Prize and of the Early Career Award, both from the APS, and has published more than 130 peer-reviewed scientific articles.

Roz Shafran, PhD, is Professor of Translational Psychology at the Institute of Child Health, University College London, United Kingdom. She is the founder and former director of the Charlie Waller Institute of Evidence-Based Psychological Treatment, Associate Editor of *Behaviour Research and Therapy*, and scientific co-chair of the British Association of Behavioural and Cognitive Psychotherapies. Dr. Shafran's clinical research interests include cognitive-behavioral theories of and treatments for eating disorders, obsessive–compulsive disorder, and perfectionism across the age range. She is a recipient of the Award for Distinguished Contributions to Professional Psychology from the British Psychological Society and the Marsh Award for Mental Health Work from Rethink Mental Illness. With more than 100 peer-reviewed scientific publications, Dr. Shafran is coauthor (with Sarah Egan and Tracey D. Wade) of the self-help guide *Overcoming Perfectionism*.

Martin M. Antony, PhD, ABPP, is Professor in the Department of Psychology at Ryerson University in Toronto, Ontario, Canada, where he was founding Graduate Program Director for the MA and PhD programs in psychology. He is also Director of Research at the Anxiety Treatment and Research Centre at St. Joseph's Healthcare Hamilton. Dr. Antony has received career awards from the Society of Clinical Psychology (Division 12 of the American Psychological Association), the Canadian Psychological Association (CPA), and the Anxiety and Depression Association of America. He is a Fellow of the Royal Society of Canada and the American and Canadian Psychological Associations, and a past president of the CPA. He has published 200 scientific articles and book chapters and numerous books, including *Handbook of Assessment and Treatment Planning for Psychological Disorders, Second Edition,* and *The Anti-Anxiety Workbook*.

Preface

Perfectionism is often thought to be a positive characteristic, involving striving to achieve high standards without experiencing negative consequences. However, in this book we focus on aspects of perfectionism that often are associated with negative consequences, such as anxiety, depression, and eating disorders. Therapists see perfectionism occurring in many of their clients—for example, the client with obsessive–compulsive disorder who has to perform her rituals in a perfect manner, and feels compelled to repeat them because she has not completed them in the "right way"; the client with social anxiety who has rigid rules about speaking perfectly in social situations, and who avoids these situations because he fears falling short of his standards; the young woman with an eating disorder who despite excelling in her academic and sporting goals, feels that she is never good enough, constantly strives to achieve a perfect weight and shape, and self-harms when she feels she has let herself or others down.

This book is appropriate for clinicians from a range of professions, and will be useful for the beginning-level clinician (including those enrolled in graduate training programs) as well as clinicians with many years of experience. Most practitioners work with clients for whom perfectionism is a large part of the presenting problem.

We focus in this book particularly on a model of "clinical perfectionism" that guides our therapeutic work. This model describes people who set extremely high standards for performance, are very concerned over making mistakes, and base self-evaluation on how well these standards are met. This judgment of self-worth on the basis of achievement is seen as a critical component of the maintenance of unhelpful perfectionism, since it causes people to persist in striving to meet their standards despite adverse consequences. Such overevaluation of striving and achievement is the basis of the collaborative conceptualization that forms the cornerstone of the cognitive-behavioral treatment of perfectionism outlined in this book. This treatment is supported by data and has been found not only to reduce perfectionism, but also to reduce a range of psychopathology, including anxiety, depression, and eating disorders. As such, the approach we outline in this book is appropriate for many clients seen in clinical practice for a range of disorders who have elevated perfectionism.

In this book we provide detailed suggestions for assessing perfectionism in your client in such a way that enhances therapeutic alliance. We describe the assessment of key maintenance factors of perfectionism, such as repeatedly setting high standards regardless of success or failure, repeated checking of performance, and cognitive biases such as dichotomous thinking and selective attention. Our approach uses a collaborative formulation as the roadmap to guide the conduct of the various treatment strategies described in this book. One of the important areas we focus on is how to develop and maintain a good working relationship with your client, and we describe how this can be challenging at times owing to the nature of perfectionism. In each chapter where we describe treatment, we pay attention to roadblocks and issues in therapy that may interfere with client engagement, and provide practical strategies for looking out for and addressing these issues with your client. The chapters describe a range of treatment strategies including self-monitoring (Chapter 9), cognitive strategies (Chapters 10 and 11), behavioral experiments (Chapter 12), strategies for reducing self-criticism (Chapter 13), tools to decrease procrastination and difficulties in time management (Chapter 14), and ways to prevent relapse (Chapter 15).

This book was written by busy clinicians for busy clinicians who need practical tools for working with clients. It includes many case studies as well as guides to other clinical resources (e.g., self-help books, referral sources, and copies of numerous perfectionism questionnaires). The book has many features to help the busy clinician easily navigate the contents, including tables, figures, troubleshooting boxes, and bulleted lists.

In summary, this book offers a framework for the cognitive-behavioral treatment of perfectionism. We believe that you take a deliberate, non-perfectionistic approach to providing treatment! We suggest if you model flexibility for your clients in working through the treatment, you will help them develop and become confident in using a range of skills that can allow them to enjoy the pursuit of their goals and dreams.

Contents

Purchasers can download and print
larger versions of the handouts
and self-report measures from
www.guilford.com/egan-forms.

COGNITIVE-BEHAVIORAL TREATMENT
OF PERFECTIONISM

CHAPTER 1

Nature and Causes of Perfectionism

What is perfectionism? As we will discuss shortly, there is no universally agreed-upon definition of the term, and even experts define it in different ways. For the purpose of this book, we focus on *dysfunctional perfectionism*—a tendency to hold excessively high standards associated with clinically significant distress or impairment. Some examples include:

- A woman who struggles to be a perfect parent, a perfect wife, and a perfect employee, often to the detriment of her own emotional and physical health.
- A graphic artist who constantly seeks reassurance that his work is of the highest quality, and that he is well respected and well liked by others.
- A student who constantly strives to meet excessively high academic standards and who is devastated when she receives a grade that is less than perfect.
- An individual who spends hours planning every aspect of every day and who becomes very distressed when things don't go according to his plans.

This guide assumes that perfectionism is a transdiagnostic process occurring across a wide range of disorders, including anxiety and related disorders, eating disorders, and depression, to name a few (Egan, Wade, & Shafran, 2011). It is generally assumed that perfectionism is a dimensional construct that can vary in severity from low to high, and recent evidence confirms this notion (Broman-Fulks, Hill, & Green, 2008). In other words, perfectionism is not something that people either *have* or *don't have*. Rather, it is something that we all experience to varying degrees.

This book provides an evidence-based framework for the psychological treatment of clinical perfectionism. It was written with the therapist in mind and is filled with summary tables, troubleshooting boxes, bulleted lists, forms, and various other resources that busy clinicians need to have at their fingertips. This guide takes a nonprescriptive approach, supporting the clinician's work within an individualized and collaborative case conceptualization framework.

This first chapter provides an introduction to the construct of perfectionism, including definitions, descriptive features, and etiology. The next three chapters review research concerning both the treatment of perfectionism (Chapter 2) and the relationship between perfectionism and various forms of psychopathology (Chapters 3 and 4). Next, the book discusses assessment of perfectionism (Chapter 5) and issues related to treatment planning (Chapter 6). The remainder of the book focuses on treatment, including cognitive-behavioral case formulation (Chapter 7); strategies for enhancing engagement in therapy, including the importance of developing a good therapeutic alliance (Chapter 8); self-monitoring (Chapter 9); cognitive strategies (Chapters 10 and 11); behavioral experiments (Chapter 12); tools for dealing with self-criticism (Chapter 13); strategies for dealing with procrastination and poor time management (Chapter 14); and methods for preventing relapse (Chapter 15). Chapter 16 provides a review of emerging treatments, including interventions for children and adolescents, and techniques involving imagery. The book also includes appendices containing a wide range of clinical resources and tools (e.g., self-help books, referral sources, handouts, and questionnaires).

This book is appropriate for clinicians from across disciplines and professions, and will be helpful to both students and seasoned therapists alike. We recommend that you use the book in the way that best serves your needs. Some therapists (e.g., those who are new to the treatment of perfectionism) may choose to read the entire book from cover to cover. Other therapists may find it most helpful to read particular chapters or sections, depending on what they are hoping to get out of this guide.

Definitions of Perfectionism

There are many different ideas about what perfectionism is and whether it is a good or bad thing, among our clients, the general public, and experts in the field. Oxford Dictionaries online defines perfectionism as the "refusal to accept any standard short of perfection" (Oxford Dictionaries, 2013). In an early psychological definition, English and English (1958) defined perfectionism similarly, as "the practice of demanding of oneself or others a higher quality of performance than is required by the situation" (Hollender, 1965, p. 94). Both of these are examples of *unidimensional* definitions, and a number of other unidimensional definitions have been proposed over the years.

Clinicians have tended to define perfectionism in terms of its negative impact. For example, in his classic *Psychology Today* article, "The

Perfectionist's Script for Self-Defeat," David Burns (1980) provided an early definition of pathological perfectionism, distinguishing *perfectionism* from the *healthy pursuit of excellence*. He defined perfectionists as "those whose standards are high beyond reach or reason, people whose strain compulsively and unremittingly toward impossible goals and who measure their own worth entirely in terms of productivity and accomplishment (p. 34). Similarly, the Obsessive Compulsive Cognitions Working Group (OCCWG) defined perfectionism in the context of obsessive–compulsive disorder (OCD) as "the tendency to believe there is a perfect solution to every problem, that doing everything perfectly (i.e., mistake-free) is not only possible, but also necessary, and that even minor mistakes will have serious consequences" (1997, p. 678).

Definitions of perfectionism all share the assumption that perfectionists hold elevated standards. However, definitions also differ in important ways. The definitions by Burns (1980) and the OCCWG (1997) focus on *pathological* or *problematic* forms of perfectionism, in which self-worth is contingent on meeting one's high standards, and in which perfectionism has negative consequences (e.g., functional impairment) for the individual. Implicit in these definitions is that pathologically perfectionistic standards are *rigid*, that is, individuals do not adjust their standards when they are unmet. In contrast to these clinically oriented definitions, neither the Oxford Dictionaries online definition of perfectionism nor English and English's (1958) definition assumes that perfectionism is necessarily a problem. For example, some very successful individuals (e.g., film director James Cameron, business magnate and television personality Martha Stewart) are self-described "perfectionists" (Antony & Swinson, 2009). Of course, it is likely that the clients seeking treatment for perfectionism and related problems are experiencing clinically oriented perfectionism, rather than a healthy pursuit of excellence.

In contrast to the unidimensional definitions reviewed earlier, other authors have suggested that perfectionism is a multidimensional construct, though there is wide disagreement regarding the number of dimensions and what the core dimensions are. The two most influential multidimensional models are those of Hewitt and Flett (1991b) and Frost, Marten, Lahart, and Rosenblate (1990). Each of these is described below, followed by descriptions of other multidimensional approaches. An understanding of the different definitions of perfectionism provides a framework with which to recognize the different forms that it may take, when it requires an intervention, and how it should best be assessed.

Hewitt and Flett's Multidimensional Model

Hewitt and Flett (1991b) define perfectionism along three dimensions: (1) *self-oriented perfectionism* (SOP; a tendency to set demanding standards for oneself and to stringently evaluate and criticize one's own behavior);

(2) *other-oriented perfectionism* (OOP; the tendency to set demanding standards for others and to stringently evaluate and criticize the behavior of others); and (3) *socially prescribed perfectionism* (SPP; the belief that significant others have unrealistic expectations, and that it is important to meet the high standards of others). Hewitt and Flett (1991b) published an initial validation study on their *Multidimensional Perfectionism Scale* (HMPS), which, along with subsequent studies, generally supported their tripartite model of perfectionism.

Frost et al.'s Multidimensional Model

Frost, Marten, Lahart, and Rosenblate (1990) defined perfectionism along six dimensions: (1) *concern over mistakes* (CM; excessive anxiety over making mistakes, in which any minor flaw is considered to represent failure); (2) *doubts about actions* (DA; doubts about the quality of one's work); (3) *personal standards* (PS; a tendency to have excessively high standards for one's own performance); (4) *parental expectations* (PE; the belief that one's parents set standards that one could not meet); (5) *parental criticism* (PC; the belief that one's parents were overly critical in response to unmet standards); and (6) *organization* (O; a tendency to overemphasize precision, order, and organization). On the surface, some dimensions (e.g., CM, DA, PS, O) appear to measure *aspects or features* of perfectionism, whereas others (e.g., PE, PC) appear to measure *causes or correlates* of perfectionism. In addition, whereas four of these dimensions (CM, DA, PC, PE) appear to be elevated in people with various forms of psychopathology, such as anxiety disorders and depression, the PS and O dimensions are typically not (though PS is elevated in people with eating disorders).

Frost et al. (1990) published an initial validation study on their *Multidimensional Perfectionism Scale* (FMPS), and there have been several subsequent studies evaluating the scale and the six-factor model underlying it. As reviewed in Chapter 6, findings suggest that O is distinct from the other dimensions of perfectionism (e.g., Frost et al., 1990), and that some of Frost et al.'s dimensions appear to be redundant. For example, items measuring PE and PC tend to load together in factor analytic studies, as do items measuring CM and DA (for a review, see Hawkins, Watt, & Sinclair, 2006).

Positive and Negative Perfectionism

There is a long tradition in the literature of distinguishing between positive and negative forms of perfectionism. For example, more than three decades ago, Hamacheck (1978) distinguished between *normal* and *neurotic* perfectionism, where a main difference between the two forms was the extent to which high standards are flexible (with normal perfectionists being more likely to allow for minor errors in their performance, relative to neurotic perfectionists). Early on, dysfunctional perfectionism was described as the "tyranny of the shoulds" (Horney, 1950). A few years later, Hollender (1965) painted the following clinical picture of perfectionism:

> The perfectionist finds it difficult to sort out items in the order of their importance or to maintain a sense of proportion. A small detail that has been missed may deprive him of gratification from a job otherwise well done. He is constantly on the alert for what is wrong and seldom focuses on what is right. He looks so intently for defects or flaws that he lives his life as though he were an inspector at the end of a production line. (p. 95)

Perhaps the most succinct description is that given by Albert Ellis, which we share with our clients with whom we have a good relationship. He simply called it "musterbation" (Ellis & Harper, 1961).

More recently, researchers have attempted to verify these two forms of perfectionism empirically. In perhaps the earliest of these studies, undergraduate students completed both the FMPS (Frost et al., 1990) and the HMPS (Hewitt & Flett, 1991b) and their responses on all nine subscales from the two measures were factor analyzed (Frost, Heimberg, Holt, Mattia, & Neubauer, 1993). Two higher-order dimensions were identified. The first of these, referred to as *Maladaptive Evaluative Concerns*, was comprised of items from Frost et al.'s CM, DA, PE, and PC subscales and Hewitt & Flett's SP subscale, whereas the second factor, referred to as *Positive Achievement Striving*, included PS and O from Frost et al.'s measure and SOP and OOP from Hewitt and Flett's measure. Whereas maladaptive evaluation concerns were found to be positively correlated with depression and negative affect (but not positive affect), positive achievement strivings were found to be related to positive affect (but not depression or negative affect) (Frost et al., 1993).

A number of subsequent studies have confirmed these findings, supporting the notion of both positive and negative forms of perfectionism, based on the FMPS and HMPS scales (e.g., Bieling, Israeli, & Antony, 2004). In addition, there have been a number of theoretical and empirical papers exploring the notion of positive (i.e., adaptive, healthy, normal) and negative (i.e., maladaptive, unhealthy, neurotic, clinical) forms of perfectionism based on other measures (e.g., Hill et al., 2004; Owens & Slade, 2008; Rice & Ashby, 2007; Terry-Short, Owens, Slade, & Dewey, 1995). For the most part, research supports the distinction between positive and negative perfectionism. For example, several studies suggest that constructs such as maladaptive evaluative concerns and dysfunctional perfectionism are more strongly related to mental health problems (e.g., obsessive–compulsive symptoms, depression, anxiety, suicidality, shame, guilt) than are constructs such as positive striving and adaptive perfectionism (e.g., Bieling et al., 2004; DiBartolo, Li, & Frost, 2008; Klibert, Langhinrichsen-Rohling, & Saito, 2005; Rhéaume et al., 2000). Of course, it is maladaptive perfectionism that is most likely to bring clients into treatment.

Dysfunctional Perfectionism

Although our clients are unlikely to want a tutorial on the various different definitions of perfectionism, it is important for the therapist to offer them a working definition of unhelpful perfectionism that will be the focus of therapy. In this book, we focus on the type of perfectionism that results in psychopathology, referred to as *dysfunctional perfectionism.*

In their paper on perfectionism, Shafran, Cooper, and Fairburn (2002) argued that it is unhelpful and confusing to use the term *perfectionism* to refer to both the healthy pursuit of excellence and the dysfunctional high standards often seen in clinical samples. They focused on one aspect of perfectionism that was often seen in the clinic. This specific form of perfectionism was termed *clinical perfectionism* and defined as "the overdependence of self-evaluation on the determined pursuit of personally demanding, self-imposed standards in at least one highly salient domain, despite adverse consequences" (Shafran et al., 2002, p. 778). According to Shafran and colleagues, the adverse consequences of clinical perfectionism may be emotional (e.g., anxiety), social (e.g., lack of social support), physical (e.g., poor nutrition from excessive dieting), cognitive (e.g., poor concentration), or behavioral (e.g., procrastination). That is not to say that they did not recognize other forms of perfectionism to be of clinical relevance, for example, it can be highly disabling to have high expectations of others that are not met, and the belief that others have high standards will also be associated with anxiety. They argued, however, that it was important for the development of effective treatment to have a narrow focus on the sort of perfectionism that is routinely seen in the clinic.

Furthermore, Shafran et al. (2002) argued that several of the constructs typically considered dimensions of perfectionism (e.g., other-oriented perfectionism, socially prescribed perfectionism, concern over mistakes, doubts about actions, parental expectations, parental criticism) are actually associated features of perfectionism but are not the core construct itself, as described in their definition. The paper by Shafran et al. (2002) generated a number of responses and considerable scholarly debate (e.g., Dunkley, Blankstein, Masheb, & Grilo, 2006; Hewitt, Flett, Besser, Sherry, & McGee, 2003; Shafran, Cooper, & Fairburn, 2003). For example, Hewitt et al. (2003) disagreed with Shafran et al.'s (2002) view that perfectionism is unidimensional, and with their definition of clinical perfectionism (e.g., their failure to incorporate interpersonal aspects into their definition). The debate regarding the definition, boundaries, and dimensionality of perfectionism is far from over, and has been a source of confusion and disagreement in the literature for as long as perfectionism has been a topic of study.

Of course, this book is focused on the *treatment* of perfectionism and is therefore concerned primarily with its dysfunctional aspects. The definition and model of clinical perfectionism that forms the basis for the treatment outlined in this book, explained in more detail in Chapter 7, is supported by the ways in which perfectionists often describe their symptoms. For example, in an effort to further understand the phenomenon of clinical perfectionism, Riley and Shafran (2005) interviewed 15 individuals who were identified as being high in clinical perfectionism and 6 individuals identified as low in clinical perfectionism. To be considered high in clinical perfectionism, participants had to endorse three core features of clinical perfectionism identified by the authors: (1) self-imposed dysfunctional standards, (2) continual striving to reach goals, and (3) significant adverse consequences resulting from continual striving for perfection. Among those who were low in clinical perfectionism, none endorsed dysfunctional standards or significant adverse consequences, though two-thirds endorsed continual striving to reach their goals. Commonly endorsed mechanisms for the maintenance of high perfectionism included self-critical reactions to failure, cognitive biases, rules and rigidity, positive emotional reactions to success, fear-driven motivation for achieving, and safety behaviors. Positive emotional reactions to success were also common among those who were deemed low in clinical perfectionism, whereas the other mechanisms were endorsed infrequently in this group. This study provides a rich description of clinical perfectionism that therapists can use when assessing and treating their clients.

There is another sense in which dysfunctional perfectionism can present in the clinic, and that is the perfectionism that is often seen in obsessive–compulsive personality disorder (OCPD). According to the *Diagnostic and Statistical Manual of Mental Disorders* (DSM-5; American Psychiatric Association, 2013), the critical nature of OCD involves being overly concerned with perfectionism, order, and control, which leads to the person becoming inefficient in completing tasks and having a lack of personal flexibility and openness. Here, perfectionism is not so much about having excessively *high* standards, but rather about having *arbitrary* standards (attention to rules, unimportant details, order, etc.) that are excessively rigid. Although this form of perfectionism can be clinically impairing and affect a wide range of life domains (e.g., work, relationships), it appears to be quite different from the perfectionism that is often seen in other forms of psychopathology (e.g., as reviewed earlier, elevated attention to organization is not correlated with other forms of perfectionism as measured on the FMPS; Frost et al., 1990).

Causes of Perfectionism

Little is known about the etiology and development of perfectionism. However, if we assume that perfectionism develops in the same ways as related forms of psychopathology, then it makes sense to turn to some of the same factors that are known to contribute to associated problems, such as anxiety and depression, where it is well established that both biological (e.g., genetics) and psychological (e.g., learning) factors play a role.

Interpersonal Influences

Most studies examining the role of interpersonal influences on perfectionism have focused on the role of parents, though virtually all studies have been correlational, and many do not include assessments of the parents themselves, instead relying on participants' impressions of their parents' behavior. For example, Enns, Cox, and Clara (2002) found that although harsh parenting (the perceived tendency for one's parents to make critical comments about the individual) and perfectionistic parenting (the perceived tendency for one's parents to have high personal standards for themselves) were both predictive of maladaptive perfectionism, only perfectionistic parenting (and not harsh parenting) was associated with adaptive perfectionism. Another study found that perceived harsh and authoritarian parenting styles were related to maladaptive, but not adaptive, components of perfectionism, in both European American men and women and Asian American women (Kawamura, Frost, & Harmatz, 2002). Although specific findings vary across studies, there is considerable evidence that perceived parenting behaviors (e.g., parental criticism, parental perfectionism) are correlated with perfectionism (e.g., Clark & Coker, 2009; Cook & Kearney, 2009; Frost, Lahart, & Rosenblate, 1991). There is also emerging evidence that adaptive perfectionists report having more balanced, cohesive, and adaptable families with nurturing parents, relative to both maladaptive perfectionists and nonperfectionists (DiPrima, Ashby, Gnilka, & Noble, 2011). Many clients report that they have always been perfectionists, or that they were driven to achieve by demanding parents. Awareness of these research findings can help the therapist to answer questions about the associations between perfectionism in parents and their children.

A small number of studies have examined the influence on perfectionism of interpersonal factors other than those stemming from parents and families. For example, one study examined the relationship between retrospective recall of emotional abuse by peers during childhood and perfectionism in adulthood (Miller & Vaillancourt, 2007). In this study, a history of perceived *indirect* peer victimization (e.g., excluding individuals from activities, gossiping, spreading rumors) was predictive of self-oriented and socially prescribed perfectionism in adults, whereas no relationship with perfectionism was found for a history of more *direct* forms of aggression (e.g., physical aggression, verbal aggression).

Learning Factors

Slade and Owens (1998) suggest that perfectionism is shaped by social contingencies, and that these contingencies may shift over time from an initial focus on positive contingencies (e.g., rewards for meeting high standards) to a focus on more negative reinforcement (negative consequences for failing to be perfect). For example, an individual who is successful at work may initially be motivated to achieve simply for the positive consequences (e.g., feelings of success, raises, promotions) but over time may become more concerned about letting people down if his or her performance starts to worsen. It is also possible that perfectionism is initially reinforcing, and that only later do its effects begin to turn negative, as various negative consequences (e.g., fatigue, falling behind on tasks, anxiety) start to occur (Shafran & Mansell, 2001). There is also evidence that when perfectionists do meet a particular standard, they respond by raising the standard (Kobori, Hayakawa, & Tanno, 2009).

Experimental research on the role of learning in the development of perfectionism is lacking, though learning (e.g., operant conditioning, classical conditioning, modeling) may help to explain the relationship between parenting styles and perfectionism, as reviewed earlier. In addition, there is considerable evidence that learning plays a role in the development of problems that are often associated with perfectionism (e.g., anxiety disorders; Craske, Hermans, & Vansteenwegen, 2006).

Genetic Factors

Very little is known about the relationship between biology and perfectionism, though emerging research with twins suggests that genetics may play a role. A twin study examining the heritability of perfectionism found that concordance rates were consistently higher for monozygotic twins than for dizygotic twins for three types of perfectionism measured by the FMPS: CM, DA, and PS (Tozzi et al., 2004). Furthermore, there was evidence that PS and CM (but not DA) shared some common genetic factors whereas DA and CM shared some common environmental factors (Tozzi et al., 2004). A more recent twin study found that anxiety and maladaptive perfectionism were both moderately heritable (heritability estimates ranging from .45 to .66), and that genetic factors mostly accounted for the relationship between anxiety and maladaptive perfectionism (Moser, Slane, Burt, & Klump, 2012). Although there is extensive research on the role of genetics in disorders associated with perfectionism (e.g., anxiety disorders, eating disorders, depression), more research is needed to better understand the ways in which genetics and environment interact in the development of perfectionism.

CHAPTER 2

Research on the Treatment of Perfectionism

Given the relatively new arrival of treatments for perfectionism, there are comparatively few efficacy or effectiveness studies compared to the wealth of literature examining cognitive-behavioral treatments of anxiety disorders, eating disorders, and depression. Thus we considered that it would be useful to summarize the studies in this chapter in order to provide an informed foundation from which practitioners can feel more comfortable about trying this treatment in their own practice. We hope this chapter will soon become outdated in the face of an avalanche of studies that evaluate the treatment of perfectionism! There is a growing body of evidence attesting to the efficacy of cognitive-behavioral therapy (CBT) for perfectionism (Egan, Wade, et al., 2011).

Review of the Evidence for the Efficacy of CBT for Perfectionism

In the literature to date, the evidence for treatment of perfectionism has been restricted to studies investigating the efficacy of CBT. Psychodynamic approaches to treatment of perfectionism have been described in the literature, but no data on their efficacy have been reported. Fredtoft, Poulsen, Bauer, and Malm (1996) reported on a group object relations approach to treating perfectionism in university students. The treatment encouraged free-floating discussion by attending to comments regarding perfectionism and dependency and using the group process to resolve conflicts; however no data were presented on efficacy. Sorotzkin (1998) reported treating perfectionism in religious adolescents in a descriptive study. Therapeutic techniques were not defined in the study, and no data were reported. Greenspon

(2008) also reported on use of a psychodynamic approach to explore one client's beliefs regarding the origins of her perfectionism and presented a case description of psychodynamic treatment, although no data were reported on outcomes. Therefore, despite arguments that perfectionism is a personality trait and as such necessitates longer-term treatment, such as psychodynamic psychotherapy (e.g., Blatt, Quinlan, Pilkonis, & Shea, 1995), there is no empirical support to date for the use of psychodynamic treatment to reduce perfectionism. Thus our review of treatment efficacy focuses on cognitive-behavioral treatment of perfectionism. We will look first at studies using nonclinical samples, and then at studies of clinical populations.

Nonclinical Samples

In the first study of cognitive therapy for perfectionism, DiBartolo, Dixon, Almodovar, and Frost (2001) investigated the use of brief cognitive restructuring compared to distraction for a public speaking task in an experimental design with 60 undergraduate university women. The participants were divided into those who scored high and low on CM on the FMPS (Frost et al., 1990). The 8-minute session of cognitive restructuring was more effective than distraction in reducing anxiety in both groups, although those high on CM reported being significantly more anxious about the public speaking task. Although the study provides some evidence for cognitive restructuring in reducing distress in perfectionists, results cannot be generalized to clinical practice, given the unrealistic nature of a short intervention in a nonclinical group (and the lack of follow-up).

In another experimental study with a nonclinical group, Shafran, Lee, Payne, and Fairburn (2006) found that performing a manipulation of personal standards resulted in changes in eating attitudes and behaviors. The community sample of women were randomly assigned to a condition of either high personal standards ($n = 18$) or low personal standards ($n = 23$) and were asked to sign a contract to guide their behavior over the next 24-hour period. The participants in the high personal standards condition were instructed to do everything to the "highest possible standard," whereas in the low personal standards condition the word *highest* was replaced with *minimal*. Examples of behavior assigned to the high personal standards group included the following: work very hard, do everything to the best of your ability, get in early to work and leave late, prepare a "to-do" list and ensure everything is completed. Conversely, the low personal standards group was instructed to take it easy at work, to leave work either on time or early, and to do activities at work such as surfing the Internet. After the 24-hour manipulation, the participants in the high personal standards condition were found to eat have eaten fewer high-calorie foods, engaged in more dietary restriction in terms of overall caloric intake, and reported higher regret after eating than those in the low personal standards condition. Although this study is not a direct test of treatment of perfectionism, it does provide evidence that manipulating standards of performance can have a detrimental impact on eating attitudes and behaviors. This suggests that it would be useful to target a reduction in personal standards, particularly in people who may be struggling with disordered eating. This is an important concept we will outline in Chapter 3: high personal standards are linked with eating disorders.

In a direct evaluation of the efficacy of CBT for perfectionism in a nonclinical sample, Pleva and Wade (2007) randomly allocated participants to either a guided self-help (*n* = 24) or pure self-help (*n* = 25) treatment based on the book *When Perfect Isn't Good Enough* (Antony & Swinson, 2009). The guided self-help group received eight weekly 50-minute sessions with a postgraduate student to help the participant work through the strategies outlined in the book, whereas the pure self-help group was given the book and a detailed information sheet outlining which areas of the book to focus on each week. The book contains four parts that focus on (1) understanding perfectionism; (2) using strategies for overcoming perfectionism (e.g., cognitive therapy and exposure-based strategies for challenging the fear of making a mistake in front of other people); (3) applying strategies for overcoming perfectionism in the context of specific problems (e.g., anger, anxiety, depression, eating problems); and (4) relapse prevention. Pleva and Wade found that both forms of self-help were effective in producing clinically significant reductions in perfectionism and symptoms of anxiety and depression, although guided self-help was superior. Specifically, 30% of the sample reported clinically significant decreases in obsessionality and depression, and 15% experienced clinically significant decreases in anxiety. These results are encouraging with respect to the efficacy of CBT for perfectionism and the delivery of this treatment using a guided self-help format, but the proportion of people experiencing clinically significant benefits is likely to be lower in a clinical sample.

In a study examining a nonclinical sample, a brief psychoeducational intervention involving feedback on emotional reactivity, symptom distress, and self-esteem was assessed in individuals with clinical perfectionism (Aldea, Rice, Gormley, & Rojas, 2010). The participants were randomly allocated to receive feedback on their perfectionism using techniques adapted from the literature (Finn & Tonsager, 1992; Newman & Greenway, 1997), or to be in a control group where no feedback was received. Feedback involved the experimenter providing information about classification of the participant's perfectionism (i.e., adaptive or maladaptive perfectionism) based on self-report measures and discussion of the results and of participants' emotional reaction to the information. Participants in the feedback condition reported significant reductions in symptoms and emotional reactivity. While not providing any direct evidence for the efficacy of treatments for perfectionism, the results highlight the possibility that psychoeducation about perfectionism may be a useful component of treatment.

Finally, another study with a nonclinical sample investigated the efficacy of an online web-based 10-week CBT intervention for perfectionism in first-year undergraduate psychology students who were randomly allocated to either stress management (SM), SM+CBT, or a control condition (Arpin-Cribbie et al., 2008). Participants in the SM condition had significant decreases in SOP and CM posttreatment but no change in anxiety or depression. Participants in the SM+CBT condition, however, also reported decreases in SOP and CM as well as socially prescribed perfectionism and depression. A more recent study has further examined web-based CBT for perfectionism in college students and also found that the treatment resulted in significant decreases in anxiety, depression, and perfectionism (Radhu, Zafiris, Arpin-Cribbie, Irvine, & Ritvo, 2012). While the results of these studies are encouraging regarding the efficacy of web-based intervention for perfectionism, it is difficult to generalize these results to clinical groups given the use of nonclinical samples.

Mixed Clinical Samples of Anxiety Disorders, Depression, and Eating Disorders

There have been a number of studies reported in the literature regarding the efficacy of CBT for perfectionism in clinical groups with mixed samples of disorders including anxiety disorders, depression and eating disorders. The literature has included case studies, single-case experimental design, and randomized controlled trials.

Uncontrolled Case Studies and Single-Case Experimental Design Series

In an uncontrolled case study, Hirsch and Hayward (1998) reported on an individual with anxiety and depression whose symptoms were maintained by perfectionism. Adding specific techniques to target perfectionism to a standard CBT treatment for anxiety and depression resulted in a decrease in perfectionism and symptoms. While no conclusions can be made regarding treatment efficacy from this case study, it does suggest that treatment of perfectionism can be added to other CBT approaches without overwhelming or confusing the client.

A number of studies have examined CBT for perfectionism in mixed anxious and depressed clinical samples using single-case experimental design series. Ferguson and Rodway (1994) were the first to report on CBT for perfectionism evaluated in a single-case experimental design series. They concluded that treatment was effective, as it resulted in significant decreases in perfectionism. Unfortunately little can be concluded from this study, as there were no details of treatment content, no objective measures of perfectionism, and no detail regarding the length of baseline, and clinical significance was not reported.

In the first well-controlled single-case experimental design series using a multiple baseline design to evaluate CBT for perfectionism, Glover, Brown, Fairburn, and Shafran (2007) reported on treatment outcome in nine individuals with a diagnosis of either an anxiety disorder or depression. The participants received 10 sessions of CBT for perfectionism, with the first 6 sessions being conducted biweekly. The treatment protocol was based on the cognitive-behavioral model of clinical perfectionism (Shafran et al., 2010) and the transdiagnostic cognitive-behavioral model of eating disorders (Fairburn, Cooper, & Shafran, 2003b). The protocol was based on selecting appropriate treatment strategies to target the relevant maintaining factors of clinical perfectionism based on the individualized, collaborative cognitive-behavioral formulation of perfectionism. Treatment consisted of a range of cognitive and behavioral strategies, including behavioral experiments to target maintenance factors including self-criticism and cognitive biases, and involved broadening the clients' scheme for self-evaluation to be based on more than achievement.

The results indicated that six participants experienced clinically significant decreases in perfectionism on the FMPS (Frost et al., 1990), the HMPS (Hewitt & Flett, 1991b), and the *Clinical Perfectionism Questionnaire* (CPQ; Fairburn, Cooper, & Shafran, 2003a). While no significant reductions in anxiety were found, three participants experienced clinically significant reductions in depressive symptoms on the *Beck Depression Inventory–II* (BDI-II; Beck, Steer, & Brown, 1996). The results of this study are encouraging, as they indicate that CBT for perfectionism is effective in decreasing perfectionism and depressive symptoms in a clinical sample, but the impact on anxiety symptoms is less clear.

Egan and Hine (2008) aimed to improve on the methodology of the Glover et al. (2007) study, which did not have a stable baseline or record outcome measures weekly, in a sample of four individuals with elevated scores on the CM subscale of the FMPS (Frost et al., 1990) and a diagnosis of either an anxiety disorder or depression. The treatment involved eight sessions of CBT for clinical perfectionism, based on the cognitive-behavioral model of Shafran et al. (2002). The results indicated there were clinically significant reductions in the FMPS total score, indicating that the treatment was effective in producing decreases in perfectionism.

Controlled Studies

The first randomized controlled trial (RCT) to evaluate the efficacy of CBT for perfectionism evaluated the 10-session treatment described by Glover et al. (2007) in 20 individuals with anxiety or depression (Riley, Lee, Cooper, Fairburn, & Shafran, 2007). The participants were randomly allocated to either immediate or wait-list treatment. The results indicated significant reductions on measures of depression (BDI-II; Beck et al., 1996), anxiety (Beck Anxiety Inventory [BAI]; Beck, Epstein, Brown, & Steer, 1988), and general symptoms (Brief Symptom Inventory [BSI]; Derogatis & Melisaratos, 1983) that was maintained at 8-week follow-up. Furthermore, 15 participants experienced clinically significant reductions in perfectionism on an unpublished clinical perfectionism interview and the CPQ (Fairburn et al., 2003a). There were also significant reductions on both the FMPS (Frost et al., 1990) and the HMPS (Hewitt & Flett, 1991b), although there were no statistically significant differences between the treatment and wait-list control group. Riley et al. also found that the number of clients with symptoms meeting criteria for depression or an anxiety disorder was halved after treatment, compared to no change in diagnostic status in the wait-list control group. This study is important as it demonstrates the efficacy of CBT for perfectionism in a controlled study, where the treatment results in decreases in perfectionism, anxiety, and depression in a mixed clinical sample.

A recent RCT (Egan, van Noort, et al., 2014) of individual cognitive-behavioral therapy of 8 weeks duration based on Shafran et al. (2010) compared face-to-face individual CBT for perfectionism to an 8-week pure self-help version of treatment and waitlist control. There were 52 individuals with elevated perfectionism of above 25 on the CM subscale of the FMPS and a range of anxiety disorders, depression, and bulimia nervosa. Results indicated that face-to-face CBT for perfectionism was effective in significantly reducing perfectionism on the CM ($d = 1.23$) and PS ($d = 0.77$) subscales of the FMPS, and symptoms of depression, anxiety, and stress on the Depression Anxiety Stress Scales—21 item version (DASS-21; Lovibond & Lovibond, 1995) ($d = 0.89$). Face-to-face treatment was also effective in increasing self-esteem ($d = 0.97$). These gains were all maintained at 6-month follow-up and the changes were all of a large effect (CM; $d = 2.11$; PS; $d = 1.77$; DASS-21; d = 1.16; self-esteem; $d = 1.16$). The self-help treatment was effective in producing decreases in perfectionism on the FMPS, which were of a moderate effect size and maintained at 6-month follow-up (CM; $d = 0.73$; PS; $d = 0.74$) but did not have a significant effect on symptoms of anxiety or depression. Finally, treatment was found to reduce comorbidity, where 21% of the sample had comorbid psychological disorders at pretreatment and only 2% had comorbid diagnoses at 6-month follow-up, supporting the idea that perfectionism is transdiagnostic and treatment can reduce comorbidity (Egan, Wade, et al., 2011).

Another recent RCT by Hoiles, Egan, Rees, and Kane (2014) compared cognitive-behavioral guided self-help for clinical perfectionism using Shafran et al.'s (2010) book with an 8-week waitlist control in 40 participants with elevated perfectionism and a range of anxiety disorders, depression, and eating disorders. Significant reductions were found in perfectionism on the CM (d = 1.6) and PS (d = 1.16) subscales of the FMPS. There were also significant large effect size reductions (d = 1.31) found in self-criticism (SC) on the Dysfunctional Attitudes Scale (Weissman & Beck, 1978), which has been used as a measure of perfectionism as well as large effect size reductions in dichotomous thinking (DT) (d = 1.22). Furthermore, there were significant moderate effect size reduction decreases in depression (d = .63) and large effect size increases in quality of life at posttreatment (d =.87). All effects were maintained at 4-month follow-up. Pre–post treatment difference scores were used to assess the mediating effect of perfectionism and related constructs (CM, PS, SC, DT) on psychopathology (depression and quality of life). Perfectionism as measured by SC was found to fully mediate the impact of treatment on well-being (a combination of depression and quality-of -life scores).

Eating Disorders

There is a very robust association between perfectionism and eating disorders (Bardone-Cone et al., 2007) with perfectionism being a well-demonstrated risk and maintaining factor in a multitude of studies (Egan, Wade, et al., 2011). Clinical perfectionism is one of the four maintaining factors included in the transdiagnostic model of eating disorders (Fairburn et al., 2003b) on which enhanced CBT (CBT-E) for eating disorders is based, that has evidence of efficacy and also effectiveness in eating disorder clinics not involved in the development of CBT-E (Byrne, Fursland, Allen, & Watson, 2011; Fairburn et al., 2009).

Shafran, Lee, and Fairburn (2004) reported a case study of CBT for clinical perfectionism based on the clinical perfectionism treatment protocol described by Glover et al. (2007) in a female with clinical perfectionism and binge-eating disorder. The client received eight sessions of face-to-face therapy followed by two telephone sessions. Shafran et al. reported that depressive symptoms, number of bulimic episodes, and symptoms of binge-eating disorder markedly decreased, and this was maintained at 5-month follow-up. Furthermore the client's score on the CPQ (Fairburn et al., 2003a) was reduced after treatment. This study is interesting as it indicates that treatment of perfectionism was associated with decreases in binge-eating disorder, although generalizations cannot be made about efficacy of treatment from this paper, as it was a case study and extraneous variables can therefore not be ruled out as an explanation for the decreases.

However, a well-controlled RCT for treatment of perfectionism in bulimia nervosa was conducted by Steele and Wade (2008), who randomly allocated 42 clients with bulimia nervosa or eating disorder not otherwise specified (EDNOS) to one of three conditions; CBT for perfectionism, CBT for bulimia nervosa, and a "dismantled mindfulness" condition. The treatment was eight sessions of guided self-help over 6 weeks, and the CBT for perfectionism was based on the self-help guide of Antony and Swinson (2009). Results at 3-month follow-up indicated that there were no significant differences between groups. However, CBT for perfectionism also produced significant decreases of large effect size in anxiety, depression, self-esteem, and eating disorder psychopathology, in addition to improvements of small effect size for bulimic behavior. Consequently, this comparison of effect sizes between treatments showed that CBT for perfectionism was more effective at addressing the associated psychopathology of eating disorders, while at the same time still resulting in a significant reduction in bulimic symptoms.

Wilksch, Durbridge, and Wade (2008) conducted an RCT prevention trial for adolescent females at high risk of eating disorders, which was determined by a high score on shape and weight concerns. Participants were randomly allocated to one of three conditions: media literacy, CBT for perfectionism, or control. They found that the perfectionism program was more effective in the high-risk group in terms of decreasing eating disorder symptomatology as well as producing a significantly lower level of CM at 3-month follow-up. This study shows that perfectionism decreases as a result of treatment (i.e., it is not a fixed trait) and opens the possibility that eating disorder risk could potentially be ameliorated by targeting perfectionism, although longitudinal research is required to assess this hypothesis.

Efficacy of Group CBT for Perfectionism

The majority of studies evaluating CBT for perfectionism have been based on delivering the therapy in an individual format, and there has been a paucity of research examining the treatment applied in group format. Barrow and Moore (1983) provided a description of how to deliver CBT for perfectionism in a group context, though no data were reported on efficacy. Kutlesa and Arthur (2008) found that an eight-session CBT group for university students resulted in significant decreases in perfectionism, anxiety, and depression at posttreatment, compared to a control group. However, as this was a nonclinical sample, it is difficult to generalize results. Egan and Stout (2007) reported pilot data using a single-case experimental design series for eight-session group CBT for clinical perfectionism in participants diagnosed with either an anxiety disorder or depression, based on the protocol described in Egan and Hine (2008). The results indicated that there were downward trends in CM, PS, and total scores on the FMPS (Frost et al., 1990), although these changes were not clinically significant. Egan and Stout reported that there were also downward trends in anxiety scores on the BAI (Beck et al., 1988) and BDI-II (Beck et al., 1996), although these changes only reached clinical significance in one participant with depression. There were two participants, however, who changed diagnostic status, no longer meeting criteria for depression at posttreatment. Although these results suggest some efficacy of treatment, few generalizations can be made from the study as the sample size was very small (n = 3), and there was only a short follow-up period of 3 weeks posttreatment. There are only two studies that have reported on group CBT for clinical perfectionism with adequate sample sizes. In the first study, Steele et al. (2013) reported on the treatment of 21 participants across two sites who received an 8-week CBT group program using a structured protocol based on the CBT self-help book *Overcoming Perfectionism* (Shafran, Egan, & Wade, 2010). CBT for perfectionism is described in detail in this book, which is an extension of protocols described in the treatment studies we reviewed earlier by these authors, and many of the techniques we present in the following chapters are based on strategies described in the book. The participants had elevated perfectionism as defined by a score above 22 on the CM subscale of the FMPS (Frost et al., 1990), and the majority had at least one psychological disorder, with principal diagnoses including major depressive disorder, dysthymic disorder, social anxiety disorder, panic disorder, generalized anxiety disorder, and OCD. Of the seven participants who did not have a diagnosis, five had previously been diagnosed with major depressive disorder but were in remission. The participants received a 4-week wait-list period, which provided a no-treatment control condition, followed by a 4-week psychoeducation condition, where they read the first four chapters of Shafran et al. (2010) on a weekly basis, and then an 8-week treatment consisting of one 2-hour group session per week. The content of the group sessions was based on Chapters 5–10 of the book, which cover areas including motivation to change, cognitive restructuring, changing procrastination, behavioral experiments, problem solving, time management, self-compassion, broadening self-evaluation, and relapse prevention. There was no change in scores over the wait-list or psychoeducation periods, indicating that perfectionism and symptoms did not change over the control period, and that psychoeducation had no effect. There was a main effect, however, from baseline to posttreatment, with significant decreases in perfectionism measures, consisting of the CPQ (Fairburn et al., 2003a), the CM and PS subscales of the FMPS (Frost et al., 1990), and the self-criticism subscale of the *Dysfunctional Attitude Scale* (DAS; Weissman & Beck, 1978). There were also significant decreases between baseline and posttreatment in depression, anxiety, and stress, based on the DASS-21 (Lovibond & Lovibond, 1995). Treatment gains in the form of reduced perfectionism, depression, anxiety, and stress were maintained at 3-month follow-up. In the second study of group CBT for perfectionism, the same 8-week protocol as Steele et al. (2013) was used to examine efficacy of group treatment in an RCT (Handley, Egan, Kane, & Rees, 2014). There were 42 participants with elevated perfectionism of above 25 on the CM subscale of the FMPS and a range of anxiety disorders (e.g., GAD, social phobia, OCD), depression, and eating disorders, compared to a wait-list control. Participants receiving group CBT for perfectionism experienced significant reductions in perfectionism with large effects on the CM subscale of the FMPS ($d = 1.23$) as well as self-criticism ($d = 1.48$). The participants also experienced significant reductions in eating disorders of a small effect ($d = 0.30$), a significant reduction in depression of a medium effect ($d = 0.74$), a significant medium effect size reduction in anxiety on the DASS-21 ($d = 0.56$) and a significant large reduction in social anxiety ($d = 0.84$). All of these treatment gains were maintained at 6-month follow-up.

The results from Steele et al. (2013) and Handley et al. (2014) support the efficacy of CBT for perfectionism that has been found in previous trials (Egan & Hine, 2008; Egan, van Noort, et al., 2014; Glover et al., 2007; Hoiles et al., 2014; Riley et al., 2007; Steele & Wade, 2008). Despite evidence to date being largely based on trials of individual treatment, there are also emerging data supporting group treatment. Additional trials on group treatment for perfectionism are welcome because group CBT has practical advantages in terms of time and cost-effectiveness (Himle, Van Etten, & Fischer, 2003). Furthermore, Bieling, McCabe, and Antony (2006) have argued that group CBT can enhance the ability to change via interpersonal learning. The unique interpersonal challenges of group therapy, as well as the benefits (e.g., opportunities for modeling of nonperfectionistic behavior by group members during behavioral experiments) will be discussed further in Chapter 5.

Effect Sizes of CBT for Perfectionism

CBT for perfectionism has produced predominately large effects, according to Cohen's (1988) criteria. The treatment has been found to have large effects in reducing perfectionism as measured by CM ($d = 1.09$; Steele & Wade, 2008), ($d = 1.72$; Steele et al., 2013), ($d = 1.23$; Handley et al., 2014), ($d = 1.23$; Egan, van Noort, et al., 2014) and by the CPQ ($d = 1.31$; Riley et al., 2007), ($d = 1.55$; Steele et al., 2013). Large effects for perfectionism have also been found on the unpublished Clinical Perfectionism Examination ($d = 1.83$; Steele & Wade, 2008). CBT for perfectionism has been found to have large effects on self-criticism on the DAS ($d = 1.46$; Steele et al., 2013), ($d = 1.48$; Handley et al., 2014), ($d = 1.02$, Egan, van Noort et al., 2014). Furthermore, while some studies have shown a small effect for PS ($d = 0.39$; Steele & Wade, 2008), ($d = 0.44$; Wilksch et al., 2008), one has shown large effects ($d = 1.91$; Steele et al., 2013). Consequently, it can be concluded from the studies to date that CBT for perfectionism can result in clinically significant reductions in perfectionism according to criteria that define treatment effect sizes as an indication of clinical significance (Kraemer et al., 2003).

In terms of psychological symptomatology, CBT for perfectionism has also been associated with large effect sizes. Large effects have been found for depression (d = 0.86; Steele & Wade, 2008), (d = 1.42; Steele et al., 2013) and eating disorder symptomatology (d = 1.73; Steele & Wade, 2008). Treatment of perfectionism has also been found to result in large effects for stress (d = 1.20; Steele et al., 2013). In terms of effect sizes for anxiety, one study has found large effects (d = 1.11; Steele et al., 2013), while another two studies have found medium effect sizes (d = 0.69; Steele & Wade, 2008), (d = 0.56; Handley et al., 2014). Large effects have also been found for social anxiety (d = 0.84; Handley et al., 2013). Large effects have also been found for a combination of depression, anxiety and stress scores on the total DASS-21 at posttreatment (d = 0.89) and maintained at 6-month follow-up (d = 1.16) (Egan, van Noort, et al., 2014). Considering these findings as a whole, it could be concluded that CBT for perfectionism has mainly large effects in terms of reducing symptoms of eating disorders, depression, and anxiety. This finding of a large effect size in terms of reducing psychological symptoms is very interesting as the treatment does not target these symptoms directly. The fact that the treatment for perfectionism produces large effects in reducing symptoms of a range of disorders has been one of the key arguments as to why perfectionism could be considered a transdiagnostic process (Egan, Wade, et al., 2011). This argument will be further outlined in Chapter 4.

Future Areas of Consideration for Research on Treatment Efficacy

While the studies reviewed have shown promising results for CBT for perfectionism, we need more research to adequately determine the efficacy and effectiveness of treatment. First, several of the studies reviewed had small sample sizes and therefore inadequate power. Future research should examine treatment in larger samples. The studies reviewed are based on a mix of single-case experimental design series, open trials, and RCTs. There is an argument that research on treatment efficacy should move from small-case single-case design to open trials through to RCTs at a later stage of treatment evidence development (Salkovskis, 2002). Given that there is now evidence across the range of earlier, small-case design studies it is important that future treatment research move to larger-scale RCTs to examine efficacy. Furthermore, only one RCT to date has compared CBT for perfectionism to another active psychological treatment (Steele & Wade, 2008). It is important therefore that future RCTs include active treatment comparison in order to enable an assessment of efficacy. Finally, the studies reviewed have generally had what would be considered short follow-up of treatment effects (i.e., 3 or 6 months' duration). It is important to establish the efficacy of CBT for perfectionism by showing that the treatment effects are maintained at longer follow-up of at least 12 up to 18 months. Finally future research should also attend to determining the *effectiveness* of CBT for perfectionism, rather than just the *efficacy* of the treatment. Efficacy research generally refers to those studies where a treatment effect is found by the researchers who developed the treatment in the center where it was developed. Effectiveness studies, however, require that the treatment be examined in multiple centers that were not involved in its development and in regular outpatient mental health services with the treatment being delivered by individuals who are not experts in it. Given that the majority of studies to date on CBT for perfectionism have been efficacy studies, it is crucial that future effectiveness research be conducted.

CHAPTER 3

Perfectionism
across Psychopathology

The link between perfectionism and psychopathology has been extensively demonstrated. Studies have shown that perfectionism is not only
correlated with but predictive of anxiety, depression, suicidal ideation,
and eating disorders. In other words, perfectionism is thought not only to
maintain various psychological disorders, but also to play a role in causing them. Hence perfectionism has been referred to as a "transdiagnostic"
process that cuts across many disorders (Egan, Wade, & Shafran, 2011). In
this chapter we will provide examples of how perfectionism manifests in
different disorders and review the many studies that have shown the link
between perfectionism and psychopathology.

Anxiety-Related and Obsessive–
Compulsive-Related Disorders

Obsessive–Compulsive Disorder

The close link between perfectionism and OCD has been recognized for
more than 100 years (Frost, Novara, & Rheaume, 2002). In 1997 the
OCCWG outlined what they thought were the key cognitive features of the
disorder, which included inflated responsibility, overestimation of threat,
overimportance of thoughts, control of thoughts, intolerance of uncertainty, and perfectionism.

The proposal that perfectionism is a central feature of OCD is not
surprising to clinicians who treat it. They can readily identify how

perfectionism manifests in clients with OCD and acts as a maintaining factor in compulsive rituals. Cleaning and checking compulsions are often maintained by individuals who need to feel that they have completed each ritual "perfectly," for example, checking a lock exactly six times to know that it is locked, or washing hands in a perfect sequence to ensure they are clean. Otherwise they must restart the ritual again due to a belief that a feared outcome may occur because they haven't performed it perfectly (e.g., harm coming to a loved one). Individuals who have OCD and perfectionism set rigid rules regarding how they meet their standards for completion of rituals. In Chapter 7 we will discuss the impact of this standard setting in maintaining perfectionism.

A clear example of how perfectionism manifests in OCD is seen in individuals who can be classified as having the OCD subtype of "not just right" compulsions. Here the individual performs a ritual, for example, brushing her hair to get it perfectly symmetrical or ordering or arranging objects in her house in a perfect and symmetrical manner. If the client feels she has not performed the ritual perfectly, the ritual may be repeated in an attempt to get it perfect so the client can experience a feeling of it being "just right." These "not just right" experiences have been shown to drive the urge to engage in compulsions (Coles, Frost, Heimberg, & Rheaume, 2003; Moretz & McKay, 2009). The role of perfectionism in OCD can be seen in the case of Jia.

Cameron believed he had to clean to a perfect standard that felt "right," or that he would contaminate others. He therefore had developed an extensive ritual around what was involved in a "clean" of his house. This task would take several hours of scrubbing floors numerous times until they were spotless and replacing many items (e.g., mops, brooms, cleaning buckets) with new and thus perfectly clean ones. He would also spend many hours ironing his shirts perfectly and arranging books and items in his house. Due to the time-consuming nature of this ritual, Cameron would procrastinate, performing his cleaning ritual only every 8 weeks and in the meantime not clean at all (including clothes, dishes, floors), which led to increasing feelings that he was contaminating others and reinforced the belief that he must scrub and arrange his house perfectly, otherwise he would be contaminating others. Cameron also performed a compulsive ritual with his daily chai latte. He visited the same coffee shop chain each day at the same time on his way home from work, and believed that if he did not get the perfect latte that felt "right" his OCD symptoms would be worse. This led to him often feeling that he had not received the perfect latte; for example, if he felt that it contained too much milk it would not taste right. Consequently, he would ask for the latte to be made again but would still not feel "right" and would spend 1–2 hours trying to mix the drink with milk at the cafe, trying to achieve a "perfect" latte.

Needless to say, these perfectionism-driven beliefs keep a person such as Cameron locked in a vicious cycle of OCD. Numerous studies have demonstrated a correlation between perfectionism and OCD. The majority of studies have utilized either the Frost *Multidimensional Perfectionism Scale* (FMPS; Frost et al., 1990), with subscales for *personal standards* (PS), *concern over mistakes* (CM), *doubts about actions* (DA), *parental expectations* (PE), *parental criticism* (PC), and *organization* (O), or the Hewitt and Flett *Multidimensional Perfectionism Scale* (HMPS; Hewitt & Flett, 1991b), which consists of *self-oriented, socially prescribed*, and *other-oriented perfectionism* (respectively, SOP, SPP, and OOP). The main finding is that PS and CM on the FMPS and SPP on the HMPS are significantly elevated in clinical OCD samples compared to controls (Antony, Purdon, Huta, & Swinson, 1998; Buhlmann, Etcoff, & Wilhelm, 2008; Frost, Steketee, Cohn, & Griess, 1994; Frost & Steketee, 1997; Sassaroli et al., 2008). It has been argued that perfectionism is a maintaining mechanism in OCD, as it interferes with treatment response (Egan, Wade, et al., 2011). In view of this conclusion, it is very essential that clinicians target perfectionism specifically, or it will continue to maintain the symptoms of OCD.

Social Anxiety Disorder

Similarly, perfectionism appears in clients suffering from social anxiety. Perfectionism has been included as a maintaining factor in cognitive-behavioral models of social anxiety (e.g., Heimberg, Juster, Hope, & Mattia, 1995). As seen in OCD, individuals with elevated social anxiety have also been shown to have significantly higher scores on CM and SPP compared to controls (Antony et al., 1998; Juster et al., 1996; Saboonchi, Lundh, & Öst, 1999).

Commonly, individuals with social anxiety disorder have beliefs about what it takes to perform to what they think is an acceptable standard in social situations. For example, take the case of Sanjeev.

Sanjeev has high standards for his social performance and has set rigid rules for himself, including the requirement that he must speak perfectly and never make an error in his speech; he must always appear perfectly relaxed and never anxious to others (e.g., by his voice shaking or being unclear); and he should always be interesting, funny, and give the right answers in meetings, or others will think he is incompetent. These beliefs lead to Sanjeev performing behaviors that maintain his social anxiety. For example, he avoids giving presentations, anticipating that he would stumble over his words. Sanjeev gives detailed descriptions of events and tells lengthy stories and jokes in order to appear funny and clever. He also ruminates over cues from others about his social performance such as interpreting a colleague looking the other way while he is speaking as evidence he is boring. These behaviors lead to Sanjeev feeling that he is failing at his goals for social performance, which further reinforces his need to try and appear "perfect" to others in social situations next time and thus reinforces the cycle of his social anxiety.

Sanjeev's example shows how perfectionism and symptoms of social anxiety can be locked in a vicious cycle of maintenance together. Beliefs about needing to be competent and flawless in social situations drive the behaviors that result in his continually feeling he is falling short, thereby maintaining his social anxiety. As with OCD, perfectionism is a particularly salient maintaining factor that, if not addressed specifically, is likely to lead to continued maintenance of social anxiety.

Panic Disorder

Studies of individuals with panic disorder have found the same pattern as in OCD and social anxiety disorder: that individuals with panic disorder have significantly higher scores on PS, CM, and SPP compared to healthy controls (Antony et al., 1998; Frost & Steketee, 1997; Iketani et al., 2002).

Many clients with perfectionism and panic disorder set rigid rules regarding the experience of anxiety symptoms. For example, someone with this combination might think, "I should never experience symptoms of anxiety; if I do, it means something is wrong with me." Many people with perfectionism and panic interpret their symptoms of panic in an all-or-nothing manner (e.g., "If I experience any anxiety at all it means I am completely out of control") due to beliefs that one should maintain "perfect" control of emotions and not experience strong anxiety states. As an example, take the case of Luca, who had panic disorder.

Luca believed any experience of anxiety was evidence that he was a "failure" at trying to control his emotional state and that this would result in him being out of control as a person. He frequently had catastrophic misinterpretations of his anxiety (e.g., that a racing heart was a signal of an impending heart attack) as is typically the case in panic disorder. However, on top of this (due to his perfectionism), he interpreted any anxious feeling as evidence that he was not meeting his standard of staying in perfect control of himself and of being a "strong" person. This interpretation further exacerbated his catastrophic cognitions regarding the meaning of panic symptoms (i.e., losing control), which in turn reinforced his belief that he must try harder to maintain perfect control of his emotional states.

The standards of emotional control that Luca set for himself interact with a typical maintaining feature of panic disorder, catastrophic misinterpretation of symptoms. It would be useful in this case not only to target the maintaining features of panic disorder that are routinely addressed in treatment (e.g., decrease catastrophic thinking and avoidance), but also to address his standards regarding "perfect" control, and the dichotomous nature of these standards, which further maintains his panic.

Specific Phobia and Generalized Anxiety Disorder

The role of perfectionism has not been well investigated in the anxiety disorders of specific phobia, generalized anxiety disorder (GAD), and post-traumatic stress disorder (PTSD). There has only been one study in specific phobia, and perfectionism was not found to be significantly higher in this group compared to controls (Antony et al., 1998). Consequently, based on the research to date, perfectionism does not appear to have a salient role in the maintenance of specific phobia.

Only one study to date has examined the role of perfectionism in a clinical GAD sample (Handley, Egan, Kane, & Rees, 2014), where PS, CM, and performance on the Clinical Perfectionism Questionnaire (CPQ; Fairburn et al., 2003a) were found to significantly predict pathological worry. The limitation of this study was that there was no control group for comparison; thus, further research is required to determine if perfectionism in individuals with clinical GAD is significantly elevated compared to controls.

Despite the lack of research with clinical samples, there have been studies that have shown a positive relationship between worry and perfectionism in nonclinical samples (e.g., Kawamura, Hunt, Frost, & DiBartolo, 2001; Stoeber & Joorman, 2001). In one study that found a positive relationship between worry and perfectionism as indicated by elevated CM and DA, it was found that experiential avoidance (i.e., avoidance of one's negative thoughts and emotional states) was a partial mediator of the relationship (Santanello & Gardner, 2007). Perfectionism may influence experiential avoidance, which in turn influences worry (i.e., that perfectionistic behaviors may be an expression of experiential avoidance). It has been suggested that worry is a cognitive process that serves the function of avoidance (Borkovec, Alcaine, & Behar, 2004). We need more research to tell us whether perfectionism is an important factor in driving the processes of worry and experiential avoidance. Clinically it makes sense that perfectionism and worry are related. In individuals with perfectionism it is common to see high degrees of worry not only over meeting their personal standards for performance, but also more generally excessive worry over everyday topics, as is seen in GAD. Although there has been no research to show that perfectionism is significantly elevated in GAD, perfectionism and worry do appear to be strongly related, and it is possible that they interact in a vicious cycle, where perfectionism drives worry and vice versa.

Posttraumatic Stress Disorder

As with GAD, little research has examined the role of perfectionism in PTSD. To date there is only one study that has examined perfectionism in a sample of 30 individuals who were in treatment for trauma experienced post-sexual assault (Egan, Hattaway, & Kane, 2014). This was not a pure clinical sample, with only 63% of the sample meeting full criteria for PTSD, yet despite this, the mean score of the sample on the *Posttraumatic Stress Checklist* (PCL-C; Weathers, Huska, & Keane, 1991) was in a clinical range.[1]

The case of Kate (adapted from Egan, Hattaway, & Kane, 2014, p. 6) illustrates the role of perfectionism as a predisposing and maintaining factor in PTSD.

> Kate described herself before the sexual assault as being a perfectionist and having very high standards across numerous areas of her life (e.g., work, appearance, musical performance), and she had always excelled in her studies and work. After the trauma she reported significant rumination over the event, focusing on why it should have happened to her, what she should have done differently, and feeling like a failure for not having done something different to avoid the attack. Kate also reported feeling that she had failed to meet her standards of being in control of her life and her emotional states, saying she viewed the PTSD symptoms she was experiencing as a sign of her failure to be strong and in control, and that she should cope better. She said she was also feeling like a failure at work, performing below her standards as she was spending a lot of time ruminating over the trauma and feeling anxious.

For Kate, we could hypothesize that perfectionism was both a predisposing and maintaining factor of the PTSD symptoms. Clearly more research is needed to clarify the importance of perfectionism in PTSD. In particular, a study with a PTSD group compared to a control is required.

Body Dysmorphic Disorder

The role of perfectionism in body dysmorphic disorder (BDD) is also an intuitive one. As clinicians who work with BDD know well, often clients are obsessed with a particular body part out of a need to appear perfect. There

---

[1]Although the study did not include a control group to which to compare levels of perfectionism, the mean level of CM (*M* = 29.7) was similar to that in studies that have examined mixed anxiety disorder samples of social anxiety disorder, OCD, and panic disorder (*M* = 21.5–27.5; Antony et al., 1998). In fact, the mean CM score on the FMPS in the PTSD sample was higher than those for all other anxiety disorders, as reported in a review (Egan, Wade, et al., 2011).

has been little research conducted on perfectionism in BDD, although two studies have found a relationship between the constructs. In a large non-clinical university student sample, Bartsch (2007) found that SOP and SPP predicted dysmorphic concerns. In the only study utilizing a clinical sample to date, Buhlmann et al. (2008) found that individuals with BDD were significantly higher on CM and DA on the FMPS compared to controls. The authors of the study gave a clinical example of the common thinking style of clients with BDD that embodies perfectionism: "As long as I don't look perfect, I won't be able to be happy" (Buhlmann et al., 2008). Given that perfectionism appears to be a major component of BDD, where clients become fixated on wanting a particular body part to appear perfect, it would be useful to determine how treatment of perfectionism impacts BDD symptoms.

Chronic Fatigue Syndrome

Chronic fatigue syndrome (CFS) has been linked with perfectionism: two studies have found that clients with CFS have significantly higher perfectionism on the FMPS subscales of CM and DA compared to healthy controls (Deary & Chalder, 2010; White & Schweitzer, 2000). Research has also found in a large sample of 192 clients with CFS that CM and DA scores are correlated with degree of fatigue (Kempke et al., 2011). The link between perfectionism and CFS is not surprising when you consider that one of the main negative physical consequences of perfectionism that clients report is exhaustion. There appears to be a "boom and bust" approach to striving and achievement in clients with CFS and perfectionism, where they describe working for intensive periods so hard and with little balance (e.g., little time for rest and lack of sleep) that they end up in a period of chronic fatigue and exhaustion. It would be useful for future research to determine if treatment of perfectionism results in significant decreases in CFS symptoms and distress.

Obsessive–Compulsive Personality Disorder

OCPD is defined in DSM-5 (American Psychiatric Association, 2013) as a disorder that has at its core perfectionism and a desire for control and order. The features of OCPD include areas such as cognitive and behavioral rigidity and inflexibility, hoarding, and preferring to save money rather than spend it. Egan, Wade, et al. (2011) have argued that OCPD and perfectionism are not necessarily the same, and as Shafran et al. (2002) stated, criteria such as difficulty discarding objects and a miserly spending style are not a part of the construct of perfectionism. However, clearly other criteria in the OCPD diagnosis, such as rigidity, are strongly related to perfectionism (Egan, Piek, Dyck, & Rees, 2007; Ferrari & Mautz, 1997). In fact, when the criteria for OCPD are examined, the majority of criteria appear to reflect what most people would think of as elements of perfectionism, for example, task inefficiency due to perfectionism, and perfectionism has been described in DSM-5 as the essential feature of OCPD (American Psychiatric Association, 2013).

There appears to be an interesting overlap between OCD, OCPD, and perfectionism. Studies that have used DSM-IV criteria have found the rates of comorbidity of OCD and OCPD to range from 23% to 32% (Coles, Pinto, Mancebo, Rasmussen, & Eisen, 2008; Pinto, Mancebo, Eisen, Pagano, & Rasmussen, 2006; Samuels et al., 2000). In the case of Cameron, described earlier in the section on OCD, criteria were met for both OCD and OCPD. In regard to the criteria of OCPD, Cameron met criteria for perfectionism interfering with task completion, as well as difficulty discarding objects, rigidity, and inflexibility regarding morals, as seen in the following case description.

> In addition to fearing contamination and engaging in extensive rituals to obtain the perfect latte, Cameron also described how he engaged in hoarding of books and newspapers. He had difficulty using his home office because it contained so many books and papers. Cameron also stated that he had strong morals which he learned through his strict Christian upbringing, which resulted in him being concerned about never swearing, and so he would speak slowly in order that he never swore or spoke any profanities against God. In therapy, Cameron also displayed cognitive rigidity. This was highlighted when discussing his rituals regarding drinking lattes, in which he reported that he could not let go of his need to get the latte just right.

In a case such as Cameron's, we can see that there are reciprocal relationships among OCD, OCPD, and perfectionism. Further research is required to examine the complex interplay between them; however it seems plausible that in such cases, treating perfectionism may be a parsimonious solution, as it is a major aspect of both the OCD and OCPD presentations, as illustrated in our case example.

Research has also examined the interaction between OCD, OCPD, and eating disorders. Halmi et al. (2005) found in 667 individuals with anorexia nervosa and bulimia nervosa that perfectionism scores (on the *Eating Disorder Inventory* perfectionism subscale [EDI-P]; Garner, Olmsted, & Polivy, 1983) were highest among those who also had a diagnosis of OCPD, and perfectionism was more closely related to a diagnosis of OCPD than OCD. Halmi and colleagues concluded that perfectionism and OCPD may be factors that predispose someone to the development of an eating disorder. This line of thought is supported by a study that found in a sample of individuals with an eating disorder that the odds ratio for development of the disorder was increased 6.9 times for every additional OCPD trait that participants reported having in childhood, in comparison to controls (Anderluh, Tchanturia, Rabe-Hesketh, & Treasure, 2003).

In summary, there is a strong link between perfectionism and OCPD, with perfectionism an important feature for the diagnosis of OCPD. While there is overlap between perfectionism and OCPD, they are not the same construct, as some of the OCPD symptoms are not necessarily associated with perfectionism. It would be useful for future research to determine if treatment of perfectionism results in change in diagnostic status of OCPD.

Eating Disorders

Most theories describing the maintenance of the disordered eating associated with anorexia nervosa and bulimia nervosa include perfectionism. The three-factor model proposed by Bardone-Cone, Abramson, Vohs, Heatherton, and Joiner (2006) suggests that an interaction between high levels of perfectionism and weight concern and low self-efficacy explains increases in bulimic behavior. In the transdiagnostic theory of eating disorders explaining the maintenance of both bulimia nervosa and anorexia nervosa, Fairburn et al. (2003b) assert that clinical perfectionism is one of four core mechanisms that can maintain eating disorder pathology, and if it were to be ameliorated, then "a potent additional network of maintaining mechanisms would be removed, thereby facilitating change" (p. 516). The other three key mechanisms included in the transdiagnostic model are low self-esteem, mood regulation problems in response to life stressors, and problems with interpersonal functioning. In the cognitive-interpersonal model of anorexia nervosa (Schmidt & Treasure, 2006), the combination of perfectionism and obsessive–compulsive personality traits is one of the four postulated maintaining factors, along with pro-anorectic beliefs (i.e., positive beliefs about the value or function of the illness or particular symptoms), avoidant temperament (i.e., avoidance of intense emotions and intimate interpersonal relationships), and responses elicited from close others. In terms of the relationships between perfectionism and eating, Schmidt and Treasure (2006) suggest:

> Individuals with these traits value perfection and fear making mistakes. They are excessively conscientious and cognitively rigid. . . . The traits (being rigidly rule-bound, striving for perfection) can facilitate persistent dietary restriction and the control of appetite. A wish for simplicity and focus on details make this type of behaviour satisfying and may lead to the . . . belief "anorexia nervosa makes me feel in control." (p. 349)

The interest in perfectionism is not recent; it has existed from when eating disorders were first being recognized and treated. Hilde Bruch (1978), a pioneer in the field of eating disorders, noted that clients with eating disorder demonstrate "superperfection" and argued that the adolescent turns to body weight as a viable source of self-definition and as a means of compensating for the lack of a clear identity and for associated feelings of powerlessness and incompetence. One of the reasons for these feelings of powerlessness and competence is the inability to completely control the environment and to be perfect. In 1978, Peter Slade developed a functional analysis of both anorexia nervosa and bulimia nervosa. Similar to Bruch, he hypothesized that, in the context of adolescent conflicts, interpersonal problems, and stress and failure experiences, the adolescent with low self-esteem and perfectionistic tendencies would feel a need to control completely, or attain success in, some aspect of life. In the case of the development of an eating disorder, the aspect of life chosen is dieting and weight loss.

As suggested in many of the theories described, eating disorders are often associated with both a desire to be perfect and low self-esteem or self-efficacy, hence producing a destructive cocktail of highly valuing achievement but feeling intrinsically unable to attain it and downplaying any achievements as being insufficient. This combination of issues is wonderfully exemplified in a quote from Catherine of Siena (1347–1380):

> Make a supreme effort to root out self-love from your heart and to plant in its place this holy self-hatred. This is the royal road by which we turn our backs on mediocrity, and which leads us without fail to the summit of perfection.

St. Catherine practiced what she preached and is often used as one of the early case studies of anorexia nervosa. Faced with the death of her sister Bonaventura in childbirth and subsequent pressure from her parents to marry Bonaventura's widower, who seemed a somewhat unsuitable husband given he had made his first wife's life a misery, 16-year-old Catherine started fasting. This behavior had the desired effect of her parents agreeing that she did not need to marry but instead could join the Dominican religious order. Over her short life, Catherine was able to realize a list of spectacular achievements given her gender and the era. Advocating reform of the clergy, she attracted a group of followers, and she dictated letters that make up a still extant body of holy writing. Despite her achievements, Catherine continued to practice holy self-hatred and ate less and less until eventually she ate nothing but the daily Eucharist. She maintained this regime even in the face of disapproval from the clergy. Catherine died in Rome at the age of 33.

A more recent illustration of this confluence of low self-esteem and perfectionism can be seen in the case of Natalie.

Natalie developed anorexia nervosa in late adolescence in part because "dieting was the only thing I could do better than the other girls." Even though she was accepted at Cambridge University, she believed that a mistake had been made and she had been sent the wrong offer, and instead was actually meant to be studying at the polytechnic down the road. Her misery was amplified when she developed bulimia nervosa ("I can't even do anorexia nervosa properly"). She felt like a fraud across all endeavors of her life, and in order "not to be found out," she had isolated herself from her friends, withdrawn from leisure and sporting activities that had once given her pleasure, decided to leave university, and was continuing to pursue dieting in a hope that this achievement would make her start to feel better.

Another example is provided by Liz Jones, a British journalist and writer for the *Daily Mail* who previously edited British *Marie Claire* magazine. She has had anorexia nervosa for over 40 years and has blogged about this in recent years, saying, "I might not have been good at anything else— sport, relationships, conversation—but I have been really good at being thin" and "that's the thing about being an anorexic: it makes you feel superior, clean, morally unimpeachable" (Jones, 2011).

While low self-esteem is not necessarily always a companion to perfectionism, it amplifies the chances that many experiences will be perceived as failure despite evidence to the contrary. Slade (1982) says that people who develop eating disorders "tend to see events and their own achievements in black and white terms, such that anything else less than idealized, perfect success or attainment represents failure and lack of success" (p. 171).

People with perfectionistic tendencies often turn to a domain of life that offers them some degree of attainment and control. Particularly for women and increasingly for men, weight loss is an achievement that is highly valued by Western society. Initial weight loss often elicits positive comments and reactions of admiration from others and can also lead to increased popularity and acceptance that produces a powerful short-term bolstering of self-esteem. While the long-term losses become quite destructive, in terms of lost self-esteem and respect, social isolation, narrowing of life, and the sacrifice of hopes and goals, persistence in this solution to a problem (e.g., loss of control) is supported in part by the typical black-and-white thinking that can accompany perfectionism. In eating disorders, this tendency, which can be assessed using neuropsychological testing (Holliday, Tchanturia, Landau, Collier, & Treasure, 2005; Lopez, Tchanturia, Stahl, & Treasure, 2008), is reflected in deficits related to flexible thinking or set shifting (i.e., taking longer to change responses in the face of a change of the rules or circumstances) and central coherence (i.e., "not seeing the woods for the trees" and focusing on the detail but not being able to easily get the gist of the whole picture). Continued focus on weight loss in people with low self-esteem results in them becoming afraid that if they no longer have a reason for not tackling the challenges in life, they will be found out as being second rate and defective in the process of trying to rise to these challenges.

In support of these theoretical positions, research consistently shows perfectionism to be elevated in people with eating disorders and people recovering from eating disorders compared to healthy controls (Bardone-Cone, Sturm, Lawson, Robinson, & Smith, 2010). While some studies suggest that perfectionism remains elevated once recovery from the eating disorder has occurred (Bastiani, Rao, Weltzin, & Kaye, 1995; Halmi et al., 2000; Lilenfeld et al., 2000), other studies have suggested that recovery, when robustly defined, is associated with perfectionism levels that are no different from those in healthy controls (Bardone-Cone et al., 2010). Although these latter findings may indicate that perfectionism is not a risk factor for eating disorders (i.e., it doesn't cause eating disorders), they are consistent with the suggestion that interventions that help decrease perfectionism may be key to making full recovery attainable (Bardone-Cone et al., 2010).

Eating disorders can be somewhat differentiated from the other types of psychopathology discussed in this chapter in that the evidence suggests that both healthy perfectionism (i.e., striving for achievement) *and* unhealthy perfectionism (i.e., self-criticism when goals are not achieved to what is considered to be an acceptable level) are associated with disordered eating (Bardone-Cone et al., 2007). Exactly why this is the case and how this works is unclear. It may be because the main domain of achievement in eating disorders becomes destructive, wreaking damage on both physical and psychological health, such that it interferes with or prevents achievement in other domains (e.g., academic studies, work, friendships, socializing, and hobbies). Thus the only achievement that remains and is valued is in the eating domain. This theory is illustrated by Liz Jones (2011), who says:

> It makes no sense, but I'd rather be thin than happy or healthy. . . . It's so pathetic to admit that a grown woman, and a fairly successful one, has her world ruled by how many calories she ingests . . . and that the only pleasures in life are to see how concave you can make your stomach, how many ribs you can count, how normal it is to feel faint, to see stars, to be so weak you can, some days, hardly stand.

Research also indicates that SPP, measured by the HMPS (Hewitt & Flett, 1991b), is significantly elevated in people with eating disorders (Bastiani et al., 1995; Cockell et al., 2002). As reviewed in Chapter 1, SPP can be defined as developing perfectionistic motivations in response to the belief that significant others expect one to be perfect. Whether this belief is based on reality can be debated, but certainly previous theorists (Bruch,

1978) have emphasized that both intrapersonal and interpersonal aspects of perfectionism are implicated in the emergence and continuance of eating disorder symptoms. Longitudinal research of 13-year-old girls found that a "wish to be thinner" and their mothers' rating on perfectionism contributed most to the prediction of disturbed eating attitudes 7 years later (Westerberg-Jacobson, Edlund, & Ghaderi, 2010). Interestingly, high self-esteem appeared to be a protective factor when the girls had a high degree of perfectionism. A study of 433 "trios" (a female with anorexia nervosa or "proband" and her mother and father) found that the most severe disordered eating in the proband (24% of the sample) was associated with mothers who also had elevations on eating disorder symptoms and anxious/perfectionistic traits (M. J. Jacobs et al., 2009). Elevated ratings on maternal perfectionism may not indicate perfectionistic pressures from the mother, but may rather indicate a genetic susceptibility that results in a more homogeneous and familial variant of anorexia nervosa. While perfectionism in the father has not been implicated to date, the importance of paternal variables in terms of contribution to risk for eating disorders has been found across a variety of longitudinal studies, including maladaptive paternal behavior (Johnson, Cohen, Kasen, & Brook, 2002), low levels of paternal care (Wade, Treloar, & Martin, 2008), paternal eating attitudes (Westerberg, Edlund, & Ghaderi, 2008), and importance of weight to father (Field et al., 2008). These latter two variables may indicate some perfectionistic pressure specific to appearance and weight from the fathers.

What evidence is there to support the earlier suggestions that interventions to decrease perfectionism may be critical to attaining full recovery from eating disorders, and that changes in perfectionism may facilitate changes in disordered eating? To date, the scant evidence available indicates that treating people with eating disorders by targeting perfectionism alone is helpful but insufficient, but treating perfectionism when it is problematic in conjunction with an evidence-based therapy for eating disorders can improve outcome. Two studies inform this conclusion.

The first, reviewed in Chapter 2, is from Steele and Wade (2008), who treated 48 people with bulimia nervosa using guided self-help (eight sessions working through a self-help book with a novice therapist) of three different types. The first was CBT for eating disorders, considered to be the gold standard treatment for bulimic disorders. The second was a perfectionism treatment (comprised of guided self-help based on Antony & Swinson's [1998] book), and the third was designed to be a placebo treatment, a form of dismantled mindfulness. At 6-month follow-up all groups had improved significantly with respect to eating disorder symptoms, and there was no statistical difference between the groups, but within-group effect sizes for the change in behavioral eating disorder variables ranged from .16 to .47 (small) in the perfectionism group compared to .21 to 1.07 in the CBT group. Of note, however, there was a greater improvement in cognitive and attitudinal scores associated with eating disorders in the per-fectionism group (2.23) compared to the CBT group (1.88), though both effect sizes are large. Only the perfectionism group experienced a large decrease in unhealthy perfectionism (while there was no change in healthy perfectionism), with a within-group effect size change of 1.25 compared to .01 and .25 in the CBT and placebo groups. The perfectionism group also experienced the largest improvements in self-esteem (1.30), depression (.94) and anxiety (.73). This suggests that perfectionism treatment can be power-ful in terms of changing the cognitive and attitudinal scores associated with eating disorders.

The second study was conducted by Fairburn and colleagues (2009) and compared two versions of an expanded form of CBT for eating disor-ders (where body mass index was greater than 17.5), one that focused on the symptoms of the disordered eating, and one that additionally focused on identified maintaining factors from the transdiagnostic model: perfection-ism, low self-esteem, or problems with interpersonal relationships. When comparing the group that focused on disordered eating and maintaining factors, it was found that the group that had problems with one of the three maintaining factors responded better in terms of reductions in their global eating psychopathology at 60-month follow-up than those people who did not experience problems in these areas. Taken together, these two studies indicate that, for those clients identified as having problems with perfectionism, adding the treatment of perfectionism to evidence-based treatments for disordered eating may lead to a better outcome for the main-tenance of reductions in disordered eating.

Depression

Clinicians can readily describe clients they have treated for whom perfec-tionism appears to be a major factor in the development and maintenance of depression. The majority of the literature has focused on the role of perfectionism in major depressive disorder, where there is extensive evi-dence that perfectionism plays an important role; however, there is some interesting recent research showing that it may also play an important role in bipolar disorder. Among the most concerning lines of evidence are the numerous studies that have shown perfectionism is linked to suicidal behavior.

Major Depressive Disorder

In many clients who present for treatment of major depressive disorder (MDD), perfectionism can be seen as a prominent feature, and they often report rumination on thoughts of being a "failure" that are linked to not meeting their personal goals and standards. Moreover, when clients present specifically for treatment for perfectionism, many report symptoms of depression. It is not surprising that people with high levels of perfectionism also report depressive symptoms. Just the impact of striving, which may include working excessively long hours and sleeping only 3–4 hours per night, can be seen as playing a role in the maintenance of depression, which is characterized by exhaustion and low mood.

Depression seems to link closely to the avoidance features of perfectionism, where individuals with perfectionism often get caught in cycles of procrastination and avoidance of tasks due to fear of not completing them well enough to meet their standards, which leads to low mood and depressive symptoms. Take the example of Asha:

> Asha had elevated perfectionism regarding her work as an accountant and her social performance. Asha reported that she needed to excel by always producing excellent reports to be given to the CEO of her company and never making mistakes in her financial reporting. She also reported that she had to have many friends, who contacted her frequently, to feel that she was meeting her important personal standard of being a social person who was well liked by others. The problem was that because of Asha's high standards for her performance (e.g., never making even a minor error in her reports), she would often procrastinate on starting her reports, and did not contact friends regularly as she was often ruminating over her work. Due to this, Asha would often leave her reports to the last minute and need to "pull an all-nighter" where she would work the entire night to get a report done. This had an impact on Asha's ability to socialize, as she would decline social invitations, either because she was working or because she was exhausted from having stayed up working the entire previous night. The problem with this strategy was that often Asha would then make very minor errors in her reports, or not feel happy with the final product, which would lead to bouts of intense self-criticism over these reports, which she perceived were "not up to scratch" and resulted in her feeling like a failure. After this, Asha would report strong periods of low mood and tearfulness. She also reported low mood centered around the idea that she did not have enough friends; however, this was often due to friends starting to contact her less frequently as she would regularly turn down social invitations due to needing to work. This all resulted in Asha feeling like she was a failure as a person because she did not have enough friends and was not achieving her standards for work. Asha was reporting low mood, tearfulness, a lack of interest in things that she used to like to do (like going for coffee with friends and going to the gym), and feeling like she was inadequate.

In this case, it can be seen that perfectionism is a strong driving factor in maintaining Asha's depressive symptoms and is therefore a very important factor to address in treatment. It is likely that if these behaviors centered on how Asha judges her personal standards are not addressed, then she will continue to experience low mood and depressive symptoms.

When one examines the literature regarding the role of perfectionism in depression, Asha's case example is in accord with the extensive evidence demonstrating the relationship between the two. Significantly, the role of perfectionism in depression has been shown not only in correlational studies, but also in studies where perfectionism has been found to predict later development of depressive symptoms (i.e., prospective studies). There have been numerous studies showing that people with clinical depression tend to have higher levels of SPP compared to controls (Enns, Cox, & Borger, 2001; Hewitt & Flett, 1991a). Studies have also found that individuals with depression have higher levels of CM than controls (Huprich, Porcelli, Keaschuk, Binienda, & Engle, 2008; Norman, Davies, Nicholson, Cortese, & Malla, 1998; Sassaroli et al., 2008). It is interesting that one study has found elevated SOP in a depressed sample compared to controls (Norman et al., 1998). As outlined earlier, in the section regarding eating disorders, SOP has been found to be elevated in individuals with eating disorders compared to controls, and in at least one study in depression, this has also been found to be the case. This highlights the fact that although some authors in the area of perfectionism have argued that measures such as SOP and PS are associated with positive states and represent a "healthy" or "positive" form of perfectionism, there is evidence that in certain clinical groups, including those with depression and eating disorders, these scales are elevated, suggesting that they are correlated with psychopathology.

While there are a range of studies that show perfectionism is elevated in people with MDD, those showing that perfectionism can predict the later development of depression are much more convincing than these data with respect to a possible causal relationship. These studies are important; although correlational studies can suggest that two variables are linked, in the end they can't give us any evidence that one variable (e.g., perfectionism) causes another (e.g., depression). Longitudinal studies, on the other hand, provide better evidence, and there are several studies that do provide evidence in large samples of people with major depression that perfectionism predicts the development of depression. In the first longitudinal study, Hewitt, Flett, and Ediger (1996) found that SPP predicted the development of depressive symptoms 4 months later. However the strongest evidence regarding the role of perfectionism in depression comes from two studies that followed a large sample of clients with clinical depression over follow-up periods of 3 years (Dunkley, Sanislow, Grilo, & McGlashan, 2006) and 4 years (Dunkley, Sanislow, Grilo, & McGlashan, 2009). It was found that the perfectionism subscale of the DAS (Weissman & Beck, 1978), which has been labeled as self-criticism (DAS-SC), was able to predict increases in depressive symptoms at both 3- and 4-year follow-ups.

Bipolar Disorder

It is not only unipolar depression in which perfectionism has been recognized as having a major role; there are two studies to date suggesting that it is also important in bipolar disorder. To measure perfectionism both studies used the DAS-SC. Jones and colleagues (2005) found that individuals with bipolar disorder had significantly higher scores on this perfectionism measure than controls. The reasons why perfectionism may play a role in bipolar disorder are not particularly well understood with little research in the area, however a recent study found that DAS-SC scores predicted the onset of hypomanic and manic episodes (Alloy et al., 2009). This suggests perfectionism may be a vulnerability factor for the onset of mood swings in bipolar disorder. This makes sense clinically in that individuals with bipolar disorder who strive for perfectionism may work all hours and engage in other behaviors that are likely to put them at risk of manic episodes. More research in the area is needed on the relationship between perfectionism and bipolar disorder, but it is an interesting area to consider for those clinicians working with clients with bipolar disorder.

Suicidal Ideation and Behavior

One of the most troubling aspects of perfectionism is the role it has been shown to have in predicting suicidal ideation and behavior. The research has found a strong relationship between perfectionism and suicide behaviors (Hewitt, Flett, Sherry, & Caelian, 2006). Correlational studies have linked SPP and suicidal ideation in clinical samples (Hewitt, Flett, & Weber, 1994; Hewitt, Norton, Flett, Callander, & Cowan, 1998). SPP has also been found to predict suicidal ideation in individuals hospitalized for self-harm (Rasmussen, O'Connor, & Brodie, 2008). Unfortunately there are some well-known examples of people who were seen as being at the top of their game and excellent in their fields who have completed suicide, and perfectionism has been pointed to as being a major factor involved in these tragic cases. Take, for example, the case of Bernard Loiseau, a top chef in France who committed suicide after criticism in the press and rumors that his restaurant might be downgraded from three Michelin stars (the best possible level) to only two. The role played by his perfectionistic nature was documented in a biography of Loiseau titled *The Perfectionist: Life and Death in Haute Cuisine*. Another tragic case linking suicide to perfectionism was that of the famous professional cyclist Marco Pantani, who won high-profile races including the Tour de France and Giro d'Italia, and held records for the fastest time riding over famous mountains often featured in the Tour, such as Alpe d'Huez. When his career ended due to declining performance (typical of athletes as they get older), he tragically took his own life, and it was reported that he had mentioned to others preceding his suicide that if he could not be the best at cycling anymore he was not interested in living. This was another sad case in which an individual was so distressed at not being the very best at achieving his or her personal standards that suicide seemed like the only option. Yet another example can be seen in the case of a client, Juanita.

> Juanita completed suicide after battling with periods of depression for several years. Unfortunately she had only recently come into contact with mental health services when she completed suicide. When reviewing the case it was found that Juanita described herself as having been a perfectionist for as long as she could remember. She had always excelled at everything, performing extremely well in college and becoming a successful dentist, as well as excelling in diving, in which she represented her state in competitions. In her personal life, she was married with a young child. In her suicide note Juanita stated that she "had never been able to shake the feeling of not being good enough," and tragically that despite the love she had received from her family and her husband, she could not go on because she felt that she was never living up to her standards, that she could never achieve what she wanted to, and that she was a failure even in taking her own life.

This sad case illustrates that in extreme cases, suicidal ideation and behavior can be an outcome of feeling that one is unable to meet personal standards and that one is "never good enough." The relationship between perfectionism and suicide illustrated by these unfortunate examples is also supported by research evidence. Though there have been correlational studies showing that perfectionism is linked to suicidal behaviors, the strongest evidence comes from prospective studies demonstrating that perfectionism can predict suicidal behavior over time. In two different studies perfectionism has predicted suicidal behavior 6 months later. Beevers and Miller (2004) found in a clinical sample of inpatients being treated for depression that DAS-SC scores could predict suicide ideation 6 months after discharge from hospital. This suggests that it is important for clinicians working with inpatients to identify and target perfectionism. Further evidence regarding perfectionism and suicidal behavior was provided by a study of 515 adolescents, in which SPP was found to predict higher levels of self-harm and depression over a 6-month period (O'Connor, Rasmussen, & Hawton, 2010).

CHAPTER 4

Perfectionism as
a Transdiagnostic Process

Definition of a Transdiagnostic Process

In Chapter 3, we presented evidence demonstrating that perfectionism is significantly higher across a range of disorders (e.g., anxiety and related disorders, eating disorders, chronic fatigue, depression, bipolar disorder) compared to healthy controls. In a recent review, Egan, Wade, et al. (2011) argued that perfectionism is a transdiagnostic process. A transdiagnostic process is "an aspect of cognition or behavior that may contribute to the maintenance of a psychological disorder" (Harvey, Watkins, Mansell, & Shafran, 2004, p. 14). As outlined by Egan and colleagues, a transdiagnostic process that is of interest and relevance to therapists is one that does not just occur across disorders, but is also either a risk or maintaining factor of disorders. It may be useful to consider targeting such a process in an attempt to ameliorate a range of symptoms of various disorders.

Based on the literature, we will explain why we think of perfectionism as a transdiagnostic process. However, the key point of this chapter is to outline why it is important to establish whether perfectionism is a transdiagnostic process *in your client*. This analysis will also include the significance of determining whether perfectionism is a predisposing and/ or maintaining factor of psychopathology. We will also consider how to determine if perfectionism is causal, correlational, or a consequence of psychopathology *in your client*, as this will enable you to decide on treatment interventions.

Rationale for a Transdiagnostic Approach

In recent years there has been an increasing interest in transdiagnostic approaches to developing theories and treatments for common underlying constructs across diagnostic categories. Among the first proponents of a transdiagnostic approach were Fairburn et al. (2003b), who put forward a theory of eating disorders that proposes core underlying transdiagnostic processes that serve to maintain eating disorders, including clinical perfectionism. The transdiagnostic theory of eating disorders has predictive validity (Hoiles, Egan, & Kane, 2012), and CBT-E, which is based on the theory, has been found to be more effective for the treatment of eating disorders than previous versions of CBT for bulimia nervosa (Byrne et al., 2011; Fairburn et al., 2009). One of the advantages of this approach has been the de-emphasis of diagnostic categories, and instead a focus on addressing the critical constructs maintaining the eating disorder, regardless of diagnostic status. Similarly, a range of other transdiagnostic treatments have been recently proposed and found to be effective. This includes the unified treatment protocol for mood and anxiety disorders of Barlow and colleagues (2011), which has emerging evidence of efficacy (Bossieau, Farchione, Fairholme, Ellard, & Barlow, 2010; Ellard, Fairholme, Bossieau, Farchione, & Barlow, 2010; Farchione et al., 2012) and the transdiagnostic treatment of anxiety disorders of Norton and colleagues (e.g., Norton & Philipp, 2008). These treatments have been based on the notion of targeting underlying transdiagnostic processes.

What these transdiagnostic approaches and treatments have in common is the rationale that targeting key, critical processes that maintain a range of disorders is likely to be more effective and efficient in dealing with comorbidity than multiple disorder-specific interventions. For example, Barlow et al. (2011) based the theoretical rationale for their transdiagnostic treatment on the wealth of data showing that the nature, etiology, and structure of disorders are more similar than they are different. Barlow et al. (2011) also argued that transdiagnostic treatments have the advantage of being designed to be effective for all disorders a person may have rather than just a single disorder. As clinicians know well, comorbidity is the rule rather than the exception in clinical practice (Kessler, Chiu, Demler, Merikangas, & Walters, 2005). One of the advantages of a transdiagnostic approach, therefore, is that it may help explain the high rates of comorbidity of disorders, and proponents of the transdiagnostic approach suggest that comorbidity occurs because disorders share maintaining mechanisms (Harvey et al., 2004). Providing a treatment that is transdiagnostic with one set of principles is easier and more efficient and will help evidence-based therapies be delivered in clinical settings. We argue that because of these outlined benefits, a treatment based on targeting underlying transdiagnostic processes (such as perfectionism) is likely to be beneficial.

Perfectionism as a Transdiagnostic Process: Treating Perfectionism Regardless of Diagnosis

In this section, we will review evidence for why CBT for perfectionism can be considered a transdiagnostic process of clinical importance, and why it needs to be addressed in therapy (for a more detailed argument, see Egan, Wade, et al., 2011).

Perfectionism Is Elevated across Disorders

As shown in Chapter 3, perfectionism is elevated across eating disorders, anxiety and related disorders, depression, and chronic fatigue compared to healthy controls. This evidence demonstrates that perfectionism is relevant to the majority of disorders, and thus it is important to consider addressing it specifically in therapy, as its presence suggests the salience of this factor across most diagnoses.

Perfectionism Is a Risk and Maintaining Factor across Disorders

Perfectionism has been recognized as a risk factor for eating disorders (e.g., Bardone-Cone et al., 2007; Jacobi, Hayward, de Zwaan, Kraemer, & Agras, 2004; Lilenfeld, Wonderlich, Riso, Crosby, & Mitchell, 2006; Stice, 2002) as well as a maintaining factor of these disorders (e.g., Fairburn et al., 2003b). Furthermore, perfectionism is a maintaining factor of numerous anxiety disorders and depression. Egan, Wade, et al. (2011) outlined the inclusion of perfectionism as an important maintenance factor in models of anxiety-based disorders, for example social anxiety (Heimberg, Juster, Hope, & Mattia, 1995) and OCD (OCCWG, 1997). It is worth reiterating that if perfectionism is considered to be a maintaining factor for mental health problems, then interventions that reduce perfectionism will impact positively on the mental health condition.

Perfectionism Has Been Associated with Treatment Outcome across Disorders

Some studies have shown that perfectionism predicts treatment outcome across multiple disorders. It may be worth taking a moment to reflect on which of your clients have responded well to therapy and which have responded less well. It may be that in your clinical practice and experience, high levels of perfectionism interfere with treatment progress. There may be a range of reasons for this, including the impact of perfectionism on engagement (see Chapter 8). On the other hand, you may believe that perfectionism does not impact negatively on treatment for mental health problems, but nevertheless you are reading this manual because perfectionism is a clinical problem that you need to address in your practice.

Perfectionism and Treatment Outcome in Anxiety Disorders and OCD

Egan, Wade, et al. (2011) reviewed several studies where perfectionism was found to predict treatment outcome in anxiety disorders and OCD. It has been found that perfectionism predicts response to exposure and response prevention in clients with OCD. Chik, Whittal, and O'Neill (2008) found that perfectionism, as measured by the DA subscale of the FMPS, predicted poorer response to treatment for OCD. Kyrios et al. (2007) found the perfectionism subscale of the *Obsessive Beliefs Questionnaire* (OBQ; OCCWG, 2001) was the only one on the measure to significantly predict treatment outcome in OCD. Similarly, Pinto, Liebowitz, Foa, and Simpson (2011) found that the diagnosis and severity of OCPD was a predictor of poorer treatment outcome to exposure and response prevention in OCD. In particular, they found that when individual OCPD diagnostic criteria were considered, perfectionism was the only one to predict worse treatment outcome (Pinto et al., 2011).

Similar findings exist with regard to social anxiety, for which several studies have found perfectionism to predict treatment response. Lundh and Öst (2001) found that those clients who did not respond to treatment for social phobia had higher pretreatment perfectionism scores. Ashbaugh et al. (2007) found that changes in CM and DA predicted symptoms of social anxiety following group CBT, even after controlling for pretreatment levels of social anxiety. Egan, Wade, et al. (2011) argued that this data provides indirect· evidence of perfectionism being a maintaining factor in anxiety disorders.

Perfectionism and Treatment Outcome in Depression

There are several studies that show perfectionism can get in the way of clients being able to successfully engage with treatment for depression (Egan, Wade, et al., 2011). The case for needing to target perfectionism in depression is strong when you consider the evidence from five studies that reported on the data from the well-known National Institute of Mental Health Treatment of Depression Collaborative Research Program trial, which compared interpersonal psychotherapy, CBT, and antidepressant medication (Elkin et al., 1989). In these studies, perfectionism was measured on the DAS-SC, and it predicted poorer response to treatment in all groups at posttreatment (Blatt et al., 1995) and 18-month follow-up (Blatt, Zuroff, Bondi, Sanislow, & Pilkonis, 1998). Perfectionism was also found to predict poorer social networks, which predicted poorer treatment outcome (Shahar, Blatt, Zuroff, Krupnick, & Sotsky, 2004). Perfectionism also predicted poor ability to cope with life stressors at 18-month follow-up after treatment (Blatt & Zuroff, 2005). One interesting factor that seemed to be related in this data was that perfectionism was related to poorer therapeutic alliance in the psychotherapy groups (Zuroff et al., 2000). The reasons for this poor alliance and how to address it will be covered later in this book; however, it is an interesting possible explanation for why those people with higher perfectionism did more poorly across treatment. Given how important it is, we have included a chapter on how to effectively enhance engagement and alliance with clients with elevated perfectionism (see Chapter 8). Indeed, as Blatt (1995) concluded, perfectionism is a destructive force in depression.

There are similar findings in the literature that has examined outcome for treatment of depression in adolescents. R. H. Jacobs et al. (2009) examined the sample of 439 adolescents who were in the Treatment for Adolescents with Depression study, which compared CBT, fluoxetine, a combination of CBT and fluoxetine, and a pill placebo. Perfectionism as measured by DAS-SC at pretreatment was found to be related to continued high depressive symptoms over the treatment program. Furthermore, the adolescents with higher perfectionism showed poorer improvement on suicidal ideation. Perfectionism was also shown to be a mediator of treatment outcome.

It is not only this data set that suggests that if perfectionism is not specifically targeted in treatment it will remain a problem in individuals with depression. Evidence from another study shows that a component score of maladaptive perfectionism comprised of SPP and the FMPS subscales of CM, DA, PE, and PC remains unchanged pre- to posttreatment of depression (Cox & Enns, 2003). Given all of these arguments, it is clear that perfectionism needs to be specifically targeted when it is elevated in individuals with major depression.

Perfectionism and Treatment Outcome in Eating Disorders

Egan, Wade, et al. (2011) also presented evidence that perfectionism predicts treatment outcome in eating disorders. This includes data showing that perfectionism as measured by the perfectionism items (EDI-P) from the *Eating Disorders Inventory* (EDI; Garner et al., 1983) is associated with poorer prognosis (Bizuel, Sadowsky, & Riguad, 2001) and higher treatment dropout in anorexia nervosa (Sutandar-Pinnock, Woodside, Carter, Olmsted, & Kaplan, 2003). As seen in similar data on depression, perfectionism appears to remain elevated posttreatment in clients who have been treated for an eating disorder (Bastiani et al., 1995; Lilenfeld et al., 2000; Nilsson, Sundbom, & Hagglof, 2008; Pla & Toro, 1999; Srinivasagam et al., 1995), despite one study that found perfectionism did not predict treatment outcome in bulimia nervosa (Mussell et al., 2000).

Treatment of Perfectionism Decreases Symptoms across Multiple Disorders

A final argument that can be made as to why perfectionism can be considered a transdiagnostic process is that data on treatment outcome indicate that without targeting symptoms of the disorder directly, CBT for perfectionism results in reductions in symptoms across a range of disorders (e.g., Riley et al., 2007; Steele & Wade, 2008) as described in detail in Chapter 2. This is not surprising if we consider the data from Bieling, Summerfeldt, Israeli, and Antony (2004), where the number of comorbid diagnoses in a sample of 345 clients was positively correlated with perfectionism (as measured by the FMPS subscales of CM, PC, and DA, and the HMPS subscales of SOP and SPP). This suggests that perfectionism may be one process that accounts for comorbidity. Given the arguments we presented earlier in this chapter regarding comorbidity being the norm in clinical practice, and the advantage of transdiagnostic treatments in being able to address this, the appeal of focusing on perfectionism as the focus of a transdiagnostic treatment is obvious. This is even more the case when considering Bieling et al.'s (2004) finding that *maladaptive evaluative concerns* (consisting of the FMPS subscales of PE, CM, and PC and the HMPS subscale of SPP) predicted higher levels of comorbidity even after controlling for current symptoms. These findings lead Bieling et al. (2004) to state a rationale for considering perfectionism as a transdiagnostic process: "Perfectionism is not associated with a single disorder or type of disorder, but may be an underlying factor across several disorders and categories of psychopathology" (p. 194). This statement effectively captures the argument that perfectionism underlies a number of disorders, thus leading Bieling et al. (2004) to conclude that treating perfectionism would lead to a decrease in symptoms across a number of areas. Consequently, directly targeting perfectionism may be more effective in patients with comorbid disorders than single-disorder-based approaches that target maintaining factors sequentially (Bieling et al., 2004).

Indeed, the data on treatment outcome to date support the argument of Bieling et al. (2004). While details of treatment outcome studies were presented in detail in Chapter 2, the findings of Steele and Wade's (2008) study are important to review here. Steele and Wade found that CBT for bulimia nervosa and CBT for perfectionism had equivalent results for reduction in bulimia nervosa symptoms, but that CBT for perfectionism had larger effects for anxiety and depression. This finding is very important as it suggests that CBT for perfectionism reduced a range of psychopathology, thus supporting the argument that perfectionism is a transdiagnostic process.

Establishing Whether Perfectionism Is an Important Transdiagnostic Process in Your Client

It is important to understand the role perfectionism plays for each individual client and, as a result, whether it warrants direct intervention. In cases where perfectionism presents as a clinical problem in its own right, then it undoubtedly should be the focus of treatment. However, a client may present with depression, anxiety, and perfectionism. In such a case, should the therapist treat the depression, anxiety, or perfectionism? In order to address this common clinical situation, it is necessary first to evaluate the role of perfectionism in the maintenance and, to a lesser extent, the etiology of depression and anxiety. It has been suggested by Egan, Wade, and Shafran (2012) that a functional analysis can help to establish the role of perfectionism in the development and maintenance of psychopathology in each individual client. This includes determining if perfectionism alone is the presenting problem or if it appears as a part of the interaction, and within the context, of particular disorders (Egan et al., 2012).

Perfectionism as the Primary Presenting Problem

When considering a functional analysis of perfectionism, in some cases it is clear that a client will present for treatment with perfectionism as their main presenting problem. Usually they present for treatment because perfectionism is significantly interfering with their work or interpersonal life due to patterns of procrastination and avoidance and repeated checking. Clients also tend to describe in the initial session the overwhelming feeling that they are "not good enough" and feel like a failure due to not being able to meet their standards. If this is the case, and perfectionism is the primary factor that is causing anxiety, low mood, and other difficulties then it should be addressed first following the strategies outlined in this book.

Perfectionism as a Predisposing Factor

It may be the case that the client's perfectionism has predisposed him or her to develop both anxiety and depression. The anxiety may have begun with a focus on performance in a range of domains, but then additional maintaining factors and low mood may have developed later. Take the example of Chloe.

> Chloe had high levels of perfectionism and was anxious about her schoolwork. She began to spend a long time on work and then worried that this was impacting her friendships. She began to feel anxious about going out and was concerned about how she would come across to others. She felt other people might notice her blushing or stammering and so avoided social situations. As she became more isolated, her belief that she was not doing well at anything intensified and her mood deteriorated. At the time she came for treatment, diagnostic criteria were met for social anxiety disorder, generalized anxiety disorder, and depression.

For Chloe, the perfectionism had clearly predisposed her to develop elevated anxiety and low mood, but it was not the focus of treatment. Her treatment goals were to feel less anxious and for her mood to improve, and treating the perfectionism would not have been the appropriate course of action. In such a case, once the anxiety and low mood were addressed using appropriate evidence-based methods (e.g., see *www.nice.org.uk* for specific recommendations), it would be worthwhile to address the perfectionism as part of a relapse prevention program. Similarly, if the decision is made after formulation that the evidence-based approach for a specific disorder will be the course of treatment either before or instead of treatment of perfectionism, the therapist may consider referral to a medical practitioner for a review of pharmacotherapy if warranted. For example, if a client is suffering from severe depression it may be useful to start medication along with evidence-based cognitive-behavioral strategies for reducing depressive mood before starting to try and change their perfectionism.

Of course, if perfectionism interfered with treatment progress for the social anxiety or depression, then direct treatment would also be warranted. Egan et al. (2012) have outlined how for many clients progress in treatment of the disorders with evidence-based protocols may be difficult due to perfectionism. Egan et al. (2012) give a common example of how clients with perfectionism may find it difficult to engage in behavioral activation because they believe that engaging in pleasant events is a waste of time as they are not using their time productively. When this is the case, we suggest that the evidence-based protocol for the disorder be put on hold and perfectionism become the target of treatment instead. Once the perfectionism has been treated then the protocol for the disorder can be resumed (Egan et al., 2012).

Perfectionism as a Maintaining Factor

In another client with multiple disorders and perfectionism, it may be that perfectionism is an appropriate focus of treatment if it is seen to play an active role in maintaining the psychopathology. Take the case of Riya as an example.

> Riya said that her perfectionism was leading her to clean the house for several hours a day. She also described low mood, triggered by a perceived failure to meet own standards, as she was only a "housewife." Riya has also experienced postpartum depression, maintained by her strong belief that she needed to be a perfect mother who was overwhelmed with love for her newborn baby.

On assessment, understanding that Riya's obsessive–compulsive symptoms and low mood were a direct result of her overvaluation of striving, achievement, and perfectionism was fundamental to the decision to use the protocol in this book. It must be emphasized that we do not do this lightly. The evidence for the efficacy for disorder-specific protocols is strong—there are multiple, large randomized controlled trials in their support—whereas the evidence for the efficacy of the treatment of perfectionism is in its infancy. It is for this reason that if it is possible and appropriate to implement an evidence-based protocol for a specific disorder, that is our preference. However, there is almost no evidence about how to treat multiple coexisting disorders. Based on the small amount of data (e.g., Craske et al., 2007), the preferred option is to implement disorder-specific protocols in sequence rather than "mix and match" protocols. It is this unhappy situation regarding how to address the clinical reality of multiple coexisting problems that has led to the development of more efficient unified approaches such as that of Barlow et al. (2011) and the transdiagnostic treatment described in this manual.

Perfectionism as Correlational and a Consequence of Psychopathology

For other clients, perfectionism may simply be a correlate of the psychopathology rather than a predisposing or maintaining factor. Someone may present with high levels of perfectionism in the domain of work or sports, as well as with PTSD and panic disorder. In such a case, there is clearly no need to address the perfectionism. Similarly, there may be clients for whom perfectionism developed as a consequence of having other psychopathology. For example, Mario had a heart attack at age 45 and subsequently developed panic disorder. To help prevent another heart attack, he took healthy living to the extreme with rigid rules about his diet and exercise. He developed similar rules about "stress" and would not engage in any activities that caused him stress. He felt that to get things wrong or make mistakes would be highly stressful for him and so began to check to ensure he did not make errors in his social or work interactions. Over time, his perfectionism became self-maintaining with his self-evaluation overly dependent on striving, achievement, and excessively high standards.

In conclusion, this transdiagnostic treatment of CBT for perfectionism is suitable for people who present with perfectionism as a problem in its own right, when it is a barrier to changing a disorder, or when there are multiple coexisting problems that appear to be maintained by perfectionism and there is no alternative, evidence-based intervention to address the multiple difficulties. Prior to starting treatment, a careful analysis should be undertaken to assess whether the perfectionism is a predisposing, causal, or maintaining factor in the psychopathology, or whether it is a correlate or consequence of it. The crucial point is that as a clinician you derive an individualized formulation of the role of perfectionism for your particular client to establish the treatment plan.

CHAPTER 5

Assessment of Perfectionism

Successful treatment of perfectionism depends upon a comprehensive, evidence-based assessment strategy. This chapter describes the process and available tools for the assessment of perfectionism. It begins with a discussion of the purpose of assessment, followed by a description of core assessment strategies, including interview-based approaches, behavioral assessment techniques, and self-report scales.

Comprehensive cognitive-behavioral assessment for perfectionism includes a number of central features. First, it should include multiple methods. There is no single tool that is adequate for the clinical assessment of perfectionism. At the very least, comprehensive assessment should include a thorough clinical interview, behavioral methods (e.g., behavioral diaries, behavioral observation), and completion of empirically supported scales. In addition, it is often helpful for the process to include multiple informants (e.g., interviews with the client, as well as with significant others). Cognitive-behavioral assessment is an ongoing process that begins before the initiation of treatment and continues throughout the course of treatment, and occasionally after treatment has ended (e.g., follow-up evaluations to assess the maintenance of gains). Which assessment tools to use depends on the goals of the assessment and the questions that the clinician is trying to answer. Table 5.1 includes a summary of the most commonly used assessment strategies.

Goals of Assessment

The assessment process (e.g., timing and types of assessment methods) is determined, in part, by the purpose of the assessment. For example, although existing self-report measures are useful for assessing the severity of perfectionism and particular perfectionism features (e.g., perfectionism-related beliefs, presence of maladaptive vs. adaptive perfectionism), they are often less helpful for establishing a diagnosis, where a semistructured diagnostic interview is more likely to be useful. In the context of clinical perfectionism, assessment typically has a number of goals:

- To assess the presence, absence, or severity of particular symptoms or behaviors (e.g., procrastination, perfectionistic beliefs).
- To assess any associated problems such as depression, eating disorders, anxiety disorders, or obsessive–compulsive and related disorders that may impede treatment, require concurrent monitoring as treatment progresses, or provide domains of intervention with respect to perfectionism.

TABLE 5.1. Components of Comprehensive Assessment of Perfectionism

Clinical interview

- May include both unstructured and structured interview methods.
- Assessment domains
  - o Diagnostic features
  - o Cues and triggers for perfectionistic beliefs and behaviors
  - o Behavioral features
  - o Cognitive features
  - o Physical responses
  - o Environmental factors
  - o Skills deficits
  - o Severity and impact
  - o Development, course, and treatment history
  - o Medical history
  - o Motivation to change

Behavioral assessment strategies

- Self-monitoring diaries can be used to assess features of perfectionism (e.g., cognitions, behaviors, triggers, consequences) between therapy sessions.
- Behavioral observation is a useful strategy for assessing perfectionistic behaviors as they occur.
- In some circumstances, behavioral approach tests may be useful for assessing fear and avoidance responses in the context of clinical perfectionism.

Self-report scales

- Assessment domains
  - o Perfectionism severity
  - o Behavioral domains of perfectionism
  - o Adaptive versus maladaptive perfectionism
  - o Perfectionistic self-presentation
  - o Associated cognitions
  - o Perfectionism in relationships
  - o Perfectionism in sports
  - o Perfectionism, eating disorders, and body image
  - o Perfectionism in adults versus children

- To assess the impact of perfectionism on functioning and quality of life at work or school, in relationships, and in other life domains.
- To facilitate the selection of symptoms or behaviors to target in treatment.
- To inform the process of collaborative case conceptualization.
- To facilitate the development of a treatment plan.
- To assess the effects of the intervention, both during treatment and after treatment has ended.

Clinical Interview

This section reviews the core domains to assess during a clinical interview focused on perfectionism and related problems.

Diagnostic Features

As reviewed elsewhere in this book, perfectionism is a transdiagnostic construct present in a wide range of psychological disorders, including eating disorders, anxiety disorders, and depression, to name a few. A comprehensive diagnostic assessment is helpful for identifying disorders that are often associated with perfectionism. Semistructured interviews provide a reliable and valid method for assessing the presence and absence of associated conditions (for a review of established diagnostic interviews, see Summerfeldt, Kloosterman, & Antony, 2010). One popular semistructured interview is the *Structured Clinical Interview for DSM-5* Disorders (SCID; First, Williams, Karg, & Spitzer, 2014). The SCID (*www.appi.org*) is among the most studied and comprehensive diagnostic interviews, and is available in a both a research version and a briefer, less comprehensive, clinician version. The *MINI International Neuropsychiatric Interview* (MINI; Sheehan et al., 1998; *www.medical-outcomes.com*) is another popular diagnostic interview that takes about 15 minutes to administer, and is currently being updated for DSM-5. To the extent that associated psychological problems are present, assessment of the core features of these disorders is warranted. For example, if a client experiences periods of depression, then a thorough assessment of the depression can be included. For information on strategies and measures for assessing psychological disorders (including those associated with perfectionism), see Antony and Barlow (2010).

Diagnostic assessments may not be engaging for some clients, and thus the timing of diagnostic interviews and the rationale presented to the client need to be carefully considered. One approach is to offer the initial assessment over two sessions, where the first session is focused on a collaborative discussion of the perfectionism and its impact, allowing for a firm establishment of therapeutic alliance, and the second session includes a diagnostic interview. While some therapists may believe that two assessment sessions are excessive, it is worth remembering that therapy begins at assessment, where the types of issues discussed, and the way that they are discussed, can already start to introduce the client to a slightly different perspective on the problems with which he or she has been grappling.

Cues and Triggers for Perfectionistic Beliefs and Behaviors

Understanding the context in which perfectionistic beliefs and behaviors occur is important for selecting appropriate treatment strategies. For example, a client whose perfectionism is triggered by social situations might be taught strategies to shift thoughts about being judged by others, and might be encouraged to confront any situations that are avoided. Examples of possible perfectionism triggers to ask about include *interpersonal cues* (e.g., receiving negative feedback from others), *other situational cues* (e.g., weighing oneself; struggling to meet a strict deadline), *cognitive cues* (e.g., intrusive thoughts that one is inadequate), *emotional cues* (e.g., low mood), and *interoceptive cues* (e.g., sweating in front of others). Cues and triggers will often come up naturally during the initial evaluation and over the course of therapy. They can also be identified through targeted questions.

Examples of questions to ask include:

> "What sorts of situations trigger feelings of anxiety, sadness, anger, or distress (especially situations in which your standards are not met)?"
>
> "Are there particular emotions or feelings that tend to activate your high standards?"
>
> "Do feelings of inadequacy ever get triggered by thoughts that pop into your head? What sorts of thoughts trigger your perfectionism?"
>
> "When you compare yourself to others, how does it affect the way you think about yourself?"
>
> "Are there physical feelings that trigger your perfectionistic standards or beliefs (e.g., a feeling of fullness in individuals with body image concerns; a feeling of shakiness in individuals who are overly concerned about always looking calm in front of others)?"

Behavioral Features

Behavioral features of perfectionism are those things that clients "do" as a result of their perfectionism. Perhaps the most important behavioral features to assess include *avoidance behaviors* (e.g., avoiding anxiety-provoking situations, such as eating forbidden foods or socializing with people who trigger feelings of inadequacy; procrastinating on a project for work or school) and *counterproductive safety behaviors* (e.g., overpreparing for a presentation or other interpersonal challenge; repeated checking to see that everything at home is organized perfectly before leaving the house; suppressing frightening thoughts). Treatment typically involves the gradual reduction of avoidance behaviors and safety behaviors (especially those that impair functioning or prevent cognitive change), so comprehensive assessment of these features is key for developing an effective treatment plan.

Examples of questions to ask include:

"Are there things that you do to prevent yourself from feeling anxious about not meeting your standards?"

"What sorts of things do you do to ensure that you meet your high standards?"

"Are there things that you do that others might consider to be perfectionistic behaviors?"

"Are there strategies that you use to prevent yourself from making mistakes that you might regret later?"

Cognitive Features

CBT involves teaching clients to identify the beliefs, assumptions, predictions, and biases (e.g., in attention and memory) that contribute to perfectionism, and to think more flexibly in the situations where perfectionism is a problem. The assessment of relevant cognitive features typically begins at the first meeting with the client and continues throughout the course of treatment. Clients may report their perfectionistic beliefs spontaneously, though it is typically most helpful to elicit cognitive features by asking about them.

Examples of questions to ask include:

"What were you thinking just before your anxiety began to increase?"

"What would it mean about you if you didn't do your best, for example, if you didn't get the highest grade in the class?"

"What are you predicting might happen if others were to notice your mistakes?"

"Do you hold others to the same standards to which you hold yourself?"

"To what degree do you define your self-worth in terms of your attaining your goals?"

Physical Responses

Clients should be asked about the physical ways in which their perfectionism affects them. For example, some clients may experience *panic attacks* (including intense arousal symptoms such as racing heart, breathlessness, dizziness, and others) upon not living up to their high standards. To the extent that panic attacks are themselves a source of concern for the client, it may be helpful to teach the client strategies for managing his or her panic attacks.

Examples of questions to ask include:

"How do you feel physically when your anxiety hits?"

"When you are unable to meet your high standards, do you experience uncomfortable physical sensations, like racing heart, sweating, or dizziness?"

"Are you frightened by any of the physical sensations that you experience when you are feeling anxious? Do you worry that they might lead to some sort of catastrophe?"

Environmental Factors

Clients should be asked about environmental factors that contribute to perfectionism. For example, perfectionistic behaviors may be encouraged in the client's relationships, at school, or in the workplace. The client's employer may pressure the client to perform at an unrealistically high level and may punish failure to meet expectations. Relatedly, perfectionistic behaviors may be reinforced through attention, praise, money, or other rewards. Another environmental factor that may exacerbate perfectionism is life stress (e.g., health problems, family stress, financial strain, work stress, interpersonal conflict). In addition to asking about life stress during the interview, clinicians may find it useful to administer a brief questionnaire to assess perceived stress, such as the *Perceived Stress Scale* (Cohen, Kamarck, & Mermelstein, 1983).

Examples of questions to ask include:

"Are there ways in which your perfectionism has been rewarded in your life? Are there others who seem to appreciate those traits in you?"

"Have you noticed a relationship between day-to-day stresses in your life and the ways in which you are affected by either your high standards or your difficulty in meeting them?"

"Does your perfectionism cause problems in your relationships with others (e.g., friendships, intimate relationship, parenting)?"

Domains of Perfectionism

Understanding the domains in which perfectionism is a problem can be helpful for identifying the contexts in which treatment strategies are likely to be practiced. The domains of perfectionism may also provide clues regarding the cognitions underlying a client's perfectionism. Examples of common domains of perfectionism include work, school, hobbies (e.g., art, music), daily activities (e.g., housework, driving), organizing, relationships, making small decisions, eating, sports/fitness, and washing/grooming (Antony & Swinson, 2009).

Examples of questions to ask include:

"Are there particular situations where your perfectionism seems to be strongest? For example, at school? At work?"
"In what areas of your life do tend to be most perfectionistic?"
"How does perfectionism affect your relationships?"

Skills Deficits

Clinicians should be mindful of possible skills deficits that may be associated with a failure to meet one's standards. For example, poor study skills may interfere with a client's ability to perform at a high level at school. Similarly, deficits in social skills, problem-solving skills, time management skills, or organizational skills may affect performance in various life domains. In these cases, treatment may include strategies for improving these skills, in addition to strategies for coping better when one's standards are not met.

A number of strategies can be used to assess skills deficits, including behavioral observation, clinical interviews, interviews with significant others and family members, and standardized psychological tests. Through behavioral observation, the clinician may note evidence of skills deficits and follow up with additional assessment as needed. For example, after noting that a client is frequently late for therapy appointments, the therapist may follow up with questions to assess whether lateness is a pattern across other life domains, and if so whether the issue is related to problems with time management (e.g., overscheduling). Clinical interviews may also generate useful information about skills deficits. For example, during an interview a client may report a long history of academic performance issues that may be related to poor study skills. The therapist should be sure to ask for objective evidence of any skills deficits reported, since perfectionism may lead clients to judge themselves as "deficient" in the absence of any evidence. Interviews with significant others or family members of the client can provide corroborating evidence of any reported skills deficits. Finally, for some types of suspected deficits (intellectual ability, memory, etc.), standardized psychological tests may provide an objective assessment of the client's skills and aptitudes.

Severity and Impact

Clients should be asked about the ways in which perfectionism impacts negatively upon their lives, including the distress it creates and the ways in which it causes impairment across a variety of areas, such as work, school, relationships, daily activities (e.g., housework), health, and other life domains. Through the assessment process, clients can also be encouraged to distinguish between standards that cause distress and impairment versus standards that are potentially helpful. Antony and Swinson (2009, pp. 88–89) provide a list of questions to facilitate distinguishing between helpful and unhelpful standards:

> "Are your standards higher than those of other people?"
> "Are you able to meet your standards? If so, at what cost?"
> "Are other people able to meet your standards?'
> "Do your standards help you to achieve your goals or do they get in the way (e.g., by making you overly disappointed or angry when your standards are not met or causing you to get less work done)?"
> "What would be the costs of relaxing a particular standard or ignoring a rule that you have?"
> "What would be the benefits of relaxing a particular standard or ignoring a rule that you have?"

Development, Course, and Treatment History

The interview should include a discussion regarding how and when the problem developed. For example, has perfectionism been a lifelong problem? At what age did the client begin to notice that perfectionism was an issue? Is the client aware of any early experiences that may have led to the problem, such as modeling of perfectionistic behaviors by significant others, external pressure to be perfect, criticism by others, or reinforcement of perfectionistic behaviors?

Establishing the course and history of the problem is also useful. For example, it is helpful to know whether there have been times in the past when the behaviors associated with perfectionism were adaptive or functional, and either how they evolved over time, or the client's situation changed over time, such that the behaviors became a problem.

Some possible questions to ask include:

> "What has the course of the problem been over time?"
> "Has the perfectionism been stable?"
> "Has it worsened or improved over time?"
> "Has it waxed and waned?"
> "Have changes in the perfectionism coincided with any major life events or other possible triggers?"
> "Was there a time when your perfectionism was helpful to you (e.g., rewarded by others)? What changed over time?"

In addition to getting a sense of the development and course of the problem over time, it is helpful to know the history of any treatment the client has received, including both psychological treatments and medications. The clinician should ask questions about what treatments were received, the duration and intensity of past treatments, and compliance with previous interventions (e.g., completion of treatment homework). If the client has received CBT in the past, the clinician should ask about the specific strategies that were used. Some clients (and therapists) may believe they're using cognitive and behavioral strategies, when in fact the most appropriate strategies are either not being used at all or are being used incorrectly.

Medical History

As with the treatment of any psychological problem, is important that the client receive a full medical examination. Some psychological symptoms that are associated with perfectionism (e.g., depression, anxiety) may stem from medical problems that require treatment. In addition, some symptoms of psychological disorders (e.g., low body weight in eating disorders) may trigger medical issues that need to be addressed by a physician.

Motivation to Change

Clients are often ambivalent about changing their perfectionism (Egan, Piek, Dyck, Rees, & Hagger, 2013) due to the perceived benefits of perfectionism. It can be useful to identify ambivalence early in the process by asking questions about the client's commitment to therapy and the perceived costs and benefits of changing. For clients who are ambivalent about treatment, engaging the individual in motivational interviewing (e.g., Miller & Rollnick, 2013) before starting CBT may be useful. In addition, the book *Overcoming Perfectionism* (Shafran et al., 2010) includes worksheets to help clients to assess their level of motivation and reduce ambivalence about treatment.

Behavioral Assessment Strategies

Compared to interviews and self-report scales, behavioral strategies can provide more objective data regarding how an individual's perfectionism affects his or her behavior. For example, completion of *self-monitoring diaries* throughout the course of treatment can provide data on relevant behaviors as they occur. Examples of variables that can be recorded on diaries include perfectionism triggers, perfectionistic thoughts, perfectionistic behaviors, and consequences of perfectionistic behaviors. Clinicians should be mindful of cases in which the data recorded by clients are overly detailed and thorough. The ways clients complete their diaries can sometimes provide important clues about the nature of the client's perfectionism, as well as possible targets for treatment.

Behavioral observation can also be useful for gathering data on the client's perfectionism. This strategy involves observing the client and noting examples of perfectionistic behaviors or other behaviors of interest. Behavioral observation may be conducted by the therapist (e.g., observing perfectionistic behaviors in the therapy session) or by others (e.g., having the client arrange for a family member to record examples of perfectionistic behaviors that occur between therapy sessions). Observation by family members is particularly useful in cases where perfectionism impacts upon family relationships.

A related strategy is the *behavioral approach test* (BAT), which often includes behavioral observation as a component. BATs involve asking a client to approach a feared situation and measuring (1) whether the client is able to complete the task, and (2) the client's response during exposure to the feared situation. BATs are used frequently in the assessment of anxiety disorders and may be useful for assessing clients for whom perfectionism is associated with anxiety, fear, and avoidance.

For example, a client who is anxious about making a mistake in front of others might be encouraged to purposely do something incorrectly (e.g., mispronounce a word; show up late for an appointment; include typos in an e-mail) and then to report on the outcome (e.g., his or her cognitive and emotional responses to the situation; safety behaviors used to manage anxiety). BATs can be helpful in cases where clients are less aware of how they actually respond in a feared situation (perhaps because they normally avoid the situation).

Although BATs can provide useful information (e.g., about the client's actual response in a feared situation), therapists should be sensitive to possible negative effects from the BAT, including (1) possible ruptures to the therapeutic relationship, particularly for clients who are reluctant to change their perfectionistic standards, and (2) clients feeling discouraged if they are unable to complete the BAT with minimal discomfort. If BATs are to be used, they should be set up carefully. Clients should understand the rationale for the BAT (as an assessment tool) and should not be coerced into doing anything they are not ready to do. BATs may be most appropriate after therapy is well under way, when clients are fully engaged in the therapeutic process and a trusting relationship between the client and therapist is well established.

Self-Report Measures of Perfectionism

This section focuses primarily on measures designed specifically for the assessment of perfectionism. A selection of the self-report measures of perfectionism discussed in this chapter can be found in Appendix 3 and can also be downloaded from the publisher's website (*www.guilford. com/egan-forms*). Scoring instructions are provided in this chapter for the 15 reprinted and downloadable measures in Appendix 3. For scales that are not reprinted in this book, information is included in Table 5.2 on where the scale can be obtained.

Note that a number of broader psychological tests have also been used to measure perfectionism, including the *Minnesota Multiphasic Personality Inventory–2* (MMPI-2; Butcher, Dahlstrom, Graham, Tellegen, & Kaemmer, 2001; e.g., Rice & Stuart, 2010); *Millon Index of Personality Styles Revised* (MIPS-R; Millon, 2004; e.g., Rice & Stuart, 2010); *Dysfunctional Attitude Scale* (DAS; Weissman & Beck, 1978; e.g., Blatt et al., 1998); and *Personal Style Inventory* (PIS; Robins et al., 1994; e.g., Shahar, 2006), to name a few.

In selecting which scale(s) to use several factors should be considered. It is important to select scales that (1) assess constructs of interest (e.g., perfectionism severity, perfectionism domains, perfectionism-related cognitions), (2) are practical to administer (e.g., brief, easy to score, easy for clients to understand), and (3) are useful for assessing change over time (if the scale is to be used for assessing outcome). All things being equal, it is also preferable to use scales with established reliability (e.g., internal consistency, interrater reliability, test–retest reliability) and validity (e.g., concurrent validity, construct validity, content validity, convergent validity, criterion-related validity, discriminant validity, discriminative validity, incremental validity, face validity, predictive validity, sensitivity and specificity, supported subscale structure). However, only the most basic types of validity and reliability have been studied for existing perfectionism measures, and each of the scales reviewed has limitations. For example, validity of these scales has, for the most part, been established by examining the correlations between these scales and other self-report measures of perfectionism. Given the overlap in content across the most popular perfectionism scales, it is not surprising that perfectionism measures tend to be highly intercorrelated. In contrast, little is known about the predictive validity of commonly used perfectionism measures (e.g., whether they actually predict the occurrence of behaviors thought to be associated with perfectionism). In fact, as reviewed in Chapter 1, there is not even an agreed-upon definition of *perfectionism* among experts.

A number of other factors should be considered when selecting scales. For example, some scales are designed for use in particular populations (e.g., children, athletes, people with eating disorders), whereas others are designed for more general use. Some scales focus only on clinical (i.e., maladaptive, unhealthy, or "bad") perfectionism, whereas others include items to assess healthy high standards (sometimes referred to as adaptive or "good" perfectionism), and some are designed to distinguish between these two types of perfectionism. Scales also differ with respect to how they define perfectionism and its components, whether they view perfectionism as a unidimensional or multidimensional construct, how well they have been validated in diverse populations, their complexity, their cost, and other important dimensions.

Although there is no perfect scale for measuring perfectionism, a small number of scales have emerged as particularly popular options, at least among researchers who study perfectionism. The two general perfectionism scales that have been researched the most have been around for more than two decades, and were both originally referred to as the Multidimensional Perfectionism Scale. To avoid confusion, we refer to them by their authors' names: the *Hewitt and Flett Multidimensional Perfectionism Scale* (HMPS; Hewitt & Flett, 1991b) and the *Frost et al. Multidimensional Perfectionism Scale* (FMPS; Frost et al., 1990). The *Almost Perfect Scale—Revised* (APS-R; Slaney, Rice, Mobley, Trippi, & Ashby, 2001) is also widely used in perfectionism research, though not nearly as much as the FMPS and HMPS. Despite their popularity among researchers for measuring perfectionism, their usefulness in routine clinical practice has been questioned. All three of these measures include items that measure both positive and negative forms of perfectionism, and not all subscales are relevant to perfectionism in clinical populations.

The other scales reviewed in this section are either less well validated, less popular, or have a more specialized focus. Nevertheless, they are potentially useful, depending on the assessment objectives. The remainder of this section provides a description of existing self-report perfectionism measures, which are summarized in Table 5.2.

Almost Perfect Scale—Revised

The APS-R (Slaney et al., 2001) is a 23-item questionnaire designed to measure three independent dimensions of perfectionism: *high standards* (i.e., a tendency to have elevated standards for one's own performance; items 1, 5, 8, 12, 14, 18, and 22); *order* (i.e., a tendency to prefer order and organization; items 2, 4, 7, and 10); and *discrepancy* (i.e., a belief that one consistently fails to meet one's own high standards; items 3, 6, 9, 11, 13, 15, 16, 17, 19, 20, 21, and 23). Items are rated on a 7-point scale ranging from 1 (strongly disagree) to 7 (strongly agree). The APS-R was designed to improve upon existing measures (e.g., Frost et al., 1990; Hewitt & Flett, 1991b; Slaney & Johnson, 1992) with four goals in mind: (1) to measure variables that define perfectionism, rather than variables that reflect causes, correlates, or consequences of perfectionism; (2) to measure both adaptive and maladaptive aspects of perfectionism; (3) to reflect commonly held views regarding the definition of perfectionism; and (4) to be empirically sound (Slaney et al., 2001).

TABLE 5.2. Summary of Self-Report Measures

Measure	Purpose	Length	Comments
General perfectionism measures			
Almost Perfect Scale—Revised (APS-R; Slaney et al., 2001)	Assesses three dimensions of perfectionism: (1) high standards, (2) order, and (3) discrepancy.	23 items	• Well researched; strong psychometric properties. • Distinguishes between adaptive and maladaptive perfectionism. • Translated into multiple languages. • Reprinted in Appendix 3 of this volume.
Behavioral Domains Questionnaire (BDQ; Lee et al., 2011)	Assesses the behavioral expression of perfectionism across five life domains: (1) housework, (2) work, (3) social, (4) hobbies, and (5) appearance.	37 items	• Assesses seven different types of perfectionistic behaviors. • Preliminary evidence supports clinical utility. • Reprinted in Appendix 3 of this volume.
Burns Perfectionism Scale (BPS; Burns, 1980)	Assesses clinical perfectionism.	10 items	• One of the first published perfectionism measures. • Widely cited but little is known about its psychometric properties. • Reprinted in the original article in *Psychology Today.*
Clinical Perfectionism Questionnaire (CPQ; Fairburn et al., 2003a)	Assesses clinical perfectionism.	12 items	• Scale has well-supported psychometric properties. • Useful scale for assessing perfectionism across sessions. • Reprinted in Appendix 3 of this volume.
Consequences of Perfectionism Scale (COPS; Kim, 2010)	Assesses perceptions of perfectionism as being either adaptive or maladaptive.	10 items	• Preliminary research supports reliability and validity. • Reprinted in Appendix 3 of this volume.

(continued)

TABLE 5.2. *(continued)*

Measure	Purpose	Length	Comments
General perfectionism measures *(continued)*			
Frost et al. Multidimensional Perfectionism Scale (FMPS; Frost et al., 1990)	Assesses six dimensions of perfectionism: (1) concern over mistakes, (2) doubts about actions, (3) personal standards, (4) parental expectations, (5) parental criticism, and (6) organization.	35 items	• One of the two best-studied and most popular scales for measuring perfectionism. • Good support for psychometric properties, except for mixed evidence regarding the number of factors. • Translated into multiple languages. • Reprinted in Appendix 3 of this volume.
Hewitt and Flett Multidimensional Perfectionism Scale (HMPS; Hewitt & Flett, 1991b)	Assesses three dimensions of perfectionism: (1) self-oriented perfectionism, (2) other-oriented perfectionism, and (3) socially prescribed perfectionism.	45 items	• One of the two best-studied and most popular scales for measuring perfectionism. • Strong support for psychometric properties. • Available from the publisher (Multi-Health Systems).
Neurotic Perfectionism Questionnaire (NPQ; Mitzman et al., 1994)	Designed to measure perfectionism in people with eating disorders, though content of items is general.	42 items	• No data on psychometric properties. • Scale is not widely used. • Reprinted in original journal article.
Perfectionism Inventory (PI; Hill et al., 2004)	Assesses eight domains of perfectionism: (1) concern over mistakes, (2) high standards for others, (3) need for approval, (4) organization, (5) perceived parental pressure, (6) planfulness, and (8) striving for excellence.	59 items	• Original journal article suggests good psychometric properties. • Not widely used or studied. • Reprinted in Appendix 3 of this volume.
Perfectionistic Self-Presentation Scale (PSPS; Hewitt, Flett, Sherry, et al., 2003)	Assesses the desire to appear perfect in front of others across three dimensions: (1) perfectionistic self-promotion, (2) nondisplay of imperfection, and (3) nondisclosure of imperfection.	27 items	• Preliminary research supports psychometric properties. • Available from Paul Hewitt's website (*http://hewittlab.psych.ubc.ca/requests.htm*).

Measure	Description	Number of items	Notes
Positive and Negative Perfectionism Scale (PANPS; Terry-Short et al., 1995)	Assesses positive and negative aspects of perfectionism.	40 items	• Psychometric support is mixed. • One study suggests that a briefer (19-item) version may be more useful. • Reprinted in Appendix 3 of this volume.
Perfectionism-related cognitions			
Perfectionism Cognitions Inventory (PCI; Flett et al., 1998)	Assesses the frequency of automatic thoughts involving themes of perfectionism.	25 items	• Preliminary research supports psychometric properties. • Available from Paul Hewitt's website (*http://hewittlab.psych.ubc.ca/requests.htm*). • Reprinted in Appendix 3 of this volume.
Multidimensional Perfectionism Cognitions Inventory—English (MPCI-E; Kobori, 2006)	Assesses cognitions associated with self-oriented perfectionism and socially prescribed perfectionism along three dimensions: (1) personal standards, (2) pursuit of perfection, and (3) concern over mistakes.	15 items	• Preliminary research supports psychometric properties. • Reprinted in Appendix 3 of this volume.
Perfectionism in relationships			
Dyadic Almost Perfect Scale (DAPS; Shea & Slaney, 1999)	Assesses perfectionistic beliefs about one's partner along three dimensions: (1) high standards, (2) order, and (3) discrepancy.	26 items	• Preliminary research supports psychometric properties. • Reprinted in Appendix 3 of this volume.
Family Almost Perfect Scale (FAPS; Wang et al., 2010)	Assesses beliefs regarding family members' standards along three dimensions: (1) family standards, (2) family order, and (3) family discrepancy.	17 items	• Preliminary research supports psychometric properties. • Reprinted in Appendix 3 of this volume.
Multidimensional Parenting Perfectionism Scale (MPPS; Snell et al., 2005)	Assesses perfectionism in the context of parenting (includes 11 subscales).	65 items	• More research needed on psychometric properties. • Reprinted in Appendix 3 of this volume.

(continued)

TABLE 5.2. *(continued)*

Measure	Purpose	Length	Comments
Perfectionism and sports			
Sport Multidimensional Perfectionism Scale–2 (Sport-MPS-2; Gotwals & Dunn, 2009)	Assesses perfectionism in the context of sport along six dimensions: (1) personal standards, (2) concern over mistakes, (3) perceived parental pressure, (4) perceived coach pressure, (5) doubts about actions, and (6) organization.	42 items	• Preliminary research supports psychometric properties. • Reprinted in Appendix 3 of this volume.
Sport Perfectionism Scale (SPS; Anshel et al., 2009)	Assesses sport-related perfectionism.	35 items	• Preliminary research supports psychometric properties, including unidimensional factor structure. • Reprinted in Appendix 3 of this volume.
Perfectionism, eating disorders, and body image			
Eating Disorders Inventory— Perfectionism Subscale (EDI-P; Garner, 1991)	Assesses perfectionism in the context of eating disorders.	6 items	• Part of the EDI-3, a popular and well-established measure for eating disorders. • Available from the publisher, PAR.
Physical Appearance Perfectionism Scale (PAPS; Yang & Stoeber, 2012)	Assesses perfectionism about physical appearance along two dimensions: (1) worry about imperfection, and (2) hope for perfection.	12 items	• Preliminary research supports psychometric properties. • Reprinted in Appendix 3 of this volume.

Perfectionism in children

Measure	Description	Items	Notes
Adaptive/Maladaptive Perfectionism Scale (AMPS; Rice & Preusser, 2002)	Assesses perfectionism in children ages 9 to 12 years, along four dimensions: (1) sensitivity to mistakes, (2) contingent self-esteem, (3) compulsiveness, and (4) need for admiration.	27 items	• Preliminary research supports psychometric properties. • Reprinted in Appendix 3 of this volume.
Child and Adolescent Perfectionism Scale (CAPS; Flett et al., 2000)	Assesses perfectionism in children along two dimensions: (1) self-oriented perfectionism, and (2) socially prescribed perfectionism.	22 items	• Preliminary research supports psychometric properties. • Available from Paul Hewitt's website (*http://hewittlab.psych.ubc.ca/requests.htm*).
Childhood Retrospective Perfectionism Scale (CHIRP; Southgate et al., 2008)	Assesses childhood perfectionism retrospectively, with an emphasis on obsessive–compulsive personality traits.	20 items	• Two versions available (20 items each)—one for the individual to report on his/her own perfectionism in childhood, and one for an informant to complete. • Preliminary research supports psychometric properties. • Reprinted in the original journal article by Southgate et al. (2008).
Perfectionistic Self-Presentation Scale—Junior Form (PSPS-JR; Hewitt et al., 2011)	Assesses perfectionistic self-presentation in children and adolescents across three dimensions: (1) perfectionistic self-promotion, (2) nondisplay of imperfection, and (3) nondisclosure of imperfection.	18 items	• Preliminary research supports psychometric properties. • Available from Paul Hewitt's website (*http://hewittlab.psych.ubc.ca/requests.htm*).

The APS-R is one of the three most widely used measures of perfectionism, and its psychometric properties (e.g., factor structure, construct validity, convergent validity, discriminant validity, internal consistency, test–retest reliability, internal consistency) are supported by a number of studies (for a review, see Slaney, Rice, & Ashby, 2002). The measure's three factors appear to measure independent constructs, with acceptable levels of internal consistency (Slaney et al., 2001).

The APS-R has been used to distinguish between adaptive versus maladaptive perfectionism. Maladaptive perfectionism is associated with elevated scores on both the *high standards* and *discrepancy* subscales, whereas adaptive perfectionists tend to have high scores on the *high standards* subscale and low scores on the *discrepancy* subscale. The APS-R has been used in both adults and in children (Vandiver & Worrell, 2002), and has been studied across a number of ethnically diverse groups (e.g., Chan, 2010; Mobley, Slaney, & Rice, 2005). The APS-R has been translated into several languages, including Chinese, Dutch, Japanese, Korean, and Turkish. An eight-item version of the APS-R was recently developed by Rice, Richardson, and Tueller (in press).

The APS-R is reprinted in Appendix 3 of this volume. Scores for each of the three subscales are generated by computing the sum of scores for items in the subscale. In a sample of over 1,500 undergraduate students, Rice and Ashby (2007) reported means and standard deviations for each subscale as follows: *high standards* ($M = 42.45$; $SD = 5.46$), *order* ($M = 21.22$; $SD = 4.63$), *discrepancy* ($M = 39.80$; $SD = 15.22$). In their comprehensive psychometric analysis, Rice and Ashby (2007) found that a score of 37 or higher on the *high standards* subscale distinguished perfectionists from nonperfectionists, and that among perfectionists, a score of 45 or higher on the *discrepancy* subscale suggested significant maladaptive perfectionism. In this study, the *order* subscale was not useful either for identifying perfectionists or for distinguishing between adaptive and maladaptive perfectionists.

Behavioral Domains Questionnaire

The *Behavioral Domains Questionnaire* (BDQ; Lee, Roberts-Collins, Coughtrey, Phillips, & Shafran, 2011) is a 37-item measure designed to assess the behavioral expression of perfectionism across five life domains: *housework* (sample item: "How often have you found it difficult to stop cleaning the house because you've been striving to complete it to your personal standards?"); *work* (sample item: "How often have you checked your work over and over for mistakes?"); *social* (sample item: "How often have you thought about past social interactions to see if your behavior met your personal standards?"); *hobbies* (sample item: "How often have you avoided group activities because you wanted to achieve the best and were afraid of being compared?"); and *appearance* (sample item: "How often have you brushed your teeth for longer than five minutes?"). Each item is rated (based on the past 4 weeks) on a 5-point scale ranging from 1 (never) to 5 (always). The BDQ assesses seven different types of perfectionistic behaviors: (1) taking excessive time over tasks (items 1, 2, 14, 17, 26, 32, and 33); being overly thorough (items 3, 4, 5, and 37); inability to stop a task once started (items 6, 15, 29, 34); checking for mistakes (items 7, 10, 12, 18, 21, 28, 30, 36); difficulties in task completion (items 11, 13, 16, and 35); safety behavior (items 8, 9, 20, 22, 24, 25, and 31); and avoidance (items 19, 23, and 27). Although internal consistency for the total score was excellent, it was generally lower for the subscale scores (Lee et al., 2011). The BDQ appears to be a clinically useful scale, though more research is needed to establish its psychometric properties.

The BDQ is reprinted in Appendix 3 of this volume. A score is generated for each of the seven behavior subscales by computing the mean of scores for the subscale (i.e., summing all relevant items and dividing by the number of items in that subscale). Therefore, each behavior subscale can have a score between 1 and 5. Means and standard deviations for individuals with elevated perfectionism were reported by Lee et al. (2011) as follows: *excessive time* (M = 1.89; SD = 0.50), *overly thorough* (M = 1.50; SD = 0.53), *inability to stop a task* (M = 1.80; SD = 0.62), *checking* (M = 2.24; SD = 0.57), *task completion difficulties* (M = 1.73; SD = 0.69), *safety behavior* (M = 2.31; SD = 0.69), *avoidance* (M = 1.90; SD = 0.64). In general, scores more than one standard deviation above or below the mean can be considered high or low, respectively.

Burns Perfectionism Scale

The *Burns Perfectionism Scale* (BPS; Burns, 1980) is one of the earliest measures for assessing clinical perfectionism, and was originally printed in David Burns's classic *Psychology Today* article on the role of maladaptive cognition in problematic perfectionism. The BPS is a 10-item measure in which each item is rated on a 5-point scale ranging from +2 (agree very much) to –2 (disagree strongly). The scale treats perfectionism as a unidimensional construct. Although the BPS is widely cited, little is known about its psychometric properties. The article containing the scale is reprinted in various places online (e.g., *www.ucdenver.edu/life/services/counseling-center/Documents/The-Perfectionists-Script-for-Self-Defeat.pdf*).

Clinical Perfectionism Questionnaire

The CPQ (Fairburn et al., 2003a) was developed to measure *clinical perfectionism*, a unidimensional, transdiagnostic construct defined as "the overdependence of self-evaluation on the determined pursuit of personally demanding, self-imposed, standards in at least one highly salient domain, despite adverse consequences" (Shafran et al., 2002, p. 778). The CPQ is a 12-item self-report questionnaire that measures the tendency to set high goals and the consequences of not meeting them (sample item: "Have you pushed yourself really hard to meet your goals?") including self-worth being based on meeting standards. Items are rated on a 4-point scale, ranging from 1 (not at all) to 4 (all of the time).

The CPQ has been used in several studies that have examined its psychometric properties in both nonclinical (Chang & Sanna, 2012; Dickie, Surgenor, Wilson, & McDowall, 2012; Egan, Shafran, Lee, Fairburn, Cooper, et al., 2014; Stoeber & Damian, 2014) and eating disorder samples (Egan, Shafran, et al., 2014; Steele, O'Shea, Murdock, & Wade, 2011). After the removal of two psychometrically problematic items, the CPQ was found to have two moderately correlated factors, each with modest internal consistency and test–retest reliability (Dickie et al., 2012): (1) *personal standards*, and (2) *emotional concerns and consequences*. A similar two-factor solution has also been found in another nonclinical sample (Egan, Shafran, et al., 2014). Furthermore, the CPQ has been shown to have good internal consistency and convergent validity in eating disorder samples (Steele, O'Shea, et al., 2011). The CPQ has also been shown to have good test–retest reliability and construct and discriminative validity, being able to differentiate between a clinical eating disorder sample and healthy controls (Egan, Shafran, et al., 2014). In another study, total scores on the full CPQ were found to have adequate internal consistency, and the CPQ was found to predict maladjustment over and above the effects of negative affect and multidimensional perfectionism (Chang & Sanna, 2012). Finally, the CPQ is sensitive to the effects of treatment (Riley, Lee, Cooper, Fairburn, & Shafran, 2007).

Preliminary studies on the CPQ suggest that this scale may be useful for assessing clinical perfectionism, particularly as a measure of treatment outcome (e.g., Steele et al., 2013). However, more research on the CPQ's psychometric properties is needed, especially in clinical samples as to date clinical research has been restricted to eating disorder clinical samples. The CPQ is reprinted in Appendix 3 of this volume. Items 1, 3, 4, 5, 6, 7, 9, 10, 11, and 12 are scored as follows: 1 = not at all; 2 = some of the time; 3 = most of the time; 4 = all of the time. Items 2 and 8 are reverse scored, such that 4 = not at all; 3 = some of the time; 2 = most of the time; 1 = all of the time. A total score is computed by summing all 12 items. In a group of treatment-seeking individuals with clinically significant perfectionism, Riley, Lee, Cooper, Fairburn, and Shafran (2007) reported a mean of 35.70 (SD = 5.07) before treatment and 28.80 (SD = 13.15) following treatment.

Consequences of Perfectionism Scale

The *Consequences of Perfectionism Scale* (COPS; Kim, 2010; Kim & Chang, 2010) was designed to measure perceptions of perfectionism as being either adaptive or maladaptive. This 10-item instrument includes 6 items describing positive consequences of perfectionism and 4 items describing negative consequences. Items are rated on a scale ranging from 1 (extremely untrue of me) to 5 (extremely true of me). The scale was shortened from an earlier 30-item version. Recent research supports the factor structure, reliability, and validity of this instrument (Stoeber et al., 2013). The COPS is reprinted in Appendix 3 of this volume. Items 2, 3, 5, and 9 (negative consequences of perfectionism) are reverse scored (1 = 5; 2 = 4; 4 = 2; 5 = 1). A total score is then computed by summing all 10 items.

Frost et al. Multidimensional Perfectionism Scale

The FMPS (Frost et al., 1990) is one of the most extensively studied scales for measuring perfectionism in both clinical and nonclinical populations. This 35-item measure assesses perfectionism across six dimensions and generates both a Total Perfectionism score as well as scores for each of the following six subscales: (1) *concern over mistakes* (CM; sample item: "If I fail at work/school, I am a failure as a person"), (2) *doubts about actions* (DA; sample item: "I usually have doubts about the simple everyday things I do"), (3) *personal standards* (PS; sample item: "I set higher goals than most people"), (4) *parental expectations* (PE; sample item: "My parents set very high standards for me"), (5) *parental criticism* (PC; sample item: "As a child, I was punished for doing things less than perfectly") and (6) *organization* (O; sample item: "Organization is very important to me"). Items are rated on a scale ranging from 1 (strongly disagree) to 5 (strongly agree), and are reprinted in the original article on the development of the scale (Frost et al., 1990). Because O does not correlate highly the other subscales, O items are not included when computing the total FMPS score (Frost et al., 1990).

Although the scale generates a total score, there are a number of reasons to question the usefulness of the total. All factor analytic studies on the FMPS suggest that the measure is multifactorial, and it is not clear that the dimensions assessed are additive. As reviewed in Chapter 1, some subscales (e.g., CM) appear to measure core features of perfectionism, whereas others (e.g., PE, PC) appear to measure causes or correlates of perfectionism. In addition, some subscales (e.g., PS and O) appear to reflect a higher-order construct of adaptive or healthy perfectionism, whereas other subscales (CM, DA, PC, PE) appear to reflect a higher-order construct of maladaptive or unhealthy perfectionism (e.g., Bieling et al., 2004; Frost et al., 1993). The total score would seem less useful, given the fact that the subscales measure such different constructs.

A number of studies have investigated the factor structure of the FMPS. Although the original paper by Frost et al. (1990) supported the proposed six-factor solution, most subsequent studies have found four factors, with the CM and DA items loading together, and the PE and PC items loading together (for a review, see Hawkins et al., 2006). Otherwise, the FMPS has good psychometric properties, including acceptable levels convergent validity, discriminant validity, and internal consistency, both for the total score and the subscales (e.g., Frost et al., 1990). It is also sensitive to treatment (e.g., Pleva & Wade, 2007). The FMPS has been translated into a number of languages, including Chinese, German, Korean, and Spanish, to name a few. There have also been efforts to develop briefer versions of the FMPS (e.g., a 24-item version; Khawaja & Armstrong, 2005).

The FMPS is reprinted in Appendix 3 of this volume. Subscale scores are computed by summing relevant items as follows: CM = sum of items 9, 10, 13, 14, 18, 21, 23, 25, and 34; DA = sum of items 17, 28, 32, and 33; PC = sum of items 3, 5, 22, and 35; PE = sum of items 1, 11, 15, 20, and 26; PS = sum of items 4, 6, 12, 16, 19, 24, and 30. O = sum of items 2, 7, 8, 27, 29, and 31. A total score can be computed by summing all of the subscale scores except O. Antony et al. (1998) reported FMPS means and standard deviations for both individuals with social anxiety disorder and a group of nonclinical volunteers. Values for the social anxiety disorder group were as follows: CM (M = 27.48; SD = 8.35), DA (M = 13.03; SD = 4.03), PS (M = 22.42; SD = 5.89), PE (M = 13.49; SD = 5.40), PC (M = 11.33; SD = 4.54), O (M = 22.03; SD = 5.19). Values for the nonclinical group were as follows: CM (M = 17.43; SD = 5.25), DA (M = 7.74; SD = 3.15), PS (M = 22.74; SD = 6.07), PE (M = 13.63; SD = 4.31), PC (M = 8.69; SD = 3.65), O (M = 22.57; SD = 4.38). Generally, scores greater than one standard deviation above the mean can be considered higher and scores less than one standard deviation below the mean can be considered lower.

Hewitt and Flett Multidimensional Perfectionism Scale

Like the FMPS, the HMPS (Hewitt & Flett, 1991b) is one of the most researched questionnaires for measuring perfectionism. The HMPS is a 45-item questionnaire designed to measure three dimensions of perfectionism: (1) *self-oriented perfectionism* (SOP; sample item: "When I am working on something, I cannot relax until it is perfect"), (2) *other-oriented perfectionism* (OOP; sample item: "Everything that others do must be of top-notch quality"), and (3) *socially prescribed perfectionism* (SPP; sample item: "I find it difficult to meet others' expectations of me"). Each item is rated on a 7-point scale ranging from 1 (strongly disagree) to 7 (strongly agree).

The HMPS has been found to have acceptable psychometric properties in both clinical and nonclinical samples, including concurrent validity, temporal stability, and internal consistency (Hewitt & Flett, 1991b; Hewitt, Flett, Turnbull-Donovan, & Mikhail, 1991). An exploratory factor analysis in a student sample supported the three-factor structure of the HMPS (Hewitt & Flett, 1991b); however, an attempt to replicate these findings in both clinical and nonclinical samples was successful only when an empirically derived subset of 15 items (five from each subscale) was used (Cox, Enns, & Clara, 2002). For the most part, SPP is most consistently associated with higher levels of psychopathology, relative to SOP and OOP (e.g., Antony et al., 1998; Bieling et al., 2004; Hewitt et al., 1991b; Frost et al., 1993). The HMPS is available for purchase from Multi-Health Systems (*www.mhs.com/product.aspx?gr=cli&id=overview&prod=mps*).

Neurotic Perfectionism Questionnaire

The *Neurotic Perfectionism Questionnaire* (NPQ; Mitzman, Slade, & Dewey, 1994) is a 42-item questionnaire designed to measure problem perfectionism. Although it was designed primarily for use in people with eating disorders, the content of the items is general (sample item: "If I do badly at something, I feel like a total failure"), and none of the items contains content specifically related to eating, body image, or weight. The authors of the NPQ provided some evidence that scores on the NPQ are related to eating disorder psychopathology, though we are aware of no published data on the psychometric properties (e.g., factor structure, reliability, validity) of the scale. The full NPQ is reprinted in the original article by Mitzman et al. (1994).

Perfectionism Inventory

The *Perfectionism Inventory* (PI; Hill et al., 2004) was developed as a comprehensive tool to capture the dimensions assessed by both the FMPS and the HMPS, as well as dimensions that are not assessed by either of these scales. The PI includes 59 items, rated on a 5-point scale, ranging from 1 (strongly disagree) to 5 (strongly agree). The PI assesses perfectionism across eight domains: (1) *concern over mistakes* (CM; items 6, 14, 22, 30, 38, 46, 53, and 57); (2) *high standards for others* (HSO; items 3, 11, 19, 27, 35, 43, and 50); (3) *need for approval* (NA; items 2, 10, 18, 26, 34, 42, 49, and 59); (4) *organization* (O; items 4, 12, 20, 28, 36, 44, 51, and 56); (5) *perceived parental pressure* (PP; items 7, 15, 23, 31, 39, 47, 54, and 58); (6) *planfulness* (P; items 5, 13, 21, 29, 37, 45, and 52); (7) *rumination* (R; 8, 16, 24, 32, 40, 48, and 55), and (8) *striving for excellence* (SE; items 1, 9, 17, 25, 33, and 41). In addition, a composite (i.e., total) PI score as well as two higher-order perfectionism scale scores (*conscientious perfectionism* and *self-evaluative perfectionism*) can be computed. Exploratory and confirmatory factor analyses by the authors of the PI support both the eight-scale structure of the PI and the two higher-order composite PI scales (Hill et al., 2004). Internal consistency and test–retest reliability were strong for each of the eight scales. Convergent validity was also strong.

The PI has not been widely used, and the original validation study is the only published investigation of its psychometric properties. The PI is reprinted in Appendix 3 of this volume. A score for each of the eight subscales is generated by calculating the mean of scores for all items in the subscale (i.e., computing the sum of the items and dividing by the number of items in the subscale). Therefore, each subscale can have a score between 1 and 5. The composite PI score is generated by computing the sum of all eight subscales. The *conscientious perfectionism* sum scale is generated by computing the sum of the HSO, O, P, and SE subscales, and the *self-evaluative perfectionism* sum scale consists of the sum of the CM, NA, PP, and R subscales. Means and standard deviations (for 508 adults, mean age 32.4 years with SD of 15.6 years; Robert Hill, personal communication, January 10, 2014) are as follows: CM ($M = 2.78$; $SD = 0.99$), HSO ($M = 3.19$; $SD = 0.90$), NA ($M = 3.30$; $SD = 0.99$), O ($M = 3.63$; $SD = 0.96$), PP ($M = 2.99$; $SD = 1.15$), P ($M = 3.96$; $SD = 069$), R ($M = 3.29$; $SD = 1.00$), SE ($M = 3.30$; $SD = 0.92$), *conscientious perfectionism* ($M = 14.08$; $SD = 2.49$), *self-evaluative perfectionism* ($M = 12.36$; $SD = 3.32$). The mean PI composite score in this sample was 26.44 (SD not available). In general, scores more than one standard deviation above or below the mean can be considered high or low, respectively.

Perfectionistic Self-Presentation Scale

The *Perfectionistic Self-Presentation Scale* (PSPS; Hewitt, Flett, Sherry, et al., 2003) is a 27-item scale designed to measure the interpersonal expression of perfectionism, namely the desire to appear perfect in front of others. It includes three subscales: (1) *perfectionistic self-promotion* (sample item: "I strive to look perfect to others"), (2) *nondisplay of imperfection* (sample item: "Errors are much worse if they are made in public rather than in private"), and (3) *nondisclosure of imperfection* (sample item: "I should solve my own problems rather than admit them to others"). The structure of the PSPS was supported by exploratory factor analysis across a number of samples, with all three subscales showing high levels of internal consistency (Hewitt, Flett, Sherry, et al., 2003). The scale also has demonstrated convergent validity and test–retest reliability and was rated at a fourth-grade reading level, though it is designed primarily for adults (as reviewed later in this chapter, a separate version of the PSPS for children was recently developed). The PSPS may be requested through Paul Hewitt's website (*http://hewittlab.psych.ubc.ca/requests.htm*).

Positive and Negative Perfectionism Scale

The *Positive and Negative Perfectionism Scale* (PANPS; Terry-Short et al., 1995) is a 40-item scale designed to measure positive and negative aspects of perfectionism. The scale is based on a reinforcement model in which positive perfectionism is assumed to stem from positive reinforcement and negative perfectionism is assumed to stem from negative reinforcement. A number of factor analytic studies have failed to support the original two-factor structure of the PANPS (for a review, see Egan, Piek, Dyck, & Kane, 2011), though one study suggests that a briefer (19-item) version of the scale may be more useful (Haase & Prapavessis, 2004). Although there is evidence supporting the internal consistency of the PANPS, evidence of validity is weaker, particularly for the positive perfectionism scale (Egan et al., 2011).

The PANPS is reprinted in Appendix 3 of this volume. Scores for the *positive perfectionism* subscale (items 2, 3, 6, 9, 14, 16, 18, 19, 21, 23, 24, 25, 28, 29, 30, 32, 34, 35, 37, and 40) and *negative perfectionism* subscale (items 1, 4, 5, 7, 8, 10, 11, 12, 13, 15, 17, 20, 22, 26, 27, 31, 33, 36, 38, and 39) are computed by adding up the scores for the items in each subscale. Egan, Piek, et al. (2011) reported means and standard deviations for the positive and negative subscales of the PANPS across three samples. For clinical participants with an anxiety or depressive disorder, means and standard deviations were as follows: *positive perfectionism* ($M = 70.20$; $SD = 10.19$), *negative perfectionism* ($M = 62.57$; $SD = 16.63$). In a sample of athletes, means and standard deviations were as follows: *positive perfectionism* ($M = 74.41$; $SD = 9.15$), *negative perfectionism* ($M = 48.24$; $SD = 10.93$). Finally, in an undergraduate student sample, means and standard deviations were as follows: *positive perfectionism* ($M = 74.35$; $SD = 10.19$), *negative perfectionism* ($M = 53.02$; $SD = 13.16$).

Domain-Specific Measures of Perfectionism

Perfectionism-Related Cognitions

Two independent instruments have been developed to assess the cognitions associated with perfectionism. The *Perfectionism Cognitions Inventory* (PCI; Flett, Hewitt, Blankstein, & Gray, 1998) is a 25-item questionnaire designed to measure the frequency of automatic thoughts involving themes of perfectionism (sample item: "I can't stand to make mistakes"). Items are items are rated on a 5-point scale ranging from 0 (not at all) to 4 (all the time). The scale appears to have a unidimensional structure, and has acceptable levels of internal consistency and test–retest reliability (Flett et al., 1998; Flett, Hewitt, Whelan, & Martin, 2007). The PCI can be requested through Paul Hewitt's website (*http://hewittlab.psych.ubc.ca/requests.htm*).

The *Multidimensional Perfectionism Cognitions Inventory—English* (MPCI-E; Kobori, 2006; Stoeber, Kobori, & Tanno, 2010) is a 15-item measure developed to assess cognitions associated with SOP and SPP, as defined by Hewitt and Flett (1991b). Items are rated on a 4-point scale ranging from 1 (never) to 4 (always), and load on three factors: (1) *personal standards* (PS; items 3, 5, 8, 10, and 14); (2) *pursuit of perfection* (PP; items 1, 2, 7, 11, and 13); and (3) *concern over mistakes* (CM; items 4, 6, 9, 12, and 15). Evidence of validity (e.g., factor structure, convergent validity) and reliability (e.g., internal consistency) for the MPCI-E is available in a validation study by Stoeber et al. (2010).

The MPCI-E is reprinted in Appendix 3 of this volume. A score is generated for each of the three subscales by computing the mean of scores for the relevant items (i.e., summing all items in the subscale and dividing by the number of items in the subscale, or five). Therefore, each subscale can have a score between 1 and 4. Means and standard deviations (for undergraduate students) were reported by Stoeber et al. (2010) as follows: PS (M = 2.90; SD = 0.66), PP (M = 2.14; SD = 0.65), CM (M = 2.52; SD = 0.68). In general, scores more than one standard deviation above or below the mean can be considered high or low, respectively.

Perfectionism in Relationships

The developers of the APS-R have also developed two scales to measure perfectionism in the context of close relationships. The *Dyadic Almost Perfect Scale* (DAPS; Shea & Slaney, 1999) is a 26-item questionnaire that measures perfectionistic beliefs about one's partner (sample item: "My significant other rarely lives up to my standards"), and is organized along the same three dimensions as the APS-R: *discrepancy* (items 1, 3, 4, 6, 9, 10, 12, 13, 15, 16, 18, 20, 21, 23, 24, and 26), *high standards* (items 5, 8, 11, 14, 19, and 25), and *order* (items 2, 7, 17, and 22). The DAPS appears to be both reliable and valid (Shea, Slaney, & Rice, 2006). It is reprinted in Appendix 3 of this volume. A score for each subscale can be generated by reverse scoring items 3, 16, and 21 (such that 1 = 7; 2 = 6; 3 = 5; 5 = 3; 6 = 2; and 7 = 1), and adding up scores for items in each subscale. Shea et al. (2006) reported means and standard deviations in a sample of 280 undergraduate students to be as follows: *discrepancy* (M = 40.27; SD = 15.47), *high standards* (M = 29.22; SD = 6.70), *order* (M = 17.33; SD = 4.80). Given the absence of any official cutoffs, scores one standard deviation above or below the mean can be considered high or low, respectively.

The *Family Almost Perfect Scale* (FAPS; Wang, Methikalam, & Slaney, 2010) is a 17-item scale designed to measure beliefs regarding one's family's standards for performance (sample item: "My family has high standards for my performance at work or at school"). Like the DAPS, the FAPS is modeled after the APS-R and has three subscales: *family standards* (items 1, 6, 10, 12, 14, and 17), *family discrepancy* (items 4, 7, 9, 11, 13, 15, and 16), and *family order* (items 2, 3, 5, and 8). The psychometric properties of the FAPS are supported in a study comparing Asian Americans and European Americans (Wang, 2010). The FAPS is reprinted in Appendix 3 of this volume. A score is generated for each of the three subscales by summing all relevant items. Means and standard deviations (in undergraduate students, as reported by Wang, 2010) for each of the three subscales are as follows: *family standards* (M = 33.74; SD = 5.71), *family discrepancy* (M = 15.34; SD = 7.66), *family order* (M = 18.80; SD = 4.56). In general, scores greater than one standard deviation above the mean suggest higher than average levels, whereas scores less than one standard deviation below the mean suggest lower levels.

In addition, there is a scale designed specifically to measure perfectionism in the context of parenting (Snell, Overbey, & Brewer, 2005). The *Multidimensional Parenting Perfectionism Questionnaire* (MPPQ) is a 65-item scale with 11 subscales related to different aspects of parenting perfectionism. Although Snell and colleagues (2005) provide preliminary support for the scale's psychometric properties in both student and community samples, the factor structure remains to be validated. Part A of the MPPQ is based on the HMPS (Hewitt & Flett, 1991b) and contains 30 items across five subscales: *self-oriented parenting perfectionism* (SOPP; items 1, 6, 11, 16, 21, and 26), *socially prescribed parenting perfectionism* (SPPP; items 2, 7, 12, 17, 22, and 27), *partner's self-oriented parenting perfectionism* (PSOPP; items 3, 8, 13, 18, 23, and 28), *partner's prescribed parenting perfectionism* (PPPP; items 4, 9, 14, 19, 24, and 29), and *partner's expected standards for parenting* (PESP; items 5, 10, 15, 20, 25, and 30). Part B of the MPPQ is based on the FMPS (Frost et al., 1990) and contains 35 items across six subscales: *concern over parenting mistakes* (CPM; items 9, 10, 13, 14, 18, 21, 23, 25, and 34), *personal parenting standards* (PPS; items 4, 6, 12, 16, 19, 24, and 30), *partner parenting expectations* (PPE; items 1, 11, 15, 20, and 26), *partner parenting criticism* (PPC; items 3, 5, 22, and 35), *doubts about parenting activity* (DPA; items 17, 28, 32, and 33), and *parenting organization* (PO; items 2, 7, 8, 27, 29, and 31).

The MPPQ is reprinted in Appendix 3 of this volume. A score is generated for each of the 11 subscales by summing all relevant items. Snell et al. (2005) reported means and standard deviations for an online sample of 960 community participants, about half (53.3%) of whom were parents, as follows: SOPP (M = 12.59; SD = 6.34), SPPP (M = 8.36; SD = 6.00), PSOPP (M = 8.85; SD = 6.38), PPPP (M = 6.16; SD = 6.29), PESP (M = 7.52; SD = 5.44), CPM (M = 9.20; SD = 7.20), PPS (M = 13.68; SD = 6.94), PPE (M = 5.02; SD = 4.79), PPC (M = 2.62; SD = 3.76), DPA (M = 3.78; SD = 3.43), PO (M = 15.32; SD = 6.36).

Perfectionism and Sports

Although general perfectionism measures are often used to measure perfectionism in athletes (e.g., Haase & Prapavessis, 2004), there are also scales developed specifically for that purpose. The *Sport Multidimensional Perfectionism Scale* (Sport-MPS; Dunn, Causgrove-Dunn, & Syrotuik, 2002) was developed as a sport-specific version of the FMPS. A revised version (Sport-MPS-2) was published more recently (Gotwals & Dunn, 2009). The Sport-MPS-2 is a 42-item measure that consists of six subscales: *personal standards* (PS; items 1, 8, 17, 21, 23, 33, and 36), *concern over mistakes* (COM; items 2, 10, 16, 24, 28, 32, 39, and 42), *perceived parental pressure* (PPP; items 4, 7, 11, 15, 19, 25, 29, 38, and 40), *perceived coach pressure* (PCP; items 6, 13, 22, 26, 30, and 35), *doubts about actions* (DAA; items 3, 12, 14, 20, 31, and 37), and *organization* (Org; items 5, 9, 18, 27, 34, and41). Preliminary research supports the reliability and validity of the Sport-MPS-2 (Gotwals & Dunn, 2009; Gotwals, Dunn, Causgrove-Dunn, & Gamache, 2010). The Sport-MPS-2 is reprinted in Appendix 3 of this volume. A score is generated for each of the six subscales by summing all relevant items. Gotwals and Dunn (2009) reported means and standard deviations for a sample of postsecondary student athletes, as follows: PS (M = 3.68; SD = 0.52), COM (M = 2.87; SD = 0.68), PPP (M = 2.11; SD = 0.71), PCP (M = 3.29; SD = 0.64), DAA (M = 2.40; SD = 0.59), org (M = 3.56; SD = 0.72). Generally, scores greater than one standard deviation above the mean can be considered higher, and scores less than one standard deviation below the mean can be considered lower.

The *Sport Perfectionism Scale* (SPS; Anshel, Weatherby, Kang, & Watson, 2009) is a 35-item unidimensional measure of sport-related perfectionism. Preliminary research (Anshel et al., 2009) supports the unidimensional structure of the scale and suggests acceptable levels of convergent validity; however, more research is needed for this relatively new scale. A number of studies by Anshel and colleagues have also evaluated multidimensional variants of this measure, including a 31-item, four-dimension measure called the *Perfectionism in Sport Scale* (Anshel, Kim, & Henry, 2009) and a 32-item, four-dimension measure (Anshel & Eom, 2002). The 35-item, unidimensional SPS is reprinted in Appendix 3 of this volume. It is scored by computing the sum of scores for each of the 35 items.

Perfectionism, Eating Disorders, and Body Image

As reviewed in Chapter 3 of this volume, there is a considerable body of research confirming a relationship between perfectionism and eating disorders. Although many of the studies on perfectionism and eating disorders have used general measures of perfectionism, there are also several perfectionism scales developed specifically for measuring perfectionism in the context of eating disorders and poor body image. The best studied of these is the *Eating Disorder Inventory—Perfectionism Subscale* (EDI-P; Garner, 1991). The EDI-P is a six-item scale designed to measure perfectionism in the context of eating disorders. Although, it was developed as a unidimensional scale, recent findings in an eating disorders sample suggest that it has two factors—one that measures SOP and one that measures SPP (Lampard, Byrne, McLean, & Fursland, 2012). The SOP items (rather than the SPP items) appear to be most closely related to eating disorder pathology (e.g., weight concern, dietary restraint) in both anorexia nervosa and bulimia nervosa (Lampard et al., 2012). In addition, the FMPS and the HMPS were found to be better predictors of eating disturbance than the EDI-P in a college sample (Chang, Ivezaj, Downey, Kashima, & Morady, 2008), calling into question the value of using the EDI-P rather than a more general scale. The current third edition of the EDI may be obtained from the publisher (PAR), at *www4.parinc.com/Products/Product.aspx?ProductID=EDI-3.*

The *Physical Appearance Perfectionism Scale* (PAPS; Yang & Stoeber, 2012) is a 12-item questionnaire with two subscales: *worry about imperfection* (items 1, 3, 5, 8, 9, 10, and 11) and *hope for perfection* (items 2, 4, 6, 7, and 12). Preliminary research supports the two-factor structure of the scale and suggests that the scale has adequate levels of convergent validity, internal consistency, and test–retest reliability (Yang & Stoeber, 2012). The PAPS is reprinted in Appendix 3. A score for each subscale is generated by calculating the mean of scores for all items in the subscale (i.e., computing the sum of the items and dividing by the number of items in the subscale). Therefore, each subscale can have a score between 1 and 5. Based on a sample of 715 undergraduate students (Hongfei Yang, personal communication, January 10, 2014), the mean and standard deviation for the subscales were as follows: *worry about imperfection* ($M = 2.53$; $SD = 0.79$), *hope for perfection* ($M = 3.57$; $SD = 1.00$). In general, scores greater than one standard deviation above or below the mean suggest higher or lower levels, respectively.

Measuring Perfectionism in Children

Adaptive/Maladaptive Perfectionism Scale

The *Adaptive/Maladaptive Perfectionism Scale* (AMPS; Rice & Preusser, 2002) is a 27-item scale developed with children ages 9 to 12. Items are rated on a 4-point scale, ranging from 1 (really unlike me) to 4 (really like me). The AMPS has four subscales: *sensitivity to mistakes* (measures negative emotions associated with making mistakes; items 2, 5, 8, 12, 15, 17, 20, 23, 26); *contingent self-esteem* (measures positive feelings and self-evaluations contingent on task performance; items 1, 7, 10, 14, 18, 21, 24, 27); *compulsiveness* (measures preference for order, organization, and careful attention to tasks; items 3, 6, 9, 13, 22, 25); and *need for admiration* (measures need for approval; items 4, 11, 16, 19). The psychometric properties of the AMPS are supported by two studies by the authors (Rice, Kubal, & Preusser, 2004; Rice & Preusser, 2002), but otherwise have not been studied widely.

The AMPS is reprinted in Appendix 3. Items 5, 10, 14, 15, 20, and 24 are reverse scored (1 = 4; 2 = 3; 3 = 2; 4 = 1). Scores for each subscale are then generated by computing the sum of the relevant items. Means and standard deviations (in 419 children ages 9 to 12; Kenneth Rice, personal communication, January 10, 2014) for each of the three subscales are as follows: *sensitivity to mistakes* (M = 19.43; SD = 6.32), *contingent self-esteem* (M = 25.11; SD = 4.76), compulsiveness (M = 14.78; SD = 5.00), *need for admiration* (M = 9.77; SD = 3.54). In general, scores greater than one standard deviation above the mean suggest higher than average levels, whereas scores less than one standard deviation below the mean suggest lower levels.

Child and Adolescent Perfectionism Scale

The *Child and Adolescent Perfectionism Scale* (CAPS; Flett, Hewitt, Boucher, Davidson, & Munro, 2000) is one of the most frequently used scales for measuring perfectionism in children and adolescents. However, despite the popularity of the CAPS, the scale remains unpublished, though several researchers (other than the authors of the scale) have published data on its psychometric properties. The original CAPS includes 22 items and two subscales (*self-oriented perfectionism, socially prescribed perfectionism*). However, the most comprehensive psychometric study to date (O'Connor, Dixon, & Rasmussen, 2009) suggests that a shortened, 14-item version (the CAPS-14) is more psychometrically sound, and that the items actually load on three factors (*self-oriented perfectionism–striving; self-oriented perfectionism–critical;* and *socially prescribed perfectionism*). The CAPS can be requested through Paul Hewitt's website (*http://hewittlab.psych.ubc.ca/requests.htm*).

Childhood Retrospective Perfectionism Scale

The *Childhood Retrospective Perfectionism Scale* (CHIRP; Southgate, Tchanturia, Collier, & Treasure, 2008) was designed to assess retrospectively the presence of past childhood traits associated with perfectionism (where the word *perfectionism* is meant in the "obsessive–compulsive personality" sense of the term; e.g., perfectionism across a number of life domains, inflexibility, drive for order and symmetry). There are two versions (each with 20 items)—one for the individual to complete with regard to his or her own behavior in childhood, and one to be completed by an informant. Preliminary findings suggest that the scale is reliable and valid, though more research is needed. The CHIRP is reprinted in the original published article (Southgate et al., 2008).

Perfectionistic Self-Presentation Scale—Junior Form

The *Perfectionistic Self-Presentation Scale—Junior Form* (PSPS-JR; Hewitt et al., 2011) is an 18-item questionnaire designed to measure perfectionistic self-presentation in children and adolescents along three dimensions: *perfectionistic self-promotion* (sample item: "I always have to look perfect"), *nondisplay of imperfection* (sample item: "Mistakes are worse when others see me make them"), and *nondisclosure of imperfection* (sample item: "I should fix my own problems rather than telling them to other people"). The subscales were well supported (e.g., robust factor structure, good internal consistency) in the original validation study, though further research and replication are needed. The PSPS-JR can be requested from Paul Hewitt's website (*http://hewittlab.psych.ubc.ca/requests.htm*).

Illustrative Assessment Case Example

Sasha, a 21-year-old college student, was referred by her family physician to an anxiety disorders specialty clinic for treatment of anxiety and depression. At her first session, she received a general clinical interview focused on identifying relevant diagnostic features as well as on her personal and family history. She also completed several self-report questionnaires to assess the severity of her depression and anxiety. Diagnostic criteria were met for a number of DSM-5 disorders including social anxiety disorder (anxiety and avoidance associated with a range of social and performance situations), dysthymic disorder (low mood over the past few years), and body dysmorphic disorder (she was convinced that she was generally "ugly," though others reassured her that she was attractive).

A theme that emerged during her interview was a tendency for Sasha to have very high standards across several life domains, and for this to be of fundamental importance to the way she judged herself. In particular, it was important for her to always be seen as attractive, intelligent, competent, and witty. Her grades not only had to be the highest in the class, but she also had to feel she had achieved her maximum potential and done the best that she could, irrespective of others. She studied constantly, spent hours making sure that she looked okay before going out, rehearsed funny stories to share with others, and continually asked for reassurance from friends and family. She worried all the time that she might be rejected by others if she let her standards slip. She also believed, more generally, that her future professional success depended on performing perfectly. Her mood was consistently somewhat low, and dipped even lower when she failed to meet her standards. Sasha described herself as a perfectionist.

Session 2 focused on a more thorough review of Sasha's perfectionism. The session covered all of the core assessment domains described earlier (see Table 5.1). For example, she identified various cues and triggers for her perfectionism, including being around other people (e.g., going to parties, engaging in conversations, sitting in class), studying for exams, completing coursework, and receiving critical feedback. As a result of her anxiety, she tended to overprepare and overcompensate in these situations. She was convinced that if she didn't meet the highest level in her performance her life would unravel. She felt that she was only good enough as a person if she was meeting her standards, which she often felt that she was not doing well, and which left her feeling like a failure.

Sasha reported a history of perfectionism going back for as long she could recall, though it didn't become a problem until about the age of 16, when her anxiety and low mood began to worsen. Although she reported being very motivated to feel better, she was reluctant to lower her standards for fear of possible negative consequences. At the end of Session 2, Sasha completed the *Clinical Perfectionism Questionnaire* (CPQ; Fairburn et al., 2003a), with a score of 42, suggesting a high level of clinical perfectionism.

The assessment process continued throughout treatment. Specifically, Sasha recorded her perfectionistic thoughts and behaviors in diaries each day, and she also completed the CPQ at the end of each week. Over time, the frequency and intensity of her perfectionistic behaviors decreased, as did her feelings of depression and anxiety. She was more comfortable with the possibility of being judged negatively by others, and was more willing to take risks that might lead to minor mistakes. By the end of treatment, her score on the CPQ had decreased to 18.

CHAPTER 6

Treatment Planning, Homework, and Supervision

In this chapter we provide an overview of how to develop a treatment plan for perfectionism. This will include considering any issues that need to be addressed before treatment can begin, setting goals, selecting treatment formats (i.e., group or individual therapy, guided self-help), assigning and using homework, and terminating successfully. Although we do not cover general issues of how to structure CBT sessions (how to set agendas, assign homework, and so on), we refer readers to one of the many CBT texts that outline this material in detail (e.g., Beck, 2011). We do, however, provide a case example where we outline session by session an example of treatment for perfectionism based on an individualized formulation. The issue of supervision is also addressed, given its importance both in helping to generate effective treatment plans and successfully provide therapy.

Pretreatment Considerations

Before an in-depth assessment of perfectionism occurs, we suggest you hold a "preassessment" meeting with the client to discuss his or her situation and whether CBT for perfectionism is likely to be a good fit. Table 6.1 lists the issues that can be helpful to cover. In the first section of the interview, an opportunity is provided for the client to discuss the issues that are most pressing to him or her, to understand goals, and to clarify whether the client is seeking treatment or whether there is pressure from others to seek treatment. For example, adolescents who present for treatment may be there due to parental or medical pressure, especially if the perfectionism

TABLE 6.1. Issues to Consider in an Initial Meeting

Client's situation

1. What has brought the client to the point of inquiring about therapy at this time?
2. Current overview of problems and their impact on the client's life.
3. Development of perfectionism in the client's life.
4. Impact and consequences of perfectionism in client's life.
   - "How does perfectionism affect your day-to-day life?"
   - "What are the types of situations where it is really important to reach your standards?"
   - "What are the consequences if you feel you don't reach your standards?"
   - "Does it affect the way you feel about yourself?"
   - "Can you please give me a recent example in detail of a time when you set standards for yourself and didn't meet them, and describe how you responded to this?"
5. Coexisting psychiatric and physical problems and history and family psychiatric and medical history

Is CBT a good fit at this time?

1. Current circumstances and plans.
2. Experiences of any previous therapy or attempts to change.
3. Treatment goals.
4. Attitude toward the requirements of treatment.
   - Committing to therapy. If individual therapy, an initial 10 sessions of 50 minutes' duration over an 8-week period, with appointments twice a week for the first 2 weeks where possible. If group therapy, eight weekly sessions of 2 hours' duration.
   - Avoiding long breaks in therapy (no more than a 2-week break).
   - Writing letters to family doctors (general practitioner) at beginning and end of treatment.
   - Coming to appointments on time.
   - Canceling appointments ahead of time if needed.
   - Working together with the therapist in a collaborative manner.
   - Completing weekly homework focused on experimenting with new behaviors—the most important aspect of therapy to incite change.

---

is impacting a domain of medical self-care such as in type 1 diabetes. Or an adult may present for treatment because a partner, boss, or coach has applied pressure to get help or make changes. Where pressure from others exists, you should explore with clients the degree to which they think that they need to change, and their willingness to at least consider, and experiment with, change in therapy.

The first section of the interview also allows for consideration of the distress caused by the perfectionism, and the context in which it is occurring (i.e., the disorders that may also need treatment). In particular, it can be useful to ask questions regarding the impact and consequences of perfectionism in clients' lives to determine the degree to which perfectionism causes interference and distress. The questions listed under item 4 of the client's situation in Table 6.1 have been used in treatment trials to determine if perfectionism is the primary presenting problem, and thus if it is appropriate to take the person into a treatment trial addressing perfectionism (Steele et al., 2013). This information allows an informed decision to be made about which treatment format would be most suitable for the client's situation (see the next section for issues to consider that can guide this decision).

Goal Setting

The other main aim of the initial session is to determine goals for treatment. This can be done using the well-known method of identifying *SMARTER* goals—that is, setting goals that are *S*pecific, *M*easurable, *A*ttainable, *R*elevant, and *T*ime-Bound and once this is specified, *E*valuating these goals and keeping the process of measurement ongoing (i.e., *R*eevaluating). Table 6.2 lists steps to consider in setting goals (see also Handout 6.1 in Appendix 2).

Once goals are set, it is useful to determine with clients how they will know when they have met the goal (i.e., how will it be measured). These typical steps in goal setting are, of course, well known but are important to attend to nonetheless to help clients be specific about what it is that they are trying to achieve by coming to treatment. This determination of goals may also feed into decision making regarding the format of treatment.

In the second section of the interview, the intent is to consider issues that may be a barrier to beginning CBT. This may simply relate to practical circumstances. For example, the client is going to be away for a long period of time in the middle of therapy or is unable to commit to at least weekly appointments. Or, there may be issues that need attention before therapy for perfectionism commences, such as suicide risk, severe clinical depression, substance misuse, and any major life events or crises that need to be resolved.

TABLE 6.2. Steps to Setting Specific Goals

- *What*: What do you want to accomplish?
- *Why*: Specific reasons, purpose or benefits of accomplishing the goal.
- *Who*: Who is involved?
- *Where*: Identify a location.
- *Which*: Identify requirements and constraints.

Expectations of therapy are also important to discuss, and this can be influenced by a number of issues, including the following:

- Whether the client thinks he or she has previously received CBT. You should always explore this assertion, in order to examine whether CBT was actually provided. In their book *Beating Your Eating Disorder*, Glenn Waller and colleagues (2010) have a useful chapter entitled "What to Look For in a Good CBT Practitioner" in which they highlight the following characteristics of good CBT: (1) a predominant focus on the present and the future, (2) developing the client's understanding of the links between thinking, feeling, biology, and behaviors, (3) a focus on behavioral change, and (4) an emphasis on collaborative therapy, where the client works hard during the week to implement changes. If you judge that CBT was not actually provided to the client previously, then it is important to be able to describe the differences between what is being provided now and what the client experienced before.
- Whether the client is expecting a therapeutic model that involves a focus on the expertise of the therapist or reliance on medication rather than a collaborative relationship that relies on the work that is completed outside of the session.
- Whether the client has attempted to change previously with little progress. Such experiences can damage self-efficacy with respect to the ability to change, and it is useful to talk to the client about change requiring both the "right time" (i.e., when the client is more motivated to change) and the "right therapist offering the right therapy" (i.e., clients won't be able to work with all therapists and not all therapies will necessarily be helpful).

The requirements of treatment should be discussed with the client in the light of this information and thus allow the client to make an informed decision about his or her ability to commit to therapy.

Treatment Format Choices

The most suitable treatment approach for the client should be decided based on the degree that perfectionism interferes with the client's life and a consideration of whether the client is ready for treatment at this time. There are various treatment approaches that can be utilized (e.g., group, individual), but each approach should be based on a cognitive-behavioral formulation of perfectionism to guide treatment for each individual client rather than rigidly following a treatment protocol (and hence mirroring our clients' perfectionism!).

The emphasis here is on parsimony in use of interventions. It is best to implement a few key interventions well rather than many poorly, flipping from one to another, or trying to include everything, as we know that some aspects of the psychopathology may improve without specific interventions. As covered in Chapter 2, various formats for treating perfectionism have been evaluated (although this evaluation is still in early stages) and you can consider the following formats, listed in order of increasing intensity: guided self-help (i.e., meeting with clients for about 8–10 sessions and helping them work through a self-help resource such as a book); treatment in a small group (around eight people with varying psychopathologies); individual therapy focused on perfectionism over 10 sessions and designed around a personal formulation; individual therapy focused on perfectionism over eight sessions based on a structured treatment protocol (as described below); or individual therapy that is focused on both a specific disorder and the perfectionism, as the latter is considered to be an important maintaining factor for the related disorder. This approach has been described previously in Chapter 3 in the section on eating disorders. Table 6.3 summarizes the issues that can help you decide which format is most suitable for your client.

Sample Treatment Protocols

Although we provide sample treatment protocols for the formats described earlier, there are several important factors that should guide protocol development:

- The format of therapy should be decided based on a functional analysis of the role of perfectionism (see Chapter 4), which should also help you decide whether to focus on treatment of perfectionism first or use the disorder-specific protocol for a particular disorder first.
- Therapy should *always* be based on the collaborative formulation of the maintaining factors of perfectionism from the cognitive-behavioral model of clinical perfectionism, regardless of the mode of intervention (this formulation is covered in detail in Chapter 7).
- The protocols presented here should not be used dogmatically.
- Maintain a general spirit of flexibility throughout treatment and be responsive to individual clinical needs and situations as they arise.
- Such flexibility should not be at the expense of adherence to the principles of the treatment.

TABLE 6.3. Deciding on the Appropriate Treatment Format

Description	Considerations for deciding whether appropriate
Guided self-help	
Typically eight 50-minute sessions working through chapters of a self-help book[a]	• Appropriate for a variety of psychopathologies. • A useful "first step" to therapy where psychopathology is mild to moderate. • May be followed up by more intensive therapy. • May be appropriate for therapists with less extensive CBT experience.
Group therapy	
Suitable for up to eight participants, eight 2-hour sessions, can be used in conjunction with a self-help book[a]	• Appropriate for a variety of psychopathologies, typically of mild to moderate severity. • Can be accompanied or followed up by individual treatment for related disorders. • Useful for modeling behavioral experiments. • May not be useful for clients whose perfectionism is directed at others.
Individual therapy using a tailored treatment plan: focus on perfectionism	
Ten 50-minute sessions (preferably twice weekly for the first 2 weeks)	• Appropriate for a variety of psychopathologies, typically with moderate to severe impairment and accompanying comorbidities. • Perfectionism is considered to be the primary maintaining factor for related disorders.
Individual therapy using a structured treatment protocol: focus on perfectionism	
Eight 50-minute sessions	• Appropriate for a variety of psychopathologies, of mild to moderate severity. • Perfectionism is considered to be the primary maintaining factor for the associated disorders. • May be appropriate for therapists with less experience in CBT than tailored treatment.
Individual therapy: focus on both a specific disorder and perfectionism	
Number of sessions depends on the length of the evidence-based treatment used for the associated disorder, where a session is divided into two parts: half focused on the disorder, and half on perfectionism.	• Appropriate for a variety of psychopathologies, typically with moderate to severe impairment and accompanying comorbidities. • Perfectionism is considered to be one of several important maintaining factors. • An effective evidence-based treatment for the associated disorder exists.

[a]*When Perfect Isn't Good Enough* (Antony & Swinson, 2009) or *Overcoming Perfectionism* (Shafran, Egan, & Wade, 2010).

The sample protocols in Tables 6.4–6.7 are followed by a case example of a treatment plan based on the cognitive-behavioral formulation of perfectionism. Note that some of the protocols suggest that clients read chapters and complete worksheets from *Overcoming Perfectionism* (Shafran et al., 2010). While this book is not necessary, it can be useful if engaging in guided self-help therapy, and for further examples of specific records that clients can keep during therapy. If you do not use *Overcoming Perfectionism*, then we suggest that you adapt the protocols in Tables 6.4 and 6.5, utilizing the record sheets in this book (which represent the majority of important ones from *Overcoming Perfectionism*) and skipping the sections that suggest reading materials for clients, or use the protocols suggested in Tables 6.6 and 6.7.

TABLE 6.4. Sample Treatment Protocol for Guided Self-Help

Session number and content focus	Examples of between-session homework
Assessment and prereading of Chapters 1–4 (psychoeducation) of OP[a]	
1. The first steps and the costs of changing OP: Chapters 5 and 6	• Read Chapters 5 and 6 and complete relevant worksheets. • Complete case formulation.
2. Identifying problem areas and psychoeducation OP: Chapters 7.1 and 7.2	• Read Chapters 7.1 and 7.2 and complete relevant worksheets.
3. Surveys and behavioral experiments OP: Chapters 7.3 and 7.4	• Read Chapters 7.3 and 7.4 and conduct one survey and one behavioral experiment.
4. All-or-nothing thinking OP: Chapter 7.5	• Read Chapter 7.5 and conduct a behavioral experiment of relevance.
5. Learning to notice positives and changing thinking styles OP: Chapter 7.6 and 7.7	• Read Chapters 7.6 and 7.7 and complete relevant worksheets.
6. Procrastination, problem-solving, time management, and pleasant events OP: Chapters 7.8 and 7.9	• Read Chapters 7.8 and 7.9 and complete relevant worksheets, including a behavioral experiment.
7. Self-criticism and self-compassion OP: Chapter 8	• Read Chapter 8 and complete relevant worksheets, including a compassion card.
8. Self-evaluation and freedom OP: Chapters 9 and 10	• Read Chapters 9 and 10 and identify priority areas in action plan to continue work on.

[a]*Overcoming Perfectionism* (Shafran, Egan, & Wade, 2010).

TABLE 6.5. Sample Treatment Protocol for Group Therapy

Content for group therapy	Examples of in-session tasks	Examples of between-session homework
	Session 1	
Perfectionism conceptualization, cost/benefit analysis	Group discussion of core features of clinical perfectionism: What is perfectionism? What are some of its features? What problems can coexist with perfectionism and what causes it?	*Tasks:* Work on pros and cons of perfectionism worksheet completed in the group to add more details.
	Why does perfectionism persist?: Collaborative formulation in pairs, then group discussion.	*Reading:* Read Chapters 1–6 of *Overcoming Perfectionism (OP).*
	Pros and cons of perfectionism: Group brainstorm of consequences.	
	Session 2	
Self-monitoring, facts versus fiction	Group discussion of domains of perfectionism: ways that perfectionism presents across life (if using *OP*, complete Worksheet 7.1.1).	*Tasks:* Complete self-monitoring worksheets (if using *OP*, refer to Worksheets 7.1 and 7.2).
	Group discussion of self-monitoring: Highlight tips for effective self-monitoring (if using *OP*, read through Box 7.1.3 as a group [explaining behaviors]).	*Reading:* Read Chapters 7.1 and 7.2 of *OP.*
	Group discussion of psychoeducation: Discuss perfectionism myths (e.g., the harder you work, the better you do).	
	Session 3	
Surveys and behavioral experiments	Introduce the purpose of surveys. Use thoughts from previous week's homework sheet to set up surveys (in pairs, then group discussion). Highlight that with surveys the idea is not to go to the complete opposite of your beliefs but to develop more functional belief systems (if using *OP*, read Box 7.3.2 [beliefs for surveys]).	*Tasks:* Complete a survey and behavioral experiment.
	Introduce behavioral experiments. Emphasize that these equip us with personalized evidence that provides information about thoughts, feelings, and behavior. Group discussion and construction of individual behavioral experiments.	*Reading:* Read chapters 7.3 and 7.4 of *OP.*

All-or-nothing thinking	Group discussion: Introduce "all-or-nothing" thinking. Plan a behavioral experiment for "all-or-nothing" thinking (if using *OP*, you can have clients work in pairs, then group discussion using Worksheet 7.5.1 [behavioral experiment for all-or-nothing thinking]).	*Tasks*: Complete behavioral experiment and continuum. Challenge rules for living by imposing time limits or doing less "perfectly" (behavioral experiments).
	Group discussion: Introduce the purpose of continua to assist clients to think more flexibly. Complete a continuum on an "all or nothing" thought. (if using *OP*, can complete Worksheet 7.5.2).	*Reading*: Read chapter 7.5 of *OP*.
	Highlight the importance of turning rigid rules into guidelines. Have participants develop list of "rules for living." Discuss acceptance of less than perfect performance and balance.	

Broadening attention, cognitive distortions, thought diaries	Group discussion: Challenging negative filtering distortion. Discuss pattern of how discounting success leads to "no win" situation.	*Tasks*: Complete homework of recording when noticing positive aspects of performance and lack of negative aspects (if using *OP*, use Worksheet 7.6.2). Complete thought diary to challenge cognitive distortions identified in thinking patterns (if using *OP*, can use Worksheet 7.7.3).
	Group discussion: Other common thinking distortions (double standards, overgeneralization, shoulds, catastrophizing, emotional reasoning, labeling, personalization, mind reading, and predictive thinking). Discuss use of thought diaries to gain awareness and assist in challenging unhelpful thoughts and formulating more rational thoughts (if using *OP*, can read Box 7.7.4 as a group).	*Reading*: Read chapter 7.6 and 7.7 of *OP*.

Procrastination, problem solving, time management, and pleasant event scheduling	Group discussion: Procrastination.	*Tasks*: Complete a behavioral experiment and thought diary to challenge procrastination, and a flash card of helpful statements to overcome procrastination (if using *OP*, use Worksheets 7.8.5–7.87 [behavioral experiment to overcome procrastination]). Engage in pleasant events (at least one during the week).
	Discuss as a group which areas of life clients procrastinate in (if using *OP*, can complete Worksheet 7.8.1). Discuss cost/benefit analysis of procrastination. Discuss developing flash cards/coping statements to assist with reducing procrastination and develop these in group. Discuss idea of developing "just do it" reminders and changing image to being able to cope with the task rather than procrastinating. Discussion of practical tasks to challenge procrastination: (small chunks, ordering chunks from easiest to hardest, highlighting that action precedes motivation).	

(continued)

89

TABLE 6.5. *(continued)*

Content for group therapy	Examples of in-session tasks	Examples of between-session homework
	Introduce problem-solving worksheet. Use example from *OP*, Box 7.8.8 (Aimee).	*Reading:* Read Chapters 7.8 and 7.9 of *OP*.
	Group discussion: Time management and pleasant event scheduling. Complete in-session time management schedule (*OP* Worksheet 7.8.11). Emphasize importance of balancing time for rest/relaxation with achievement.	
	Session 7	
Values, reducing self-criticism	Group discussion: Self-criticism, what self-criticism is, and why it can be destructive. Emphasize that it is about trying to decrease frequency and strength of self-critical thoughts. Introduce coach analogy and discuss as group.	*Tasks:* Record diary to help identify compassionate thoughts (if using *OP*, use Worksheet 8.4). Summarize compassionate voice responses on index "flash cards" as reminders that can be used when the self-critical voice is loud.
	Work through as a group how to identify the self-critical voice (if using *OP*, refer to Worksheet 8.1).	
	Work through decreasing self-criticism and increasing compassion: identifying the compassionate voice (if using *OP*, refer to Worksheets 8.2–8.4).	*Reading:* Read Chapter 8 of *OP*.
	Work through decreasing self-criticism and increasing compassion: how to react to the critical voice when it starts speaking up.	
	Session 8	
Expanding self-evaluation, goals, relapse prevention	Group discussion: Weakening the link between your judgment of yourself as a person and your achievements. Work on developing self-esteem based on other factors rather than solely on achievement; avoid the use of strict and inflexible rules and instead encourage realistic and flexible goals, noticing equally what you do well and what you can improve (if using *OP*, can complete Worksheets 9.1 and 9.3).	*Tasks:* Further goal setting. Behavioral survey of goals for expanding areas of life that contribute to self-worth. Continue to use behavioral experiments and other strategies introduced during treatment.
	Set goals for the next 6 months that expand areas of life and contribute to self-worth (if using *OP*, use Worksheet 9.4). Discuss plan to conduct, as homework, a survey to test the appropriateness of the goals that are set.	*Reading:* Read Chapters 9 and 10 of *OP*.
	Relapse prevention: Group discussion of how to deal with potential setbacks/relapse prevention; develop an action plan to deal with relapse.	

Note. Based on the protocol developed and evaluated by Steele et al. (2013).

TABLE 6.6. Sample Treatment Protocol for Eight-Session Structured Individual Therapy Focused on Perfectionism

Session number and content focus	Examples of between-session homework
1. Individualized collaborative formulation of perfectionism and enhancing motivation to change perfectionism See Chapters 7 and 8 (this volume)	• Add to list of pros and cons of perfectionism, focusing on negative consequences.
2. Self-monitoring and psychoeducation See Chapter 9 (this volume)	• Complete self-monitoring worksheets.
3. Surveys and behavioral experiments See Chapters 9 and 12 (this volume)	• Complete survey and behavioral experiment.
4. Challenging dichotomous thinking via behavioral experiments and continua See Chapters 11 and 12 (this volume)	• Complete behavioral experiment and continuum.
5. Challenging cognitive biases See Chapter 10 and 11 (this volume)	• Complete thought diary and complete diary of noticing positive aspects of performance.
6. Procrastination, time management, and pleasant events See Chapter 14 (this volume)	• Complete chunking task to overcome procrastination, complete time management schedule, and engage in pleasant events.
7. Self-criticism and self-compassion See Chapter 13 (this volume)	• Complete diary of compassionate thoughts.
8. Self-evaluation and relapse prevention See Chapter 13 and 15 (this volume)	• Continue utilizing behavioral experiments and other techniques learned in therapy.

Determining the Most Suitable Treatment Format

You should determine which treatment plan to use in cognitive-behavioral treatment of perfectionism based on the foundation of a thorough assessment of perfectionism and associated problems (i.e., comorbidities). As noted in Chapter 4, as yet the research regarding the use of CBT for perfectionism as a treatment for psychological disorders is in its infancy, so if you discover in the assessment that the primary problem is another disorder that is interfering most with the client's life, rather than perfectionism, then you should first intervene using an evidence-based treatment protocol for that particular disorder. If problems remain after treating the other disorder, then the focus of treatment may shift to CBT for perfectionism.

TABLE 6.7. Sample Treatment Protocol for 10-Session Individual Tailored Therapy Focused on Perfectionism

Session number and content focus	Examples of between-session homework
1. Assessment and motivation to change: Pros and cons of changing perfectionism See Chapters 6 and 8	• Complete worksheets on increasing motivation to change.
2. Cognitive-behavioral formulation See Chapter 7	• Think about formulation diagram and add any relevant information or other examples noticed.
3. Psychoeducation and self-monitoring See Chapter 9	• Complete self-monitoring worksheets with perfectionistic thoughts, emotions, and behaviors (performance checking, avoidance, counterproductive behaviors).
4. Checking, avoidance, and counterproductive behaviors, behavioral experiments and surveys See Chapters 10 and 12	• Based on idiosyncratic behaviors identified in session, complete surveys and behavioral experiments to combat perfectionism-related behaviors.
5. Dysfunctional scheme for self-evaluation See Chapter 13	• Based on "pie chart" created during the session, complete experiments to expand domains of self-evaluation.
6. Rigidity, rules, and extreme standards See Chapters 11 and 12	• Complete behavioral experiments aimed at challenging rigid rules and dichotomous thinking, doing things less than perfectly and reducing time spent on tasks.
7. Cognitive biases: behavioral experiments including pleasurable activities, refocusing attention, cognitive restructuring, and thinking errors See Chapters 10, 11, and 12	• Complete pleasant events and thought diaries.
8. Problem solving (including relaxation/ time management strategies/ procrastination) See Chapter 14	• Complete behavioral experiments aimed at making time for relaxation, rest, and nonproductive pleasant events (e.g., sitting in cafés reading paper, watch "trashy" TV), and devise relevant strategies most suited to the client to overcome procrastination.
9. Self-criticism and self-compassion See Chapter 13	• Complete diaries to increase compassionate thoughts.
10. Relapse prevention See Chapter 15	• Continue to complete behavioral experiments and other strategies after treatment ceases.

Furthermore, if perfectionism is interfering with the treatment for a particular disorder, the disorder-specific protocol can be put aside and CBT for perfectionism used until the perfectionism has been reduced to a level at which the client can reengage with treatment of the particular disorder, if still required. If, however, you find that the client is describing perfectionism as the most prominent and impairing problem, and that perfectionism is a maintaining factor across a range of psychological disorders, then you would be well served to utilize CBT for perfectionism. Finally, if you find that perfectionism and a particular psychological disorder are interfering equally, it is best to first treat the psychological disorder and then move to the treatment of perfectionism. An exception might be individuals with eating disorders in which clinical perfectionism is seen to be a major maintaining factor. In these cases, you may wisely employ enhanced CBT (CBT-E) for eating disorders (Fairburn, 2008). However, many times when we have recruited clients specifically for the treatment of perfectionism in research studies (e.g., Steele et al., 2013), we have also found that they prefer to receive treatment for perfectionism, and this should also be taken into consideration when you decide on a treatment format. Often clients have received previous treatment for one or more psychological disorders and have presented wanting to attempt a different treatment, well aware that perfectionism is a major part of their difficulties. As outlined in Chapter 2, studies have shown that perfectionism remains after treatment of a particular anxiety or eating disorder using treatment protocols designed for specific psychological disorders.

Finally, as we pointed out in Chapter 4, there is a rationale for the use of CBT for perfectionism as a transdiagnostic treatment when the client has a number of comorbidities, as there are no evidence-based guidelines for which treatments to employ when the individual has numerous diagnoses. Clearly, if perfectionism is found to be a maintaining factor across a number of diagnoses, then you should consider employing CBT for perfectionism. An example of what this looks like in clinical practice is detailed below.

Example of a 10-Session Individualized Treatment Plan Focused on Perfectionism

Zahara presented for treatment after seeing an advertisement for treatment of perfectionism in her local paper. She was a 45-year-old woman who was single and worked as a professor of architecture. Zahara reported that she had always been a worrier, and was very hard on herself. On assessment, criteria were met for generalized anxiety disorder, major depressive disorder (mild severity), and binge-eating disorder. She stated that she had also been a perfectionist for as long as she could remember, and that she had excelled in her studies and career, gaining a professorship at a young age relative to her peers. Zahara recalled to her therapist that despite winning numerous awards and being constantly recognized for her excellence in her work (e.g., being the youngest person ever in her university to receive tenure as a professor), she reported that she always had the creeping feeling of "not being good enough" and felt that she was not up to scratch and should be trying harder despite this recognition. She said she spent a lot of time comparing the number of design awards that she had received with "the best in the world" and felt that no matter how hard she worked she would never be as good as some of the most famous people in her profession.

Zahara said that she worked very long hours, often into the early hours of the morning, and would often engage in binge eating at these times, as she felt intensely tired and her mood was low. Zahara berated herself for this, and felt that she should do something about her eating as she was slightly overweight, yet could not find the time as she was constantly working. She also reported to the therapist that she felt very sad and teary at times, as she felt that she should be doing better in her work. For example, last year she had been runner-up for an international design award that she had previously won. She ruminated on this and her other worries a great deal. Zahara also stated that she worried about not being in a relationship, and while she often felt lonely and that she would like to have a partner, she could not justify the waste of time involved in trying to meet someone when she was so busy with her work.

Session 1: Assessment and Motivation to Change

One of the most important guides in the initial session that can start to give you an idea about choice of therapy approaches is the client's response to the initial question asking what has brought the person in to therapy at this time. In response to this question, Zahara stated that she thought she had a deep-seated problem with perfectionism and that she did not feel good enough; hence when she had seen that treatment was being offered to reduce perfectionism she thought it might be worth finding out about. Zahara stated that she was also ambivalent about treatment, however, because while she knew that in many ways her perfectionism was problematic (e.g., making her unhappy with her work, resulting in overeating, and preventing her from being in a relationship), she also liked achieving and did not want to end up as a "slacker" or not maintaining her tenure as a professor due to poor performance. The therapist used this opportunity to engage in a discussion regarding the goal of therapy, namely that it is not about reducing standards, as there is nothing wrong in striving itself. Rather, therapy is about reducing the self-criticism that accompanies striving and reducing the degree to which self-worth is based on achievement. Zahara seemed more interested in this, especially after she and the therapist had discussed the pros and cons of perfectionism, and it became apparent that for Zahara one disadvantage was that she was spending a lot of time checking over her work and comparing herself to other professors on the Internet, which took up time she could be spending being more productive. The therapist suggested that they could try and experiment with doing things differently, which might result in Zahara potentially becoming more productive, and she was very interested in this idea. The homework set for the session was to read Chapters 1–6 of *Overcoming Perfectionism* and for Zahara to complete a worksheet on the long-term costs and benefits of perfectionism.

Session 2: Cognitive-Behavioral Formulation

In this session the therapist engaged in a collaborative formulation with Zahara to come up with a diagram of what kept her perfectionism going. Zahara could see very strongly how she based her whole sense of self-worth on achievement, in particular at work, and that this led her to set rigid standards (e.g., "I must win more design awards than my colleagues"), leading her to judge herself in a dichotomous manner (e.g., "Being a runner-up in the international design competition is evidence that I am such a failure"). Zahara also could see with the guidance of the therapist how she set her goals even higher after success (e.g., "I need to win every award"), and even when she did win awards she downplayed them (e.g., "I might be the youngest professor at my university, but then I am not at Harvard so it's no big deal"). The therapist also helped Zahara to see how the sorts of counterproductive behaviors she engaged in, such as checking her work over and over, and comparing the number of awards she had received with those won by other top professors for many hours on the Internet, continually reinforced her view of her self-worth as being dependent on achievement. They also discussed how critical Zahara was of herself, how she constantly had an internal monologue saying she was "useless, a failure, pathetic" and how this also reinforced self-worth being based on achievement as she said to herself in response to this, "Well, you just have to keep trying harder." The homework assigned in this session was for Zahara to go away and think over the formulation and note further examples of counterproductive behaviors that she noticed over the next week.

Session 3: Psychoeducation and Self-Monitoring

In this session, the therapist asked Zahara what her beliefs were about some common ideas that people hold, for example, "The harder you work the better you do." Zahara agreed with this and with many of the other "perfectionism myths" (see Chapter 9), and this was useful in starting a Socratic dialogue regarding the disadvantages of perfectionism that Zahara had previously identified (i.e., it was costing her a great deal of time and perhaps leading her to be more inefficient). This helped Zahara see that perhaps sometimes she was overworking, and to introduce the notion of behavioral experiments aimed at putting less time into tasks and finding out what happened as a result. The therapist also introduced to Zahara the idea of starting to become more aware of her perfectionism, and assigned self-monitoring worksheets for homework, in particular to focus on recording her self-talk and counterproductive behaviors.

Session 4: Behavioral Experiments

As Zahara's homework from the previous session indicated that she was engaging in numerous counterproductive behaviors, such as checking her work and comparing herself to others, this session was spent setting up a range of behavioral experiments for Zahara to try where she put in less time than usual and decreased her unhelpful perfectionism-related behaviors. One experiment that was discussed in session and then assigned for homework was to submit a paper after only checking it briefly with a specified time limit (1 hour), compared with her usual standard of spending up to a week checking a paper before she could submit it. Another experiment was to contrast days spent checking the Internet and comparing herself to other professors and days refraining from the behavior (e.g., 2 days of the week spent comparing, and 2 days of the week not spent comparing) and comparing the impact on a range of outcomes rated 0–100 (mood, binge eating, productivity).

Session 5: Broadening Self-Evaluation to Be Based on More Than Achievement

Zahara reported success with her behavioral experiments. She found that she felt better and was more productive on the days when she did not spend hours checking her work and comparing herself to colleagues, though she admitted that she was very worried about the outcome of the paper she had submitted after only checking it briefly. She reported that "I couldn't deal with confirming I am a failure as a person" if her paper was rejected. The therapist used this as an opportunity to discuss the topic of how Zahara based her sense of self-worth almost entirely on her performance at work, and together they drew a pie chart on the whiteboard to illustrate this (see Chapter 13 for details), and another pie chart for how her self-evaluation might look if she were more balanced in her life. Zahara identified areas of her life that she had neglected due to striving (e.g., intimate relationships, friendships, physical health, fun, hobbies), and they agreed that it might be useful to design some experiments to test ways to enhance these areas. For homework, she decided to try a behavioral experiment involving looking at Internet dating sites during the time that she would have previously spent comparing herself to colleagues on the net.

Session 6: Rigidity, Rules, and Extreme Standards

In this session the therapist discussed with Zahara the many rules that she had for herself (e.g., "I must never go to bed before finishing my work I have set myself for the day" and "Only winning an award is useful; anything else indicates I am a failure." They discussed trying to reframe her rules as *guidelines* (e.g., aiming to complete some of the tasks on her to-do list but not having to complete them all each day), and the use of continua to see the "shades of gray" in her performance regarding awards (see Chapter 11).

Zahara decided that for homework she would engage in more behavioral experiments aimed at doing things less than perfectly (e.g., giving a paper draft to her colleague with a minor error in it and judging her performance in a nondichotomous way).

Session 7: Challenging Cognitive Biases

After completing numerous behavioral experiments in therapy so far, it was apparent that Zahara was to some degree still engaging in noticing her performance flaws and ignoring her successes. For example, she even did this following the outcome of a successful behavioral experiment saying, "It was no big deal" and "I should have gotten over this problem years ago." The therapist introduced thought records to challenge Zahara's unhelpful thinking styles (see Chapter 10), and they discussed how Zahara held a double standard (e.g., that it was okay for others to struggle with perfectionism, but she should have been able to get over the problem earlier). They completed a thought diary in session to challenge this belief, and for homework Zahara planned to complete some thought diaries as well as a diary to record her successes.

Session 8: Pleasant Events and Scheduling Time for Relaxation and Rest

Zahara stated that she had completed several thought diaries during the week and was engaging in numerous behavioral experiments. She was proud that she was now more easily reducing the time spent on tasks because she was not doing as much checking. However, it was obvious to the therapist that Zahara had been spending a great deal of time on her therapy homework. In fact, she had even retyped the thought record and brought in the new version for the therapist "as a gesture of thanks." She explained that "the new record was more accurate as it listed all of the unhelpful thinking styles in detail." The therapist thanked Zahara for her efforts but used this as an opportunity to revisit the formulation. Zahara appeared to be applying her perfectionism to therapy, and they agreed that Zahara would carry out a behavioral experiment where she limited her time spent doing homework and used a pencil to complete records rather than type them. This was also a good opportunity for the therapist to discuss a time management schedule with the purpose of introducing time for rest and relaxation and addressing some of the areas of life that Zahara was trying to expand in order to broaden her self-evaluation (i.e., relationships, hobbies). To address this for homework, Zahara decided to do a behavioral experiment where she challenged her idea that pleasant events were a waste of time, and while she could not agree to watch a reality TV show that the therapist suggested, she did agree to watch some episodes of a different show, *Grand Designs*, that focused on architecture and that she never had made time to watch in the past. Zahara also decided to spend time meeting old university friends for coffee, which she had avoided in the past due to her busy schedule.

Session 9: Self-Criticism and Self-Compassion

Over the course of therapy the degree of Zahara's self-criticism and use of negative labels such as "failure, screwup, useless" had appeared to decrease; however, Zahara reported that in the past week she had been plagued by an episode of self-criticism and calling herself a failure over an interaction she had with a colleague where the colleague had questioned one of her reports. In the session, the therapist introduced the notion of self-compassion, having Zahara identify values she used to treat her colleagues, students, and friends (e.g., respect, care, politeness) and asking how she might use these values for herself in considering this recent experience. Together they worked on challenging the idea that Zahara was a "failure," and on how they could turn down the volume of her negative, self-critical thoughts and increase her self-compassionate thoughts (e.g., "everyone has problems with that colleague; if I am kind to myself, I can see that I did a good job on the report, that I am good at my job overall, and that I am a good person").

Session 10: Relapse Prevention

In the final session, the therapist and Zahara agreed that she had come a long way over the past couple of months. For example, she was now getting more sleep, her mood had improved, she was socializing with others, she was much less self-critical, and she was getting more done at work, as she was spending less time checking and comparing herself to others. They discussed the main ways that Zahara could keep these changes going, including continuing to conduct behavioral experiments aimed at doing things less than perfectly, reducing the time she spent on work tasks, and broadening her self-evaluation by continuing to engage in new activities she had been ignoring, such as pleasant events and socializing. The therapist also emphasized the importance of Zahara keeping her self-critical voice in check, and when they developed an action plan to combat possible slips, this was an important area that Zahara decided she needed to look out for. If she had periods of "calling herself names," this was a sign she needed to pull out some of her therapy materials and complete some compassionate voice records (see Chapter 13).

Homework

Homework between sessions is considered to be an essential component of CBT, and one of the most important drivers of change. Some principles of homework setting include ensuring that:

- The amount of homework assigned is manageable.
- Homework instructions are unambiguous.
- The homework rationale is clear to the client.
- The therapist and client are confident that the homework can be completed.

- The therapist and client agree on the homework collaboratively, and within the guidelines of the treatment protocol. Be sure to set plenty of time (e.g., 10 minutes) for this collaborative discussion near the end of each session.
- There is a clear expectation that the agreed-upon homework will be completed.
- The next session will begin with a review of the previous week's homework.
- If the homework has not been completed, an explanation will actively be sought in a nonjudgmental way.
- Much of the homework is progressive (additive); in other words, issues introduced earlier may be continued as a theme for homework throughout therapy.

Troubleshooting: Doing Homework Less Than Perfectly

As mentioned in Chapter 8, the client who has perfectionism can be likely to either avoid doing homework (because it can't be done well enough) or to try to do it perfectly e.g., pages of typed diaries in excruciating detail, reading ahead and doing more homework than negotiated in session. With respect to this latter issue, several approaches can be useful:

- Reflect to the client, with some humor, the way perfectionism is showing up even in his or her therapy homework and brainstorm ways to do homework less perfectly, setting this up as a behavioral experiment (e.g., use pencil to complete diaries, commit at least one typographical mistake per entry, spill food or juice on one of the pages, write as messily as possible while still retaining legibility).
- Set clear guidelines for homework completion, include a maximum amount of time that can be spent on it and the level of detail required, and remind the client that the rationale of the homework is to help him or her test out beliefs about perfectionism, not to impress the therapist.

Termination

While treatment should end with a summary of past achievements in therapy and with a focus on the future, there will be a number of additional issues to cover when terminating therapy. In terms of the past, you should express appreciation for the client, for both the personal qualities (e.g., sense of humor, honesty, courage) that he or she has bought to treatment, and your enjoyment in working together. At this stage, you can congratulate the client for persisting with therapy even when it was very difficult, and for the hard work invested in changing a domain for which there may have been significant ambivalence at the start of treatment. As part of relapse prevention (which will be covered in Chapter 15), you will have already asked the client about the important changes made during therapy, and it is vital at the termination phase to remind the client that these were changes he or she caused to happen, not changes were produced by you.

In terms of future orientation, it is appropriate to explore feelings about termination, and to normalize any apprehension about "going it alone." At this stage it is also good to be clear about any follow-up contact and whether follow-up appointments are to be scheduled in advance or requested by the client as needed. Given the way perfectionism works, it is good practice to schedule in a follow-up appointment, as the client may feel that requesting one represents a failure. Ask the client to anticipate possible challenges between the final therapy visit and the follow-up appointment and ensure that specific goals are in place. Emphasize the client's ability to choose and change, and express your own optimism in the client's future based on specific observations you have made over the course of therapy.

Supervision

While the topic of supervision is not directly related to treatment planning, it is a relevant topic that should be considered at the start before embarking on treatment and throughout the treatment process; hence we have included it in this chapter. Some therapists will have ongoing supervision and many therapists will also be providing supervision. The question of how to make best use of supervision and the best methods for providing supervision are therefore highly pertinent to the process of treatment planning.

Making the Best Use of Supervision

The increased use of supervision models, standardized assessment tools (e.g., the *Cognitive Therapy Rating Scale*), and video recordings of sessions have changed the nature of supervision. These are important considerations, though the fundamental principles of supervision, like the fundamental principles of psychotherapy in general, have not changed. Fundamentally, supervision provides a context in which the therapist can safely reflect on the therapeutic intervention being provided, and where the supervisor and therapist can share ideas on both the nature and process of therapy. Typically, the supervisor is more experienced than the therapist who is being supervised. In other cases, a model of peer supervision may be more appropriate. The supervisor shares his or her knowledge and experience with the therapist, and the therapist shares his or her knowledge of the specific client. As well as being a teacher and consultant, the supervisor also provides general support.

As with therapy sessions, the better prepared one is, the better one can expect the session to go. Many therapists arrive for supervision relatively unprepared, whereas they would never dream of being unprepared for a client. It is the role of the supervisor to set up expectations of supervision and to convey the importance of supervision as an activity that requires as much consideration, reflection, and work as a therapy session. In our view, failing to prepare properly for supervision does a significant disservice to the client and is both unacceptable and unethical. It is the role of the therapist being supervised to contribute to the establishment of a supervision plan, to take responsibility for specific learning goals, to disclose openly about therapeutic practice, and to provide feedback on supervision.

CBT Supervision Models

There are several CBT supervision models. For those particularly interested in supervision, we suggest that you follow the burgeoning literature on the topic (e.g., Hawkins & Shohet, 2000; Milne, 2009; Padesky, 1996). Our supervision structure is almost identical to that of a therapy session in the format; an agenda is set collaboratively and should include a review of homework, any clients in crisis, and the discussion of any particular therapeutic issues. It ends with agreed upon-homework and a summary of the supervision session. In groups, it may be the case that each member of the group has equal time each week to discuss the difficult cases. Alternatively, you may find it works better to rotate, with one member of the group having a longer period of time to discuss a case in more depth in each session. It may also be useful to encourage having suggestions made not only by the supervisor but by fellow group members to encourage learning and model peer supervision. In keeping with the principles of CBT, we would encourage you to try different formats, obtain data from the supervisees about which they prefer, and then find a format that is most effective for your particular group.

Providing Supervision

The same principles of providing supervision apply when supervising therapists working with people with perfectionism as when supervising therapists working with people with other mental health problems. One key difference, however, is that you are working transdiagnostically and there will be times when disorder-specific issues are raised. For example, when working through this manual it may be apparent that the perfectionism is particularly problematic in the social domain. The therapist may want advice as to whether it is acceptable to "dip into" a specific evidence-based protocol for social anxiety disorder (e.g., to conduct a behavioral experiment on other people's reactions to social failure). There is nothing in this protocol that precludes the use of techniques from protocols for specific psychological disorders if you and the therapist see that it fits within the formulation. Your role as the supervisor is to help adapt the intervention so that it is of therapeutic value in changing the factors maintaining the perfectionism rather than straying to deal with a particular disorder.

Assessing Your Own Supervision

You may want feedback on your own supervision. This can be done informally with or without the use of video or audio feedback on the supervision session. It can also be done formally with the use of supervision measures such as the *Supervision Adherence and Guidance Evaluation Scale* (see Milne, 2009). Becoming a skilled supervisor is likely to require additional training, experience, and reflection, but the therapists, clients, and your own practice are likely to reap the benefits.

CHAPTER 7

The Cognitive-Behavioral Model of Perfectionism and Collaborative Formulation

In order to devise an effective treatment plan, a therapist and client need to develop a collaborative, cognitive-behavioral formulation of the maintaining factors of perfectionism. The process of case formulation is crucial, as it is the foundation on which treatment is based. Treatment will look different for each person, depending on the individualized collaborative formulation that is derived, though in general it will target the specific maintaining factors informed by the cognitive-behavioral model of perfectionism that was originally outlined by Shafran, Cooper, and Fairburn (2002), and more recently updated (Shafran et al., 2010). The collaborative formulation is an essential step to help guide the client's and therapist's understanding of what keeps the client's perfectionism going, and consequently which particular factors need to be targeted in treatment. The cognitive-behavioral model of perfectionism can be a useful guide for formulation, but you should apply the model in a flexible manner, depending on the features of each individual client's perfectionism.

The Cognitive-Behavioral Model of Perfectionism

The cognitive-behavioral model of perfectionism (Shafran et al., 2002) arose when clinicians observed that perfectionism was a salient factor in eating disorders and thus needed to be addressed, yet there were no cognitive-behavioral models of the factors that maintained perfectionism. Instead the literature had been dominated by multidimensional models (Frost et al., 1990; Hewitt & Flett, 1991b) that provide little information about what to do in treatment. At that time, Shafran and Mansell (2001) demonstrated in a comprehensive review that perfectionism was elevated across a range of clinical disorders. They argued that a model was therefore required that could account for the maintenance of perfectionism across many presenting problems, as it was not only of relevance to eating disorders.

The Original Cognitive-Behavioral Model of Perfectionism

The model of Shafran et al. (2002), as seen in Figure 7.1, is based on their definition of clinical perfectionism as "the overdependence of self-evaluation on the determined pursuit of personally demanding, self-imposed standards in at least one highly salient domain, despite adverse consequences" (p. 778). Clinical perfectionism involves continual striving to achieve self-imposed standards despite negative effects, and basing self-worth on how well people feel they are achieving their standards.

Fundamental to the definition of clinical perfectionism is that self-esteem is based on how well a person thinks he or she is doing at meeting important standards. It is not the goals and standards that are a problem in themselves, but evaluation of self based on meeting one's standards. For example, if someone thinks he or she is a failure for not meeting a standard (e.g., getting a B on an exam rather than an A), then thinking that one is a failure overall as a person after getting a B on an exam indicates clinical perfectionism. The definition of clinical perfectionism involves a person striving to meet demanding standards despite this having negative consequences, and even upon meeting those standards discounting them as not being difficult enough. The model included a number of core maintaining factors, including rigid standard setting, dichotomous evaluation of standards, cognitive biases, self-criticism, avoidance, and resetting standards higher when a person thinks a standard has not been met. An implicit component of the model was that people with clinical perfectionism engage in what we refer to as "performance-checking behavior" (e.g., comparing one's performance to that of others, seeking reassurance). The model was revised recently by Shafran et al. (2010) to explicitly include these behavioral components. The revised model also expanded on the emotional aspects of clinical perfectionism.

The Revised Cognitive-Behavioral Model of Perfectionism

The updated model of clinical perfectionism (Shafran et al., 2010) is presented in Figure 7.2 (see also Handout 7.1 in Appendix 2).

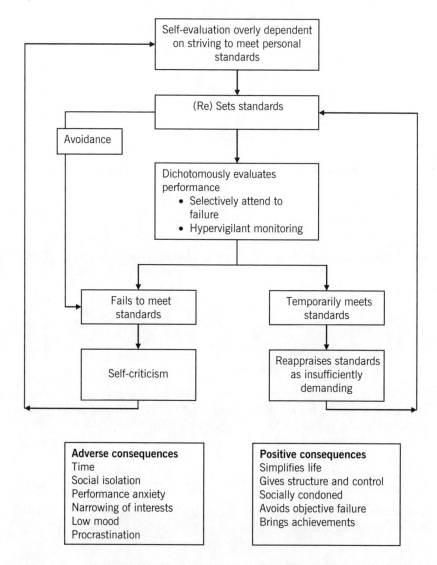

FIGURE 7.1. The original cognitive-behavioral model of clinical perfectionism. From Shafran, Cooper, and Fairburn (2002). Copyright 2002 by Elsevier. Reprinted by permission.

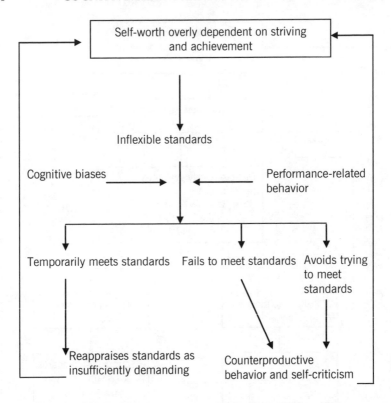

FIGURE 7.2. The updated cognitive-behavioral model of clinical perfectionism. From Shafran, Egan, and Wade (2010). Copyright 2010 by Constable & Robinson. Reprinted by permission.

Maintaining Factors

The major maintaining factors of clinical perfectionism that are outlined in the model are as follows.

SELF-EVALUATION OVERLY DEPENDENT ON STRIVING AND ACHIEVEMENT

At the top and center of the model in Figure 7.1 is the phrase "self-evaluation overly dependent on striving to meet personal standards." This is what Shafran et al. (2002) defined as the core problem in the original model, and it drives all other factors that maintain clinical perfectionism. Essentially perfectionistic individuals only see themselves as having worth if they feel they are achieving their personal standards. Self-evaluation being dependent on achievement leads the person to set inflexible standards for performance.

INFLEXIBLE STANDARDS

The high, inflexible standards set by people with clinical perfectionism are operationalized as rigid rules they set for themselves about how they should perform (e.g., "I must always receive high honors at school," "I should always speak perfectly in social situations").

COGNITIVE BIASES

Dichotomous Thinking (All-or-Nothing/Black-and-White Thinking). Individuals with clinical perfectionism constantly evaluate how well they meet their rules in a dichotomous manner, for example, believing that one has not met one's standard if one has received a grade of 79% on an exam. This results in intense self-criticism and overgeneralization, which further reinforces self-evaluation being dependent on striving (e.g., "I am a failure as a person because I got 79% on the exam"). This then leads the person to reset his or her standards even higher (e.g., "I must do better next time on my exam and get over 85%"), which restarts the cycle. Consequently, clinical perfectionism is maintained in a vicious loop.

"Shoulds" and "Musts." Self-statements involving "shoulds" and "musts" feed into the maintenance of clinical perfectionism. These statements are often the operationalization of the rules and can be used to push individuals to meet their standards or berate themselves if they feel they have not met a standard (e.g., "I should always be working on weekends and not waste time socializing," "I should have done a better job on the report"). As reviewed in Chapter 1, Albert Ellis called this thinking style "musterbation" and "shoulding on oneself," and Horney (1950) described perfectionism as the "tyranny of the shoulds." It can be helpful to discuss these terms with clients to illustrate how their rules and thinking styles are linked to their perfectionism.

Selective Attention (Noticing the Negative and Discounting the Positive). This cognitive bias is characteristic of clinical perfectionism and involves an individual focusing in on every mistake and error no matter how small (e.g., "One spelling mistake in an e-mail is evidence I am not good enough at work"). It is also typical for individuals to ignore positive aspects of their performance (e.g., ignoring that in the last meeting they had with their boss that they were praised for their good work). To illustrate the process of selective attention when deriving the formulation with clients, it can be helpful to ask them to do an experiment where they rate how itchy their head is before and after selectively attending to its "itchiness." This type of experiment is a simple way of demonstrating the role of selective attention.

Overgeneralizing. This is another characteristic thinking style that maintains clinical perfectionism, in which a person takes one instance to indicate something about him- or herself overall (e.g., "Because I made a small error in the monthly report it means I am a failure as a person").

Double Standards. This is a thinking style often reported in clinical perfectionism, involving holding a different set of standards for oneself than for others (e.g., "It's okay for other people to make spelling mistakes in their e-mails, but I should never make a mistake").

Evaluation of Standards

Individuals with clinical perfectionism strive to meet multiple personal standards on a daily basis and constantly try to judge whether their standards have or have not been met. Some perfectionistic individuals may also avoid trying to meet their standards, as follows.

FAILURE TO MEET STANDARDS

Individuals with clinical perfectionism more often than not feel they have not met their standards, resulting in intense self-critical thinking (e.g., "I am a failure"). A consequence of this self-critical thinking is the reinforcement of the notion that self-worth is dependent on striving, and the conclusion that the individual is only worthwhile as a person if he or she is meeting standards.

TEMPORARILY MEETING STANDARDS

Even when individuals with clinical perfectionism meet their standards, they discount their successes and see them as "no big deal" or conclude, "Anyone could have done it." As a result, they often reset their standards higher and try to do even better next time. In this way, even when clients think they have met their standards, they do not feel satisfied, and their self-evaluation based on striving and achievement is again reinforced, leading them to reset standards higher, creating a vicious cycle. Reinterpretating standards as not demanding enough (after meeting them) results in the person never feeling good enough, and instead feeling like a failure.

Many people with clinical perfectionism describe feeling relief for having avoided failure (as opposed to a sense of accomplishment) when they meet standards. In this way they become locked in a cycle of never being able to enjoy their successes or reflect on their achievements, and instead thinking about how the bar can be set even higher next time (e.g., "Even though I received a standing ovation for my musical performance, I know I didn't play the piece perfectly and need to improve for my next performance").

AVOIDANCE OF MEETING STANDARDS

Another outcome of evaluating standards is giving up and avoiding trying to meet one's inflexible rules because of the intense worry and anxiety over whether they can be met. Typically, this can also include avoidance of situations that may test one's performance (e.g., avoiding an exam). This avoidance behavior results in intense self-criticism and thoughts that one needs to try harder to meet one's standards, again reinforcing the idea that self-worth should be based on meeting standards. Procrastination can also be seen as a form of avoidance behavior and is very common in clinical perfectionism.

Performance-Related Behavior

People do a range of things to check out how well they are meeting their standards or to help them achieve their goals. Four main areas of performance-related behavior in clinical perfectionism include:

- *Goal achievement behaviors*, where clients engage in performance-related behaviors to meet their goals (e.g., spending hours flipping through a thesaurus trying to find the perfect word when writing an essay).

- *Testing performance*, which involves testing out how well individuals think they are doing at a task.

- *Comparisons*, which involve measuring one's performance against that of others. For example, a person might compare the number of people who were looking at her when she gave a presentation at work compared to when her colleague presented. The problem in clinical perfectionism is one of "upward social comparison" or comparing oneself to others who are perceived as much better (e.g., a woman comparing her body shape to those of models in fashion magazines, or an individual comparing his or her performance to that of the most senior person in the office).

- *Reassurance seeking*, or trying to check out how well one is meeting standards by asking others for their impressions (e.g., a student might repeatedly ask a teacher questions regarding the same piece of feedback to feel reassured about his or her performance). The problem with excessive reassurance seeking is that it creates only a fleeting feeling of assurance and contributes to the maintenance and possible strengthening of anxiety about performance.

Counterproductive Behaviors and Self-Criticism

Counterproductive behaviors are what individuals do to reduce their concerns about performance or to feel more at ease about their performance. Counterproductive behaviors are similar to what are often called "safety behaviors." They are idiosyncratic and need to be assessed for each individual. Examples of counterproductive behaviors include list making (e.g., making multiple lists at work in an attempt to guard against not performing to one's standards), overpreparing (e.g., staying up all night the night before a presentation preparing and rehearsing, such that fatigue leads to poorer performance), and being overly thorough (e.g., spending too much time on tasks, and being late for appointments as a result). The reason we use the term "counterproductive behavior" rather than "safety behavior" is to distinguish safety behaviors that are unhelpful (and therefore appropriate targets for treatment) from those that may be therapeutic when used judiciously (Rachman, Radomsky, & Shafran, 2008).

In addition to engaging in counterproductive behaviors, clients with clinical perfectionism often engage in intense self-criticism when they think they have not met their goals. Often people report that they self-criticize with the purpose of ensuring they do not make the mistake again, or to "up their game." Regardless, self-criticism clearly maintains the vicious cycle of clinical perfectionism. This is because it leads to clients thinking they are failures, which reinforces their belief that self-worth should be based on achievement, and leads them to again strive to achieve higher standards, thus staying locked in the cycle of clinical perfectionism.

Evidence for the Cognitive-Behavioral Model of Clinical Perfectionism

In support of the model, Egan et al. (2013) recently found that a clinical group high in negative perfectionism reported that they would reset standards higher following failure, compared to a group low on negative perfectionism, who stated they would set standards lower following failure. Evidence that individuals with clinical perfectionism reset standards higher after successful achievement of their goals has also been found in an experimental study (Kobori et al., 2009).

There is also a range of other studies that have supported predictions of the model. Riley and Shafran (2005) found individuals with clinical perfectionism reported setting rigid rules, avoidance, and self-criticism following failure, which supports numerous aspects of the model. There are also quantitative studies finding support for the model. In a study involving three different samples (a clinical group, students, and athletes), Egan et al. (2007) found that dichotomous thinking accounted for significant variance in negative perfectionism. This lends support to the prediction that individuals with problematic perfectionism judge their standards in a dichotomous manner. Stoeber, Kempe, and Keogh (2008) found that self-oriented and socially prescribed perfectionism were associated with higher shame and guilt following failure in a task. This finding is consistent with the model, in that individuals with perfectionism are assumed to be intensely self-critical following failure, and shame and guilt may be the emotional sequela of this self-criticism.

Example of the Cognitive-Behavioral Model of Clinical Perfectionism

To understand what the cognitive-behavioral model looks like in action, consider the case of Ines.

Ines is a 26-year-old woman who works in a busy advertising firm and has been in a relationship with her boyfriend for the past 2 years. Ines described herself as having very high standards and goals. One of the main areas she pushes herself to do well in is work. She expects that she should come up with new and innovative ideas each week in order to get noticed by her boss and eventually get promoted. Ines believes that the only way she can achieve this is to work 12-hour days and on weekends. Ines also has very high standards for her weight and appearance (e.g., anything over 110 pounds is overweight, and her hair and makeup must be perfect). She engages in a range of behaviors such as restricting her food intake, checking her weight daily, and repeatedly checking her body shape for fat.

Ines also stated that she is very house proud and likes to have things look perfect when her boyfriend or friends visit her. If she perceives her house as messy, she avoids having others visit her because she doesn't want them to think she is a "lazy pig." In the past, she enjoyed entertaining friends on weekends and making special "restaurant quality" meals for them, though lately she has been avoiding doing this because having the house perfectly clean and preparing the meal to her high standards leaves her feeling exhausted. She also said that she feels socializing can be a bit of a "waste of time" and that she should not spend her time socializing when she could be working or fitting in a class at the gym.

Ines stated that she judges herself in terms of how well she is meeting her standards and rules, and that she often focuses on her mistakes, like sending the wrong version of a sample ad to a client via e-mail. Despite recognizing the error within 5 minutes, resending the correct version, and being reassured by her friend that it was "no big deal," she still berated herself, thinking, "How could I be so stupid? I am such a failure." When instances like this occur, Ines feels that she has failed, and as a result experiences feelings of low mood, high anxiety, and panic. She recalled a recent time when she noticed a single grade less than an A on an old university transcript and was extremely anxious. She believed that she had wrecked her perfect record and she could not help focusing on how she had "screwed it up."

Ines feels that she is not doing well at meeting her goals. Even when she succeeds at something (e.g., when her boss comments that she is doing well), she discounts her success (e.g., ignoring her boss's feedback and brushing it off by saying, "He probably says that to everyone; I need to try harder"). Ines often focuses on all of the areas in which she perceives herself to be behind, even though she has often received positive comments about how much she achieves at work. Even when Ines does achieve her goals, she does not enjoy the success, and instead thinks about what she is not doing well. This type of thinking keeps Ines in a cycle of believing that she is never good enough and feeling bad about herself as a person.

Ines clearly had many features that were consistent with clinical perfectionism, and many associated negative consequences, including anxiety, depression, and exhaustion. Ines based her sense of self-worth on how well she achieved her goals at work, and on eating, body shape, weight, appearance, cleanliness in her home, and entertaining her friends. As a result, Ines set a range of rigid rules regarding achievement in these domains (e.g., never making mistakes at work, weighing no more than 110 pounds, not leaving the house without her hair and makeup looking perfect, and not having others over unless the house and food are perfect). Ines also evaluated how well she met these standards in a dichotomous manner. For example, she saw a minor error at work as a complete failure and then engaged in intense self-criticism over her mistake. She sought reassurance from a work colleague about the mistake, compared herself to others at work, and concluded that she was a failure. Even when her boss praised her presentation and referred to her as "my star performer," she brushed it off as no big deal, thinking that she could do a better job next time. She was instead focused on the error she had made, thinking "I am a screw up." She felt panicky and discouraged. She ruminated on the thought "I just have to try better next time," which further reinforced her assumption that self-worth should be based on striving and achievement.

In considering Ines's clinical perfectionism, guidelines for useful questions and how to engage the patient in a collaborative formulation are outlined below. Figure 7.3 provides a summary of how to conceptualize Ines's case using the revised cognitive-behavioral model of clinical perfectionism (Shafran et al., 2010).

How would a case such as that of Ines be approached in developing a collaborative formulation of the factors maintaining her clinical perfectionism? The first step would be to engage Ines in thinking about the behaviors and thoughts that keep her locked in the cycle of clinical perfectionism. It is useful at the start the formulation session to ask the client a question such as "How might it be useful to understand what keeps your perfectionism going?" This question begins the process of guided discovery using

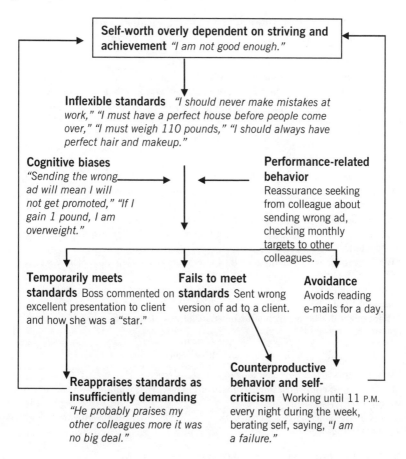

FIGURE 7.3. Example of a collaborative formulation based on the revised cognitive-behavioral model of clinical perfectionism (Shafran et al., 2010).

Socratic questioning, in which the therapist asks questions to help the client discover the cognitive and behavioral processes that keep him or her locked in a vicious cycle of clinical perfectionism. As cognitive-behavioral therapists know well, the process of understanding, collaboration, and change often comes from a line of effective Socratic dialogue in which the therapist helps the client to achieve understanding rather than telling the patient in a didactic manner what he or she "should" be thinking. Table 7.1 includes examples of questions that can help to assess aspects of the model. It can be useful to ask the client these questions in the context of a recent example of clinical perfectionism.

The following sections provide more detail regarding the areas to assess as outlined in Table 7.1.

TABLE 7.1. Sample Questions to Help Derive a Collaborative Cognitive-Behavioral Formulation of Clinical Perfectionism

1. High standards and striving

- "In what areas do you set high standards?"
- "In which areas of your life do you push yourself and feel that you have to excel?"
- "Of these areas, in which is it most important for you to achieve your standards? How would you order them from most to least important, or are they equally important?"

2. Adverse consequences of clinical perfectionism

- "What impact do you think your striving has on your life?"
- "What negative consequences occur as a result of pushing yourself in the areas you have mentioned?"
- "What effect does your striving have on your mood [e.g., sad, stressed]?"
- "What effect does it have on your social relationships [e.g., no time to socialize due to striving]?"
- "What effect does it have on your intimate relationships [e.g., partner gets angry because you never make time for him or her]?"
- "What effect does it have on your thinking [e.g., rumination over mistakes, poor concentration]?"
- "What effect does it have on your behavior [e.g., counterproductive behaviors, reassurance seeking]?"

3. Self-evaluation overly dependent on achievement

- "What factors affect how you judge yourself as a person?"
- "How much of your self-esteem is made up of how well you are meeting your high standards?"
- "Do you base your sense of self-worth on what you do, rather than who you are as a person?"

4. Setting of inflexible standards and rules

- "Do you change your standards and rules when you discover that they cannot be met?"

5. Cognitive biases

- "Do you tend to perceive your standards as being either completely met or not at all met?"
- "When you think about your performance, what do you tend to focus on?"
- "How much do you notice mistakes in performance?"
- "How much do you notice successes in your performance?"
- "How do you react to positive aspects of performance?"

6. Performance-related behaviors

- *Testing performance*—"Do you tend to check repeatedly to assess how well you are doing at things?"
- *Comparisons*—"Do you compare your performance to that of others?"
- *Reassurance seeking*—"Who do you ask for reassurance about your performance?"

(continued)

TABLE 7.1. *(continued)*

---

7. Evaluation of standards

- "Can you think of recent examples where you have met a goal, and also where you did not meet a goal?"

Failure to meet a standard

- "What do you think when you fail to achieve a goal or standard you have set?"
- "What does it mean about you when you fail to achieve a goal or standard?"
- "What is the worst part about failing at a goal?"
- "What do you do when you don't meet a goal?"
- "Do you often fear that you will fail at your goals?"

Reaction to meeting goals and resetting standards

- "How do you feel when you meet a goal or standard?"
- "Do you feel satisfied? Not satisfied? How long does the feeling last?"
- "When you meet your goals, do you discount them as being too easy [e.g., 'anyone could have done that!']?"
- "After you meet your goals, do you set even higher goals for next time? Do you set lower goals, or are your goals more or less the same?"

8. Avoidance of meeting standards

- *Avoidance*—"What do you avoid doing due to worry about your performance [e.g., never inviting friends over for dinner for fear that you won't make a good meal]?"
- *Procrastination*—"What do you put off or delay due to your perfectionism? Do you leave things until the last minute so you will have an excuse if you don't do well? Would you rather delay a task than face doing it less than perfectly? Do you ever delay starting tasks because you know they will take a long time due to your high standards?"

9. Self-criticism and counterproductive behaviors

- "Do you criticize yourself over your performance?"
- "How do you feel when you make a mistake?"
- "What do you say to yourself when you are critical about your standards?"
- "What is the result of self-criticism? What effect does it have?"
- *Counterproductive behaviors*—"Is there anything else you do to reduce the impact of your worry about performance [e.g., always making lists before starting work for the day]"?

High Standards and Striving

It is useful to begin by discussing with clients the life domains in which they have high standards and those in which they don't. This discussion will set the scene for the formulation and will help both the therapist and client to understand which particular domains are affected by clinical perfectionism. The specific domains will differ depending on the particular client. For example, a client may strive for perfectionism in one main domain (e.g., work), whereas another may strive for perfection across numerous domains, as in the case of Ines, where her perfectionism affected the domains of work, appearance, weight, and home. It is useful to have the client number the domains from most to least important. Often, clients will have difficulty ranking the importance of their domains, instead reporting that "all areas are important." It is worth persisting, however, to see if the client can identify some domains that are particularly important (e.g., Ines rated work and her weight as equally important, followed by appearance and home as least important). This can give the therapist some clues about areas that are most central to target in treatment. It can also be useful when starting behavioral experiments to have the client achieve success in areas that are lower in importance (e.g., Ines might be willing to begin with experiments aimed at doing things less than perfectly in the domain of entertaining before conducting experiments in the domain of work). It can also be useful at this point for the therapist and client to understand areas in which the client is not a perfectionist (if there are any), and the reasons why he or she is less perfectionistic in these domains. This can help the client see that perfectionism is not an unchangeable personality characteristic affecting everything, but rather a way of thinking and behaving in particular areas, which can help him or her to engage with the approach.

Adverse Consequences of Clinical Perfectionism

Asking questions at the beginning of the session about the impact of perfectionism can help to set the stage for the formulation process and help the client understand some of the negative consequences of striving. This can be particularly useful for clients who focus on the perceived positive aspects of their perfectionism (e.g., beliefs about how it helps them to achieve). It also is useful as a lead-in to asking about what we see as the main core of the formulation and main problem in clinical perfectionism, namely self-evaluation based on striving and achievement.

Self-Evaluation Overly Dependent on Achievement

A critical idea for clients to understand during the formulation session is that judging oneself to be "good enough" only when achieving one's standards is the core problem, and that it drives the other cognitive and behavioral factors that maintain clinical perfectionism. Shafran et al. (2010) suggested that of the many questions used to determine whether clients have clinical perfectionism, the single most important one is "Do you base your self-esteem on striving and achievement?" (p. 18). For example, a therapist could say, "Ines, it sounds like you spend a great deal of time trying to do well across the areas we just discussed. Can you tell me how important it is to your self-esteem that you achieve in these areas? What happens to your self-esteem if you feel you are not achieving, for example, at work? Do you think you base your self-esteem on achievement of your goals?" It is useful to then ask the client about the impact that basing self-worth on achievement has on him or her, which can lead nicely to questions about setting standards. It may also be useful at this stage to draw a pie chart showing how much the client bases self-esteem on striving and achievement (see Chapter 13 for further details). This can help to bring home to the client how dependent his or her sense of self is on striving and attainment of goals.

Setting of Inflexible Standards and Rules

It is useful here to ask the client a question such as "Okay, Ines, we seem to have found that you base your self-esteem on striving and achievement. Because of this, do you think you set any particular rules that need to be met in order for you to achieve those standards?" Basically, the goal of the therapist is to uncover examples of rigid rules and standards the individual holds. In the example of Ines, she had many rigid rules, for example that she must weigh no more than 110 pounds and never make mistakes at work.

Cognitive Biases

It is useful at this stage to ask for a specific recent example of when the person felt that he or she did not meet one of the standards just discussed. In the example of Ines, the therapist knew that work was one of the most important domains of achievement and therefore asked the following questions:

THERAPIST: Ines, given you have a rule that you should never make mistakes at work, is that rule hard to meet sometimes? Can you think of any recent examples of when you made a mistake at work that we could use to understand together what keeps this problem of perfectionism going?

INES: Yes, recently I sent the wrong ad to a client and I thought that it was absolutely terrible to have made such a mistake, I felt like a complete failure.

Using this example, the therapist was able to identify with Ines her *dichotomous thinking* (i.e., that she was a complete failure for making the mistake), *overgeneralization* (i.e., that she would never be promoted), and *selective attention* (i.e., ruminating over the mistake and ignoring positive feedback from her boss).

Performance-Related Behaviors

To assess performance-related behaviors, it can be useful to ask the general questions illustrated in Table 7.1, but it can often be most fruitful to continue asking about the example that has already been raised using Socratic dialogue—for example, "Ines, when you felt like you had really screwed up by sending that e-mail, did you do anything to feel better about it later (e.g., asking others if they thought it was a big mistake)?"

Evaluation of Standards

According to the model of clinical perfectionism as outlined, there are three main reactions clients can have regarding standards: judging that they have failed to meet the standard, judging that they have met the standard, or avoiding trying to meet the standard.

Failure to Meet Standards

In the case of Ines, her therapist asked questions about her reactions to making a mistake at work to help her understand the impact of her evaluation of not meeting the standard, which led to self-criticism and counterproductive behaviors: "Ines, so it sounds as though when you felt you had made this mistake at work, it ended up with you being really hard on yourself, and calling yourself a 'screw-up.' You also thought you had better work really late all week to make up for it."

Meeting a Standard

To determine a client's response to the perception of having met a standard, it can be useful to ask about the domain discussed in the example being followed for the formulation. In the case of Ines, the therapist asked a question about work:

> THERAPIST: Ines, can you think of any recent examples where you felt that you had achieved your goals at work?
>
> INES: Not really, I don't ever really feel like I am doing well enough at work.
>
> THERAPIST: Okay, so it sounds as though you feel you never achieve your standards at work. I wonder, though, if you can think of a recent example where someone might have commented that you had done well at work and you brushed off this comment?

Based on this questioning, the example of Ines's boss giving her a lot of praise for her presentation was uncovered. However, this example was initially difficult for Ines to generate, as she was engaging in selective attention and dismissing the positive feedback. Bringing to light such an example is very useful for the formulation process, as the therapist can use this as an opportunity to ask the client what he or she thinks the impact of ignoring positive feedback is, and what impact it has on goal setting:

> THERAPIST: Ines, given that you brushed off this positive feedback from your boss, what impact do you think that had on how hard you push yourself at work and on your standards?
>
> INES: I just think I have to do even better now and set my goals even higher. Even though he gave me positive feedback, I still feel like I have to try harder at work.

Avoidance of Meeting Standards

Many clients with clinical perfectionism have periods of procrastination and avoidance that are linked to their fears about performance. Therefore, it is useful to uncover examples of clients engaging in avoidance with respect to meeting their standards. In Ines's case, a question was asked as follows:

> THERAPIST: Given the mistake you felt you had made at work, did you avoid thinking about the mistake, or did you avoid any of your work?
>
> INES: Yes, I was so worried about it that I avoided opening my e-mail for a day after the mistake because I was afraid that I would have an e-mail from my boss asking me to explain the mistake or an angry e-mail from the client.
>
> THERAPIST: Oh okay, so it stopped you opening your e-mails for a day because you were so concerned, and did you get an e-mail like that from your boss or client?
>
> INES: No.

These types of questions can also be a useful point at which to discuss with your client the role of predictive thinking and examples of how they have made negative predictions that did not end up occurring.

Self-Criticism and Counterproductive Behaviors

The questions asked by the therapist regarding failure to meet standards will flow naturally to questions about the impact of not meeting the standards, in terms of self-criticism and counterproductive behaviors as reviewed earlier. Sample questions can be found in Table 7.1.

Troubleshooting: Individualizing the Formulation and Being Flexible about the Model

While the cognitive-behavioral model of clinical perfectionism can be a guide to the formulation, you do not need to adhere rigidly to the model or the suggested questions in this chapter to derive the model. A range of questions may be useful in helping guide the collaborative formulation session; however, this will vary, and exact questions will be different for each individual client based on his or her situation. In this way, the formulation is truly individualized. It can be useful to have a blank copy of the model to use as a guide, along with a range of questions. These questions can be used to help guide you in asking about the maintaining factors of the model. You can use the formulation template flexibly, drawing in extra boxes for maintaining factors not in the model (such as family or relationship factors) and omitting others that are not relevant. It is useful to think about any factors that may be personally relevant to the client and include these in the formulation. It can also be useful to think about any other issues that may need to be included, for example, societal expectations about achievement and striving and the impact of the client's own cultural background on his or her perfectionism.

Linking Evaluation of Standards Back to the Notion of Self-Worth Being Based on Achievement: Discussing the "Vicious Cycle" of Clinical Perfectionism

Once it was determined in the session that Ines's evaluation of herself as not meeting her standard led her to be even harder on herself and work very late all week to make up for it, the therapist asked a range of questions to highlight how she gets locked in the "vicious cycle" of perfectionism:

> THERAPIST: Ines, given that you beat yourself up over the mistake, what do you think that does to how you see yourself as only being good enough when you are achieving (the part we put at the top of the model, here)?
>
> INES: Well, I guess it just keeps reinforcing my idea that I am only good enough when I am doing well.
>
> THERAPIST: Okay, so it sounds like your self-worth is based on doing well. What does that do to setting goals and standards?
>
> INES: Well, each time I make a mistake, I think I just need to try harder next time and I set myself even harder goals to achieve.

The model can be illustrated using Socratic dialogue to show the client how she is trapped in a cycle of continual reinforcement of the idea that self-worth should be based on achievement, influencing the goals she sets, making her more likely to engage in self-criticism, and starting the cycle over again. The same can be true when a client feels he or she has met a standard. For example, Ines's therapist asked her about the impact of discounting successes:

> THERAPIST: So, Ines, even when you felt that you had met a standard by receiving positive comments from your boss, you thought that was no big deal and had to try even harder at work. What do you think that does to your belief that your worth is based on achievement?
>
> INES: It just keeps it going, I suppose, so my self-esteem is always based on achievement.

This process is repeated for each maintaining factor in the formulation diagram so that it is clear for the client how each of the factors reinforces self-worth being based on achievement.

At the end of the formulation, the client should have an understanding that he or she has been locked in a vicious cycle of perfectionism, in which the belief that self-worth is tied to striving and achievement is maintained, regardless of whether the client has met the standard, failed to meet the standard, or avoided opportunities to meet the standard. Once this point is reached, it is useful for the therapist to ask the client a question like "So, Ines, given everything we have found together today with this diagram, what things do you think we might want to target together to attack this problem of perfectionism?" This provides an opportunity to explore the maintaining factors that need to be changed to help break out of the vicious cycle and leads to developing an individualized treatment plan.

CHAPTER 8

The Therapeutic Alliance and Engagement

W hen writing a therapist's guide, it's tempting to skip over discussion of the therapeutic alliance. After all, most therapists understand the importance of the alliance and engagement. However, emerging literature is throwing new light on the role and meaning of the therapeutic alliance and engagement that is important to consider in terms of maximizing the effectiveness of treatment. When working with the client with perfectionism, special attention should be paid to the therapeutic alliance as this impacts on reductions in maladjustment and self-critical perfectionism. There should be open discussion about ambivalence toward tackling perfectionism, and attention should also be paid to building up self-efficacy with respect to change.

The therapeutic alliance and engagement are particularly important for disorders where there is ambivalence about treatment. It is frightening for the client to let go of established behaviors and strategies that are perceived to have important benefits despite the problems they generate, in order to experiment with new strategies that have an unknown benefit and some possible costs. The treatment of perfectionism is typically associated with a large degree of ambivalence on behalf of the client, and it is important that the therapist not only understand this, but be prepared for it and, indeed, preempt it. Further, there is wisdom in overtly welcoming ambivalence in the client, framing it as an opportunity for the client to consider the possible costs as well as the benefits of treatment, and to be aware from the start of the hard work that is involved in change. Therefore, this chapter examines general issues related to the therapeutic alliance and engagement, as well as specific issues of relevance to perfectionism.

What Is the Therapeutic Alliance?

The therapeutic alliance is typically viewed as being associated with three factors (Bordin, 1979). The first is the presence of shared goals, or a sense of common goals and purpose, between the client and the therapist. The second is an accepted recognition of the tasks that each person is to perform in the relationship, which engenders a sense of safety and trust in the therapy process. The third factor is referred to as an attachment bond, or simply how comfortable the client feels with the therapist. While the therapeutic relationship is seen as a multifaceted phenomenon, the major focus in recent years has been on the alliance between the therapist and the client (Zuroff & Blatt, 2006).

Taken in context, the therapeutic alliance is only one of many factors influencing the effectiveness of therapy with any one individual. In a helpful overview of the factors that contribute to clinical improvement in cognitive therapy, Dimidjian and Dobson (2004) discuss four important domains. The first is therapist factors, which involve adherence to the CBT model, competence and experience (which are not necessarily the same thing), and personal characteristics, perhaps best captured in the *Cognitive Therapy Scale—Revised* (Blackburn et al., 2001) as "interpersonal effectiveness" (e.g., creativity, insight, and inspiration). The cognitive model can be misunderstood by therapists as aiming to help clients be more rational. Adherence to the model is insightfully summarized by Paul Salkovskis (1996) as being:

> not necessarily about thinking more rationally, nor about thinking more positively . . . the aim is not to persuade the person that their current way of looking at the situation is wrong, irrational, or too negative; instead, it is to allow them to identify where they might have become trapped or stuck in their way of thinking and to allow them to discover other ways of looking at their situation. In this way, the therapist seeks to empower clients by broadening the choices they make about the way they react to their situation and by helping them to discover information that allows them to decide between the available choices in an informed way that is consistent with their beliefs and values. (pp. 49–50)

The second domain includes theory-specific factors that are necessary for therapeutic change. In cognitive therapy this relates to cognitive and behavioral interventions, and the ongoing discussion about whether cognitive interventions are important elements of cognitive therapy or whether cognitive change is mainly driven by behavioral experiments. The third domain that influences clinical improvement in cognitive therapy is client factors, which can range from sociodemographic variables, social support, and current environment to past life events and problem type (e.g., we know that the binge–purge subtype of anorexia nervosa is associated with higher dropout and poorer outcome than the restricting subtype of anorexia nervosa).

Finally, nonspecific factors, including a strong therapeutic alliance, are seen to be of importance for producing good clinical outcome. Literature reviews typically assign an overall effect size of between 0.22 and 0.26 to the association between alliance and outcome (Castonguay, Constantino, & Holtforth, 2006), which is small but significant (we typically expect good treatments to have an effect size greater than 1.00). Particularly in more structured therapies such as cognitive therapy, the therapeutic relationship is seen to be necessary for a good clinical outcome, but it is not sufficient (Waller, 2012). For example, in cognitive therapy for depression, the extent to which a positive therapeutic relationship influenced change across a range of outcomes (such as depression and social adjustment), independent of early clinical improvement in the first four sessions, was associated with a small effect size at posttreatment (Zuroff & Blatt, 2006).

While we have a common understanding of what the therapeutic alliance is, we have a more divided idea about how it is formed. This can roughly be represented by two schools of thought. The first and perhaps most commonly held understanding is that the therapeutic alliance is something that has to happen before psychotherapies can be effective (Bordin, 1979). The second and emerging understanding is that the therapeutic alliance really gets going after the client has started to apply the therapeutic techniques and is benefiting from them (Webb et al., 2012). In other words, the therapeutic alliance is based more on collaborative work and its results than on a warm relationship. Holtforth and Castonguay (2005) refer to the therapeutic relationship being in continuous interaction with technique.

Therefore, when working with ambivalent clients, *it is important to balance change consideration techniques such as motivational interviewing (which is discussed later in this chapter) with early collaborative work and experiments that explore new strategies and behaviors that can build the client's confidence for further change as well as the strength of the therapeutic alliance.*

Why Is the Therapeutic Alliance Particularly Important When Working with the Client with Perfectionism?

Perfectionism has been shown to predict poorer outcome in the treatment of bulimia nervosa (Steele, Bergin, & Wade, 2011) and depression, where there are numerous studies showing this effect. The effect of perfectionism on acute treatment outcomes was explored in a randomized controlled trial of 439 clinically depressed adolescents (R. H. Jacobs et al., 2009). Predictor results indicated that adolescents with higher versus lower perfectionism scores at baseline, regardless of treatment, continued to demonstrate elevated depression scores across the acute treatment period. In the case of suicidality, perfectionism impeded improvement. Treatment outcomes were partially mediated by the change in perfectionism across the 12-week period. An online survey posted on the Black Dog Institute website in Australia, completed by 3,486 respondents reporting a history of treatment for depression, showed that self-criticism was retrospectively associated with a poorer response to most treatments (Parker & Crawford, 2009).

The Treatment of Depression Collaborative Research Program (Elkin, 1994) has been examined on several occasions with respect to the impact of perfectionism on the treatment of depression. Pretreatment perfectionism was a significant predictor of diminished therapeutic change as assessed by all primary outcome measures (Blatt et al., 1995). The strength of the therapeutic alliance significantly predicted longitudinal perfectionism change, and perfectionism significantly predicted the rate of depression change throughout therapy (Hawley, Ho, Zuroff, & Blatt, 2006). *In other words, clients who perceived their therapist as providing high average levels of positive regard, empathy, and genuineness experienced more rapid reductions in both overall maladjustment and self-critical perfectionism* (Zuroff, Kelly, Leybman, Blatt, & Wampold, 2010).

Factors That Enhance the Therapeutic Alliance and Engagement

When you are working with clients to experiment with CBT techniques and apply them to their specific situation, a number of other factors can enhance this process and therefore strengthen therapeutic alliance and engagement. Five such factors are worth special consideration when working with clients who experience high levels of unhelpful perfectionism: collaboration, structure and flexibility, validation, therapist beliefs about therapy, and tracking beliefs and mending ruptures. This section includes a discussion of each of these factors.

Collaboration

Collaboration is the cornerstone of cognitive therapy. The therapist and client work together as a team, jointly choosing therapy goals, constructing a meaningful conceptualization of the problem, and developing plans for change. The client is expected to be active outside the session as an observer, reporter, and experimenter, and the therapist treats the client as an expert on his or her own life, where the client's input is crucial in generating behavioral experiments. The client and therapist pool their wisdom to forge a pathway ahead.

When working with people who are perfectionists, it is worth considering how their all-or-nothing and black-and-white thinking styles may impact on collaborative work. Such clients may have the following assumptions: "If I can't fix the problem by myself, then I am worthless," "If I need help, then I am weak," "If I can't come up with the right answer, then others will think less of me." Clients often feel shame for just attending therapy, and may expect the therapist to see them as a failure. There are some helpful strategies to consider when first starting work with the client.

First, the initial session should include questions about what has brought the client into therapy, how the client feels about coming to therapy, and the types of thinking that drive that emotion. From the start, encourage open sharing of feelings and thoughts that may otherwise derail therapy, and discuss them in a matter-of-fact and accepting manner.

Second, use metaphors for the change process that emphasize how collaboration can be more helpful than a solo approach to problem solving. When discussing the collaborative nature of the therapy, it is useful to say such things as "We find that when people are trying to change a long-term way of behaving that is associated with a high level of emotion it is very difficult to make changes all by themselves. It seems to work best having another person alongside who can help generate some different ideas. Indeed, often it is useful to have more than one person to bounce ideas off. For instance, when elite athletes prepare for the Olympics, we don't expect them to do all their preparation on their own. We expect that their performance will be better when they work with a coach and have the encouragement of a team around them. As we work together, it may be useful to see me as a coach who can work alongside you, and it will be useful for us to consider at some stage whether there are other people that you know and trust who can provide some ideas or encouragement from time to time."

Third, judicious therapist disclosure is useful as it is likely that the client sees the therapist as "a success," and so admissions that the therapist also finds it useful to have others to bounce off ideas can be helpful. This is also clearly displayed in the therapist–client relationship, where the therapist does not present as "the expert" but relies on the client's ideas to formulate useful strategies. As part of this approach, when discussing possible behavioral experiments with the client, it can be useful for therapists to "embrace their ignorance" and say "I don't exactly what will be most helpful, but I know a way to find out" (Waller et al., 2007). Communicating the importance of being willing to try something to see how it works, and of trial and error as the pathway to reaching workable strategies, is a good precedent to set up early as the client may initially feel uncomfortable with the idea of "not getting it right the first time."

Structure and Flexibility

Padesky (1996) states that "the ideal cognitive therapist is capable of being highly structured in therapy, comfortable with tracking a number of tasks within a session, and yet sensitive to adapting therapy structure to individual clients in order to maximise collaboration and a positive therapeutic relationship" (p. 271). The ideal encapsulated in this quote can be seen as rather a difficult task for most therapists, but it is absolutely essential to model for the perfectionistic client. Structure is an essential part of good cognitive therapy that allows the process of therapy to be transparent to clients so that they can develop an understanding of how to develop helpful strategies for themselves. However, people struggling with perfectionism may already embrace too much structure in their lives (e.g., living by lists, drawing out plans for every aspect of life, focusing on ticking off the next task to the detriment of time that can be spent on self-care).

Therefore, it is particularly important that the therapist temper structure with flexibility, modeling the use of guidelines rather than rules when conducting therapy, and paying attention to adapting any of the strategies discussed in this book to the individual requirements of the client. This starts with the agenda setting at the start of each session, where the therapist doesn't just inform the client about what will be covered, but invites clients to add their own ideas about what should be covered. Another important way of exhibiting therapist flexibility to the client is collaborative case conceptualization, where the therapist shows that he or she does not have a fixed and preconceived understanding of what is going on for the client but recognizes that each client is different with respect to what maintains the perfectionism and how the consequences of perfectionism are experienced. Guided discovery is also important in terms of exhibiting flexibility, where the therapist provides a context in which clients can safely explore new ways of approaching a problem, resulting in clients making their own contributions toward therapeutic discoveries. The client is encouraged to develop alternative hypotheses and experiments that can lead to potential solutions without the therapist presenting such ideas on a plate. The stance of the therapist is one of interest and curiosity, a willingness to learn from the client, a respect for the client's insights, ideas, and views, and a willingness to ask questions to help the client generate ideas. At times it is appropriate to suggest particular worksheets or exercises and this should be introduced first by asking permission (i.e., "Is it all right if I show you something that others have found helpful and may give us ideas about the way forward with this issues?"), followed up with "Of course, for it to be helpful for you, we will need to think about how it can best be adapted for your circumstances."

Validation

Validation or compassionate conceptualization (Linehan, 1993) is used to balance change strategies. In this process, the therapist (1) explores the benefits and costs of the current behavior associated with perfectionism, (2) communicates to the clients that their current responses make sense within their current and past life experiences and the perceived benefits of the perfectionism, and (3) helps the client to consider alternative responses that may achieve goals with fewer costs and more benefits. Validation does not involve: (1) pointing out that a response was functional in the past but not now, or (2) trying to make clients feel good about their current behavior. This approach is essential in creating a nonjudgmental atmosphere in which to explore the possibility of change where clients feel very uncertain about changing their perfectionism, for fear of possibly negative consequences.

A simple "parable" can be used to illustrate the point that the client's current situation has pros and cons, and that an alternative approach may also offer benefit once the hard work of change is negotiated, as well as helping the client to get closer to life goals that may have been overshadowed by perfectionism. For example:

> "Imagine you are crossing over a large steel arch bridge when you lose your footing and by some miracle end up sitting halfway up on one of the supporting pylons. You quite like it here and feel that you have come across a wonderful strategy for achieving a happy life: it is safe, and less tiring than walking across the bridge; it quickly becomes familiar; it is beautiful weather; the views are great; people are happy to hand you down food so you can survive. However, there are some major drawbacks: lack of company, difficulty finding a comfortable sleeping position, and lack of privacy. Also, you can see the shoreline where you had wanted to head, and over time you realize that you are not quite living the life that you wanted, so you decide to try to climb back up the pylon. Each time you do, you get nervous and retreat back to your familiar place. You keep persisting, practicing ten, twenty, then one hundred times a day, and eventually you are able to leave the pylon and get back on the bridge and continue your journey."

Therapist Beliefs about Therapy

Therapists can be just as much influenced by perfectionistic thinking as their clients, and these beliefs are associated with higher levels of burnout that will ultimately impair the therapeutic relationship (D'Souza, Egan, & Rees, 2011; McLean, Wade, & Encel, 2003). When controlling for demographic, workplace, and personal resource variables, therapist beliefs about control (e.g., "I need to fully understand what happens in therapy in order to help the client," "I must work at peak efficiency at all times") are associated with higher levels of emotional exhaustion, and beliefs about control and inflexibility (e.g., "If I just stick to one therapeutic model it will solve the problem for me," "If I deviate from the clinical model then I've failed") are associated with lower levels of personal accomplishment (Emery, McLean, & Wade, 2009).

In particular, confronting clients with high expectations who expect things to be done "right" can trigger unhelpful thoughts in therapists that can impede collaboration. (Some of these are outlined in Table 8.1.) Consideration of the consequences for the client of acting on these thoughts can be a helpful exercise, as can receiving regular supervision for one's own beliefs in therapy and how they can impact on our own emotional health and effectiveness as therapists.

Tracking the Alliance and Mending Ruptures

Research would suggest that therapists, whether novice or experienced, are not always good at knowing what their clients are experiencing (Geller, 2002; Hannan, Lambert, Harmon, Nielsen, Smart, et al., 2005). We have

TABLE 8.1. Consideration of the Impact of Therapist Beliefs on the Client

Assumption	Behavior	Consequence for the client
"If my client is in distress, then I should relieve that distress."	When the client is distressed, change the topic to something less challenging; don't let the client leave the office until he or she is calmed down.	The client believes that distress was getting out of hand, and that unless the therapist had stepped in, it would have been unbearable.
"If I am too structured, then I'll miss important client revelations or appear unfeeling."	Express lots of empathy and explanations before developing an intervention with the client.	Not enough time is set aside for developing the intervention, and thus it is less effective than it might otherwise have been.
"If my clients do not get better, then people will know I am no good as a therapist."	You talk too much, provide the answers to your own questions, and devise all the homework strategies.	Guided discovery can't occur, and thus clients have difficulty in developing the appropriate skills to help themselves.
"My client expects me to be perfect."	You overprepare for sessions, fill them with content, run out of time to cover everything.	The client can't absorb so many different ideas and explore how they fit with his or her own life, and may feel overwhelmed.

all experienced surprise when we thought we were doing so well with a client who just stops turning up. One way of increasing the chances that a client will stay in therapy for the optimal number of sessions is by using regular evaluation of the client's functioning over the course of therapy. In an interesting line of research, 49 university counseling center staff with a variety of treatment orientations saw 1,020 clients who all completed weekly measures of psychological dysfunction but were randomized to two conditions: one where the therapist had access to that information and one where therapists did not have access to it (Lambert et al., 2002). The results showed that when feedback was provided to the therapist, clients stayed in treatment longer and outcomes were better for the client. Nearly twice as many clients in the feedback group experienced clinically significant change compared to the other clients, and fewer experienced deterioration. Lambert and colleagues advocate introducing simple feedback systems in routine clinical practice so that outcomes for poorly responding clients can be enhanced. One simple example of such a feedback system is the *Outcome Rating Scale* (Miller, Duncan, Brown, Sparks, & Claud, 2003), a brief measure consisting of four visual analogue scales assessing well-being in the previous week (overall, personal, interpersonal, social). This scale has been found to have good reliability and validity (Miller et al., 2003), and can be downloaded from *http://scottdmiller.com/performancemetrics*. This scale can be administered at the beginning of each session and used to guide discussion around client progress. In the United Kingdom, disorder-specific measures are used every session in the Improving Access to Psychological Therapies (IAPT) service, and can be downloaded from *http://iapt.nhs.uk*.

Another way to encourage a client to stay in therapy is to acknowledge and address therapeutic ruptures as they occur. Research suggests that such ruptures in themselves do not cause problems, but rather the damage is caused by not acknowledging and dealing with them; repairing weakened therapeutic relationships can indeed strengthen the therapeutic alliance (Safran, Muran, Samstag, & Stevens, 2001). It is suggested that metacommunication skills be used to discuss such ruptures (Safran & Muran, 2000). In other words, invite the client to talk about alliance, and explore the client's experience of the ruptures. You also need to take responsibility for your contribution to the rupture moment, acknowledge it openly with the client, and cultivate accepting and nonjudgemental attitudes to these ruptures. While we are often aware of those moments in therapy were we have "lost" the client, for whatever reason, we can also be blissfully unaware of such moments. Evidence suggests that client and therapist views of alliance diverge, especially during the initial stages of therapy, where the client's perspective is actually more predictive of outcome. Thus, regular feedback on the therapeutic alliance is advocated (Castonguay et al., 2006). This can be achieved by the use of the *Session Rating Scale* (Miller et al., 2003). This process also shows the client that you do not expect to be perfect and are comfortable dealing with your own imperfections.

Troubleshooting

Some perfectionistic clients feel that they are letting the therapist down or that the therapist thinks poorly of them when they are not improving as quickly as they think they should. It is important to use metacommunication skills to discuss this issue: (1) allow the client to discuss his or her thoughts and feelings, (2) applaud the client's courage and honesty in discussing such difficult issues, and (3) ask that the client feed back to them any therapist behaviour that they consider as communicating disapproval or disappointment. It can also be helpful to ensure that time is spent in each session highlighting the small changes that the client is making and their significance. Some images can be useful to discuss with the client that illustrate the importance of small changes—for example, that most avalanches are started by one small, pebble dislodging; that one pebble starts a large ring of ripples in a pond; it just takes one small push to get a heavy satellite circulating around the earth to change its path.

Enhancing Motivation to Engage in Treatment

In the treatment of perfectionism, ambivalence about change is often the norm. A recent qualitative study found that in a clinical group with elevated perfectionism, many participants reported feeling ambivalent about change, and that given the choice between changing or staying perfectionistic, they would choose to remain a perfectionist (Egan et al., 2013). The reasons for this ambivalence can be varied, and it is important to explore them with the client. Some fears about becoming less perfectionistic that were expressed by one of our clients (and are common across many of our clients) include: "fear of not being good enough," "fear of being mediocre," "people will think less of me," and "I may not push myself hard enough."

When we work with the client to enhance motivation to change, we do not just focus on the *importance* of change (i.e., how important it is to the client to change; the pros and cons of change), but also the *confidence* in one's ability to change (i.e., self-efficacy). These can be rated differently by the client (i.e., one can be high while the other is low), and of the two it is self-efficacy that can be the most important predictor of change in therapy (Steele et al., 2011). There are a number of approaches that can be used to increase motivation to change. The remainder of this chapter discusses several of these strategies: developing shared goals, challenging myths about perfectionism, and openly discussing motivation to change.

Developing Shared Goals and Common Aims in Therapy

We already know that developing shared goals facilitates a good therapeutic alliance, and it is helpful to discuss the goals of therapy for perfectionism at some length with the client. Clients often fear that tackling perfectionism will result in decreased performance and that they will no longer be able to pursue excellence. In other words, they fear that the goal of therapy is for people to become ordinary. Such a goal would appeal to very few people, whether they were perfectionists or not. *It is important to emphasize to the client that this is not the goal of treatment; rather, the goal of treatment is to help clients pursue excellence in a different way that has a less aversive impact on their quality of life.* The work of Joachim Stoeber and colleagues (e.g., Stoeber, Harris, & Moon, 2007) can be discussed with the client. This study compared people who had high standards, expected the best of themselves, and had a strong need to strive for excellence ("healthy perfectionists"), people who were often frustrated about not meeting their goals and were never satisfied with their accomplishments ("unhealthy perfectionists"), and people who were not perfectionists. These three groups of people completed a task, the outcome of which was suggested to be an indication of whether they had qualities important for success in life. In actual fact, the participants were randomly assigned to receive feedback that they had "done well" or "not done well" on the task (which had nothing to do with predicting success in life). The results showed that, compared to nonperfectionists, healthy perfectionists experienced more pride when told they had done well, and fewer negative emotions when told they had done poorly, and compared to healthy perfectionists, unhealthy perfectionists experienced less pride when told they had done well, and more negative emotions when told they had done poorly. *In other words, wishing to achieve and taking pride in this is not necessarily problematic—it becomes problematic when the achievement is never good enough or when there is an overly critical evaluation of whether one's best is good enough.*

It can also be helpful to refer to the self-compassion work of Paul Gilbert (2010), who refers to three types of affect regulation systems that have been of evolutionary importance. These include *drive* (the need to achieve and pursue goals), *threat* (the need for safety and protection), and *content* (the need for soothing and kindness). All three are required for balance and happiness in life. For example, our prehistoric cousins needed to be vigilant to threat (or else be eaten by the most ravenous beast on the block), able to pursue achievement that would lead to improvements in lifestyle such as discovery of fires and wheels, and able to pursue times of soothing and winding down or else risk burnout. Like our prehistoric cousins, we have these same drives, but clients with perfectionism may have almost totally switched off content, and swing between drive ("I must achieve") and threat ("I can't achieve to the standard that is acceptable or that will impress others"). The goal of therapy is to turn down the threat, maintain the drive, and rediscover a place in life for content, which will involve enjoyment and celebration of achievements, no matter how small they may seem.

Busting the Myths about Perfectionism

There are many widely held myths about how to achieve high standards that can maintain unhealthy perfectionism. Perhaps the two most insidious are "the more effort you put in the better it gets" and "more critical and aggressive feedback gets a better performance out of a person than more balanced and constructive feedback." There are various ways to tackle myths and to help the client arrive at an alternative statement that can then be tested using a combination of psychoeducation, self-monitoring, and behavioral experiments. For more information, see Chapter 9.

Discussing Motivation to Change Openly

Motivational interviewing (MI) is a form of collaborative conversation for strengthening a person's own motivation and commitment to change, paying particular attention to the language of change (Miller & Rollnick, 2013). The scant evidence to date examining the use of MI with psychological disorders suggests that use of MI can reduce dropout (Westra, Arkowitz, & Dozois, 2009; Wade, Frayne, Edwards, Robertson, & Gilchrist, 2009) and also increase homework compliance (Westra et al., 2009), thus potentially improving outcome. While the transtheoretical model from which MI emerged is not considered by all to be an adequate description of the process observed when dealing with complex psychopathologies (Freeman & Dolan, 2001; West, 2005; Waller, 2012), there is a large body of evidence suggesting that higher initial levels of importance and confidence to change predict greater gains over therapy (e.g., Dray & Wade, 2012). MI gives the therapist important principles and strategies to discuss motivation to change in an open and nonjudgmental context.

When looking to increase importance and confidence to change, it is important to remember not just to talk about change but to encourage clients to experiment with change so that they can be informed about its possible impact as they are making up their mind about change, and also so that they can build up a sense of confidence about their ability to change. A number of strategies can help with clarifying the importance of change, including the following:

- Having a discussion about the degree of importance to change on a 10-point Likert scale, and asking "Can you tell me what reasons for change mean that your score is not 0? Can you tell what keeps you from giving yourself a 10?"
- Developing from this discussion a list of pros and cons of staying the same and of change.
- Asking clients to write down how they would expect life to look across different domains (e.g., work, study, intimate relationships, relationships with family, relationships with children, relationships with friends, leisure pursuits, spirituality, hobbies, athletic activities, finances, community involvement, emotional health) in 12 months' time if perfectionism continues on its current trajectory, and then if it is transformed into a healthy pursuit of achievement (6 months' time can be used with adolescent clients, and with adults sometimes it may be more powerful to use a 5-year time frame, depending on their stage in life). An example of a worksheet considering the long-term costs and benefits of perfectionism is shown in Figure 8.1, completed by a 24-year-old medical student, Amir (see also Handout 8.1 in Appendix 2). He had come into therapy for perfectionism because he was not enjoying his life or studies. He saw getting below 80% as a personal failure even though anything above 50% was a pass at his university. If he achieved above 80% he would analyze why it hadn't been a higher mark, and believed that the lecturer was an easy marker.
- Developing a summary paragraph based on this work that clients can keep where they will come across it often, about the reasons for sticking with unhelpful perfectionism and the reasons for experimenting with a more helpful way of achieving goals (e.g., "It is understandable that I want to keep perfectionism in my life because . . .; however, there are some important reasons to try to achieve my goals differently and this includes. . . ."). It is worth exploring the idea that sticking to the old ways of doing things does not mean that things will remain the same, but rather that the client's perfectionism will continue on the same trajectory that bought the client into therapy in the first place (i.e., the perfectionism will continue to become more intrusive and damaging to the client's quality of life and life goals).

Confidence to change can be low simply because the person has never known any other way to approach achievement and therefore can't imagine doing something differently. A number of strategies can help with imagining how things would look different and for developing confidence in one's ability to make these changes, including the following:

In 1 year's time . . . still having perfectionism	
Area of life	*What will have happened in this area?*
My social life	Become more withdrawn
My work/education	Will still be going through the motions
My emotional health	Will care less, enjoy life less
My relationship with my partner	Nothing—will still be single
My relationship with close friends	Telephone contact, maybe go out occasionally
My relationship with family	Phone contact only
In 1 year's time . . . no longer having perfectionism	
Area of life	*What will have happened in this area?*
My social life	Go out more
My work/education	Progress through medical school
My emotional health	Feel better about life
My relationship with my partner	Possibly nothing—may meet someone
My relationship with close friends	Desire to interact more, will see them more
My relationship with family	May see them a bit more

FIGURE 8.1. Long-term costs and benefits of perfectionism. Adapted from Shafran, Egan, and Wade (2010). Copyright 2010 by Constable & Robinson. Adapted by permission.

- Return to the exercise described earlier on life in the future across the different domains if clients are involved in a healthy pursuit of achievement, and imagine exactly what this means about the sort of person they will be and what they will be doing. Based on a body of research, Holmes and Mathews (2010) have suggested that images appear to act as an emotional amplifier for both positive and negative information. The use of imagery for focusing on the advantages of change may increase positive emotion around the goals of therapy and decrease fear of change.
- Use of behavioral experiments that test out the predictions about the impact of change; the best way to help clients imagine doing something differently is for them to do it! In the early phases of therapy, experiments should start off small, with possible consequences that the client can manage easily. Clients with perfectionism often either avoid homework (because it can't be done well enough) or do more than they were asked to do (because they devalue small goals), and so starting off small allows the therapist to test the water on the client's approach to homework, and to make changes accordingly.
- Use of an achievement log, where the client writes down daily achievements involving the courage to try new approaches, is useful on two fronts. First, it trains clients to look to the small steps and to recognize their value and importance. Second, it moves the focus from achievement being measured by the completion major tasks to achievement being measured by the willingness to try a task despite the risk of failure, with the intent of learning and growing. The log can include information about what was tried, the level of difficulty, and the outcome (e.g., what was learned), and should be reviewed each week with the therapist.

CHAPTER 9

Self-Monitoring, Psychoeducation, and Surveys

Once you have established a solid working relationship with your client, you can shift the therapy toward targeted interventions. In Chapters 10 and 11 we will delve into detail about specific cognitive and behavioral techniques. Here, we introduce the building blocks of CBT with self-monitoring and psychoeducation, which are essential to discuss with clients early on, as they set the stage for the rest of the treatment and can also have therapeutic effects. We also discuss surveys; while they can be used throughout treatment of perfectionism, surveys can be useful to incorporate early in treatment, particularly to gain relevant information for psychoeducation regarding clients' specific beliefs regarding perfectionism.

Self-Monitoring

Self-monitoring is used to increase a client's general understanding and insight into perfectionism. It is distinct from session-by-session monitoring, which is used to assess symptoms on a regular basis. Here we aim to train clients to pay attention to, or monitor, particular cognitions, emotions, or behavior.

The Value of Self-Monitoring

Many therapists ask their clients to engage in self-monitoring but then give up when their clients come back saying they didn't monitor. There are many reasons why both therapists and clients give up on monitoring, but fundamentally it boils down to neither appreciating the full value that regular monitoring can bring. When you first introduce the notion of self-monitoring, discuss the rationale for self-monitoring given below and encourage clients to stick with it, even when it is hard to do.

Research Evidence

Research evidence shows that some people can make significant improvements from simply monitoring their symptoms. For example, Ehlers and colleagues (2003) found that 12% of people with PTSD symptoms following a traffic accident recovered sufficiently after 3 weeks of daily monitoring of their intrusions that they no longer met diagnostic criteria for PTSD. The effectiveness of low-intensity therapies such as guided self-help for anxiety disorders and depression (Coull & Morris, 2011) can be attributed, at least in part, to the monitoring of symptoms. Recent research trials are increasingly using self-monitoring as an active comparison condition because of its efficacy (e.g., Shawyer et al., 2012).

Evaluating the Formulation

One of the first functions of self-monitoring is to help establish the validity of the case conceptualization and collaborative formulation (see Chapter 7). It is all very well for you to sit in the office with your client and use the model to arrive at a collaborative formulation that makes sense to both of you. However, how does it operate in the real world? One of the goals of treatment is to help provide clients with an alternative, more benign explanation of their difficulties or particular situations. This is only helpful, however, if such an explanation is consistent with reality. In the treatment of perfectionism, the formulation should help clients understand the reasons they drive themselves as hard as they do, and why they are unable to relinquish their striving for success. Arriving at a formulation that is not consistent with their real-world experiences will be of limited benefit. Asking the client to monitor the key variables in the formulation; noticing the areas in which perfectionism is expressed, as well as thoughts, feelings, behaviors, rules, and self-criticism, will give a good indication of whether the formulation matches with the client's reality.

Increasing Objectivity

The mechanisms by which self-monitoring can help alleviate symptoms are not known. It may be that monitoring operates by helping clients obtain distance from their thoughts, emotions, and behaviors and view them more objectively. CBT for perfectionism, like other cognitive-behavioral interventions, aims to help clients see that it is not events, per se, that cause the emotional distress but their interpretations of events. Similarly, the vicious cycles that are keeping clients locked into perfectionism can be understood by viewing some behaviors more objectively—although the behaviors (e.g., checking) were designed to be helpful, they often become counterproductive (see Chapter 7). When clients engage in self-monitoring, it slows down their thinking because they need to write down their experiences; it helps them to step back from their emotions in order to identify them accurately, and it helps them consider what behavioral responses may be helping keep the perfectionism going. In this way, self-monitoring increases objectively and helps clients begin to see that there may be an alternative way of viewing the situation.

This is why *regular* monitoring is important. Simply recording thoughts, feelings, and behaviors on one occasion may be helpful for understanding what is going on, but regular self-monitoring is more than that—it is a tool for change. It is important to emphasize that you are not asking clients to complete these forms for research purposes, but because they help provide information in real time about what is going on. Completing the forms retrospectively will mean that all sorts of cognitive biases come into play—in particular, overgeneralization for clients with low mood and self-critical thinking. Completing the monitoring as experiences happen enables an unfiltered, more objective analysis of what is going on in the moment for the client.

Patterns

One of the most obvious benefits of regular self-monitoring is that it can help reveal patterns of thinking, feeling, and behavior. For example, people with chronic fatigue syndrome and perfectionism often take a "boom or bust" approach to managing their lives. Regular monitoring can help such clients see that when they try to get everything done to the highest possible standard when they feel less fatigued, this has the counterproductive effect of making them more tired the next day. At times when they take a less "all-or-nothing" approach to getting tasks done, they are likely to see that this results in less perceived tiredness.

What to Monitor?

Clients can be asked to monitor the variables in their formulation, or it may be more useful to ask them to monitor other variables, such as the domains in which their perfectionism is expressed, their rules, or their reaction to failure. In order to maximize the benefit of self-monitoring, it is helpful to personalize the monitoring forms. Standard forms are included in this chapter, but we would encourage you to personalize them either by giving examples to help clients identify the particular thoughts, feelings, and behaviors, or by adding a column of particular relevance such as "self-critical thoughts."

Exactly what is being monitored may vary according to the specific goal and individual formulation for the client. Figures 9.1–9.3 provide examples of monitoring sheets you can use to help clients understand what to monitor. It can be useful to change the monitoring sheets according to your client's needs. The exact format of these handouts does not need to be used, and the formats vary between handouts. The important point is that you ask your client to monitor relevant thoughts, behaviors, and emotions regarding perfectionism. Note that asking clients to monitor "avoidance" can be difficult—after all, avoidance is the absence of a behavior rather than a specific concrete behavior that can be monitored easily. In such cases, it is a good idea to be as specific as you can about what you think would be helpful for your client to monitor.

Date and perfectionism area and situation	Perfectionism thoughts (rate 0–100% how much you believe them at the time)	Perfectionism behaviors	Feelings (rate 0–100%)
May 7 Home—making the bed	It has to be smooth with no wrinkles and "hospital corners." The pillow must be in the right position. If it is not, then I will worry about it all day.	Spend 30 minutes making the bed.	Anxious (75%)

FIGURE 9.1. Monitoring sheet: Example 1. Adapted from Shafran, Egan, and Wade (2010). Copyright 2010 by Constable & Robinson. Adapted by permission.

Perfectionism area and situation	Rules (rate 0–100% how much you believe them at the time)	Self-critical thoughts	Feelings (0–100% intensity)	What do you do? (rate 0–100%)
Work—completing a presentation	There must be no mistakes in this; each word must be perfect on each slide.	It's taking me so long; I can never find the right word. I'm stupid.	Anxiety (100%)	Use thesaurus on the computer to find the best word possible

FIGURE 9.2. Monitoring sheet: Example 2 (see also Handout 9.1 in Appendix 2). Adapted from Shafran, Egan, and Wade (2010). Copyright 2010 by Constable & Robinson. Adapted by permission.

Thought	Emotion	Avoidance	Procrastination	Performance checking	Safety behaviors
I need to win this chess competition	*Fear, anxiety*	*Not moving my pieces for a very long time and considering every single possibility for every move (I ran out of time and lost the game for that reason even though I was up a pawn).*	*Putting out your hand to touch the piece, then withdrawing it*	*Replaying the last move over and over in my mind*	*Going over the game in between breaks rather than going for a walk*

FIGURE 9.3. Monitoring sheet: Example 3. Adapted from Shafran, Egan, and Wade (2010). Copyright 2010 by Constable & Robinson. Adapted by permission.

When to Review Self-Monitoring

Many guides to CBT advocate that the first thing therapists should do is to set the agenda and to then go through the homework. However, in their work on eating disorders, Fairburn and colleagues (2009) recommend that the homework be reviewed in the first 5 minutes of the session and used to set the agenda. The thinking behind this is that many of the agenda items that come up are likely to be related to the homework. We also think that sessions run more smoothly with this structure and suggest using it. An additional benefit is that reviewing self-monitoring as the very first agenda item gives the message that this work is of paramount importance, and its value is therefore communicated implicitly to complement the explicit messages that you will have given above.

Troubleshooting Difficulties in Self-Monitoring

Many therapists start self-monitoring with gusto and enthusiasm. However, in many cases this soon wanes. Clients have a number of legitimate concerns about self-monitoring that should be addressed prior to starting. These concerns include the sheer hassle factor of having to keep track of thoughts, feelings, behaviors, and rules. If you have never experienced monitoring, we suggest you try it yourself for a couple of weeks to help you understand the commitment that it requires. You can use the forms provided earlier, or you can design your own to monitor a particular situation or emotionally relevant thoughts and behaviors (see Figures 9.1–9.3).

Clients will present a range of obstacles to monitoring, and suggested ways to address them are provided below.

Obstacles to Self-Monitoring

Practicalities

Monitoring in real time is difficult. Unsurprisingly, the majority of clients will not want others to see what they are doing, or to draw attention to themselves in any way. Suggesting that clients complete the forms somewhere private, such as a bathroom, may work for some people. Others may be able to pop outside, or use a particular notebook that looks as though they are recording something work related. Some clients may find writing difficult. In such circumstances it is possible to suggest recording orally. Although this may work for some people and also allow them to "buy time" and see their thoughts, emotions, and behaviors objectively, it can sometimes be harder to see patterns of change. If a client prefers to type on a smartphone or tablet rather than write on paper, that is fine too. The example of Felix is provided below:

> Felix was a 50-year-old, highly intelligent man with severe dyslexia. He had been told by his mother that he should never write anything down because people would think he was stupid due to his difficulties in spelling. At the time of coming for therapy, Felix reported problems with social anxiety, health anxiety, and OCD. His self-evaluation was highly dependent on striving and achievement, and he was a perfectionist. When self-monitoring was suggested, Felix said he would much prefer not to write due to his dyslexia and the fear that the therapist would regard him as stupid. He thought that seeing his writing in black and white and noticing his own spelling mistakes would reinforce his view that he wasn't achieving what he should. Although it was highly tempting for the therapist to agree for the sake of engagement and collaboration, she also felt that Felix was suffering from having a multitude of thoughts constantly whirring around in his head and that giving him a method to externalize them and see them written down might help alleviate them. Felix agreed to use the monitoring form and to write his thoughts, feelings, and behaviors for the first few days of therapy. The therapist agreed that she would not judge his intellect based on his monitoring records; nor would she pay any attention to his spelling. The next session was only 3 days later. Felix could not believe the relief he felt from recording his experiences on paper, and he continued to monitor throughout treatment.

Doing It "Perfectly"

When one of our clients promised one of us that she would be the "best patient ever," the therapist's heart sank. Many clients engage in monitoring in an overly thorough, detailed way. They may write reams and reams, and use color-coded highlighters. Some will inevitably be tempted to write out or type up their monitoring to make it neater. All of these issues should be preempted rather than responded to afterward, as clients can interpret such comments as critical and as a sign that they have done it "wrong." Emphasizing that there is no "right way" and "wrong way" to do self-monitoring serves an obvious dual function—it helps immediately to establish that this activity is not "black and white" and it also helps clients view the task primarily as one aimed at helping them rather than for achievement purposes. Such emphasis is also important for those perfectionists who err on the side of avoidance and procrastination. Reiterating the value of self-monitoring and emphasizing that it does need to be done as close to the time as possible will help give clients the experience of not delaying. Such an experience can then be referred to later in therapy.

Other Common Objections

Many clients are concerned that monitoring will make their concerns worse, or that seeing things written down will make their problems more "real." In such cases, the best response is to say that while there is a chance that may happen, it may not be as bad as the person thinks, or the increase in preoccupation will ordinary only be temporary. At times, we have responded with a discussion about what clients have to lose—very often their preoccupation is at an extraordinary high level in any case. We have occasionally tested objections to self-monitoring in a more formal way with a behavioral experiment—this is a far better option than simply giving up.

Reaction to Clients' Not Monitoring

If clients return to therapy saying they have not monitored, your response should be quizzical rather than critical; it is the first item on the agenda. It is up to you to fully understand why the client has not monitored, and you should assume the responsibility for failing to explain it clearly enough, for not emphasizing its importance, or for not anticipating the difficulties in the first place. Working together to overcome the difficulties is of paramount importance, even if it takes the entire session or the entire next two or three sessions. A key tenet of treatment is that it is better to do a few things well than many things half-heartedly. People with perfectionism can relate to this concept very well indeed! In our view it is fundamental to the success of therapy that clients engage in self-monitoring.

The majority of cognitive-behavioral protocols involve self-monitoring. Self-monitoring is an essential component of therapy although it is not always easy to do. Personalizing the monitoring, anticipating difficulties, and ensuring that it is given pride of place on the agenda can all help ensure maximum therapeutic benefit.

Psychoeducation

Many of your clients will have particular beliefs about perfectionism that can be addressed using a combination of strategies, including behavioral experiments. There are many myths that will require refuting, and this is important to address along with other strategies used to help motivate the client to engage in therapy (see Chapter 8). Examples of these myths include "the harder I work, the better I will do," "to be good at something, you need to dedicate your entire life to it," "practice makes perfect," and "you can do anything you want to if only you want it badly enough." Having the information to address these beliefs is a fundamental first step to refuting them, and it is also relevant to the therapeutic alliance. By now it should be clear that the goal of therapy is not for people to "lower their standards" but instead to help broaden their self-evaluation so that it is less dependent on striving and achievement (see Chapter 13). A key component of this is to help clients obtain objective information about the way their world works, and what works best for them. Is it the case that they do better when they focus exclusively on a particular task? Or is it actually better to put in a reasonable amount of work and then to relax, have a drink with a friend, and an early night? Behavioral experiments will follow from examination of some of the myths and the provision of psychoeducation.

Troubleshooting: Why to Avoid Referring to "Lowering of Standards" with Clients

It is important to discuss with clients at the psychoeducation phase that the emphasis in therapy is not about lowering standards. In our experience if you talk about the idea of lowering standards, then they do not engage in treatment as they fear that they will become a "mess" or "lazy" and not achieve. The essence of therapy is about broadening domains for self-evaluation. If this occurs, then inevitably along the way the client will have choices to make about what is more important—focusing on striving and achievement to the exclusion of other areas or introducing time to relax. What we have found happens is that clients overestimate the impact that relaxing will have on their objective achievement, and that the process of psychoeducation and behavioral experiments lead clients to conclude that they can maintain their standards and achievement without the extreme effort they have been putting in. Sometimes clients find that they will do better if they put in another few hours of work but that the incremental gain is not worth the striving. In that case, they will decide to reevaluate or modify their standards so they are more in their control and work better for their overall functioning. A large part of what we do in treatment in behavioral experiments is to get clients to spend less time on standards; however, it is important not to discuss this as "lowering" or "reducing" standards. It is best to avoid such language and instead talk about "modifying" of standards, because "lowering standards" acts as a red exit flag for some clients. For example, in anorexia nervosa, it is usual in therapy to discuss "regaining nutritional health" rather than "weight gain" as it reduces clients' negative emotional reactions to the idea of weight gain and makes the idea of change easier.

This could be seen as a matter of semantics; however, language is critical. For example, if someone finds out through a behavioral experiment that spending an extra 6 hours on a task gives them an extra 1 percent in terms of performance but chooses to do the extra work, then we might want to talk to them in therapy about modifying their standards. As therapists, we want our clients to have other things in their lives, so they reach the conclusion that it is not worth it to spend the extra 6 hours to give them that extra percentage; alternatively, we would want to help them have the ability to decide to spend the extra 6 hours in one situation but not in another, so they have flexibility. Consequently, we are likely to attract people to therapy and help keep them there if we say therapy will not be about lowering standards but may involve adopting different standards or different ways of achieving these standards.

One of the key points we hope clients understand from discussing one of the myths presented below—"If a job's worth doing, it's worth doing well"—is that not every job is worth doing well. If the client has been trying to do every job well, then we may ask him or her to decide which jobs are important to do well on, but the client can still have high standards for some goals. We would not refer to this as lowering standards, as it gives the impression that we want them to do a second-rate job, and certainly clients with perfectionism have no interest in that. There is also the issue of unrealistic goals (e.g., "I must get an A for every bit of work I hand in"). This is out of their control to some extent, and dooms them to failure at some point. Therefore the different standard we might ask them to work with is "I will give my best effort to everything I hand in," and then that is reviewed with the client as to what a best effort looks like given the circumstances. Again, we would not mention lowering standards—this is not an accurate way of describing the process—but modifying the standards so they are more under their control.

The concept of achieving standards in different ways is easier to introduce: if someone has to do 10 drafts before they can produce a product, we ask them to approach this differently and do 3 drafts, and see if it actually makes a difference to the quality or not. This is explored further in Chapter 12.

Useful Facts for Therapists

When refuting a client's unhelpful beliefs about performance and perfection, it's useful to have some general facts at hand.

Yerkes–Dodson Law: The Relationship between Arousal and Performance

For more than a century it has been known that performance increases with arousal, but that this relationship is not infinitely linear. The Yerkes–Dodson law (Yerkes & Dodson, 1908; see Figure 9.4) tells us that when levels of arousal become too high, performance deteriorates.

The graph in Figure 9.4 can help clients recognize that there is a zone of optimal performance. Clients, like the rest of us, are keen to work out where their "zone of optimal performance is" or where they are working most efficiently. People with perfectionism in particular hate to waste time or effort that could be spent more efficiently. Within this graph it is explicit that if they are operating beyond the zone of optimal performance, then they are, at best, wasting effort and, at worst, actually being counterproductive in terms of their achievement. In our experience, performance rarely seems to deteriorate in the way the graph would indicate it should, but our patients do discover that their performance does not continue to improve in direct proportion to the effort that they put in. Stoeber (2011) found strong evidence that there is a negative relationship between perfectionist strivings and efficiency (defined as "accuracy divided by time invested in the task"). Since many people with perfectionism hate to waste time and strive to be efficient, sharing this information can be helpful.

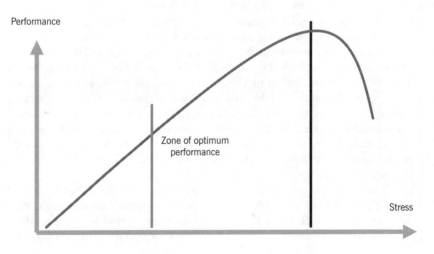

FIGURE 9.4. Illustration of the Yerkes–Dodson law.

The psychoeducation needs to be adapted for the particular domain of perfectionism and the individual. For example, a triathlete who overtrains does not do as well as if she trained an optimal amount (that is, less) due to physiology. On the other hand, a musician who practices too much may not perform well because practicing too much has robbed her recital of its emotional component.

What Makes "Success?"

Many people believe hard work is the key to success. Their evidence for this includes the famous quote by Edison that genius is "1 percent inspiration and 99 percent perspiration." In fact, people who are highly successful, such as entrepreneur Richard Branson, do certainly work hard, but they also play hard. Successful athletes tend to be the ones who played a range of sports when they were younger rather than exclusively focusing on one from a very early age (with some notable exceptions, such as gymnastics). There are many factors that go into being successful—intelligence, personality, and drive, as well as opportunities, luck, and good mentoring.

The Relationship between Success and Mistakes

Albert Einstein had a different perspective from Edison. He suggested that "anyone who never made a mistake never tried anything new." In Chapter 11 on cognitive strategies, orthogonal continua will be used to directly address the belief that to be a success means never making a mistake. To lay the groundwork for that, it is helpful to plant the seed of doubt that *success* and *flawless* are synonyms by some discussion around how progress is made, and some examples of successful people who have made mistakes in the past and learned from them.

If I Don't Do Something Perfectly, I Will Be Anxious All Day

Psychoeducation in the treatment of anxiety disorders includes a large component involving education on the nature of anxiety. For example, clients are often told that panic attacks peak within 10 minutes and then die down naturally within about an hour. Such information is also highly relevant to clients with perfectionism, who fear that they will remain anxious throughout the day if they make a mistake or leave something that has not been done correctly.

Self-Criticism Helps People Work Harder and Achieve More

Theories and research literature actually link self-criticism with lower goal achievement. Self-determination theory (Deci & Ryan, 2000) distinguishes between autonomous and controlled motivation. In the former, goals and decisions are self-generated or generated freely; in the latter, goals are controlled by external or internal pressures, such as self-criticism (i.e., if you can't achieve this goal then you are useless). Research across a number of studies has shown autonomous motivation to be associated with more successful goal attainment, better quality of life, and lower levels of self-criticism than controlled motivation (Powers, Koestner, & Zuroff, 2007). Self-criticism is also associated with lower levels of self-reported "present goal progress" and "future goal expectations" (Shahar, Kalnitzki, Shulman, & Blatt, 2006). Higher levels of self-criticism are associated with lower levels of goal progress in university students with respect to academic and social goals (Powers et al., 2007), and in athletes and musicians (Powers, Koestner, Lacaille, Kwan, & Zuroff, 2009). You should invite clients to examine the evidence from their monitoring and also to review their lives so that they can come to a conclusion about how useful self-criticism is to them.

Countering Myths

Below are some alternatives to the myths that you can help your clients test using behavioral experiments.

Myth	Alternative
1. *The harder people work, the better they will do.*	Hard work is necessary but not sufficient; overwork can be counterproductive.
2. *To get ahead you have to be single-minded and give up all outside interests.*	Getting ahead requires dedication, but if you're overly focused, you may lose the "big picture."
3. *Clever people have to work less than stupid people.*	It's true that clever people pick things up quickly, but some tasks require time no matter how clever the person may be.
4. *The more you put into something, the more you get out of it.*	This can be true but isn't always. Think of vacuuming —is it true that you get a lot more satisfaction if you spend the entire day doing it than if you spend an hour? Especially when your carpet soon gets dirty again.
5. *People notice every little detail and are quick to form critical judgements.*	Studies on "change blindness" at Daniel Simons's laboratory (*www.simonslab.com*) found that people often fail to notice large changes to visual scenes; for example, if a person they were talking to was

	surreptitiously replaced by a different person during a brief interruption. It is very unlikely that your friends will notice a bit of mess in your house.
6. *People can't be happy if they're not successful.*	Whether people are "successful" depends on lots of things, but mostly on their own beliefs about success. Perhaps it is the other way around—people can't be successful if they are not happy?
7. *If I avoid it, then it tends to sort itself out.*	This may be true in some areas (such as responding to e-mails immediately), but not in others (such as paying taxes).
8. *If a job's worth doing, it's worth doing well.*	This may be a general principle, but it doesn't apply to everything. If you do everything very well, you may simply get asked to do more.

Example of Psychoeducation

Jez was a successful ballet dancer with the New York City Ballet. It had been necessary to overcome a lot of obstacles to achieve his success, including the disapproval of his father, who felt that ballet was not an appropriate career for his son. His father had relented when he realized how dedicated his son was to his chosen career. Jez had attended ballet classes since the age of 5 and had never missed a class for any reason. He had refused to go on vacation with his parents from the age of 10 so that he did not miss any rehearsals, and even if he was ill he still practiced. He won numerous awards for both his dedication and his achievements, and in Jez's mind his dedication was the fundamental reason for his success. Jez had referred himself for treatment because he was unable to sustain a relationship. Although this did not bother him per se, he felt he needed to experience true love and heartbreak in order to be able to express it appropriately through his dance.

It was clear that Jez would not be able to sustain any type of relationship while he dedicated himself to his ballet in the way that he was doing at the time of referral. This presented him with a dilemma—in order to be a successful ballet dancer and experience life in the way that was necessary for his dancing, he would have to reduce the hours spent practicing the technical aspects of his work. Discussion of the Yerkes–Dodson law was helpful in encouraging Jez to take the risk of reducing his practice time so he could have interests outside ballet. Although the original motivation had been to have a relationship to improve his ballet, he soon found value in simply having a relationship for its own sake.

Psychoeducation is an important component of the treatment of perfectionism. Helping clients separate fact from fiction will help engage them and encourage them to try to establish a different perspective and alternative beliefs that can be evaluated using cognitive and behavioral strategies.

Surveys

Your Own Beliefs as a Therapist

As a therapist you are likely to hold many beliefs about the "right" way to do a task, and the "wrong way." You may think it is absolutely disgusting not to brush your teeth each morning and night, and you may think people who don't wash their hands after using the toilet are the scum of the earth. On the other hand, you may be the type of therapist to think that one good brush a day is sufficient, and that urine is sterile so there's no need to wash your hands after using the toilet. You may believe that some germs are good for you, so in fact it's best to get rather dirty. There is huge variability in beliefs about every single area in life, and it is vitally important that you do not let your own beliefs about standards, mistakes, failure, achievement, and striving interfere with the therapy. Being aware of how they can interfere is the first step to ensuring that they don't.

Your beliefs as a therapist can interfere with therapy in a number of ways. As discussed in the previous chapter, the therapeutic alliance can be affected by your perfectionism and beliefs, and such beliefs are also associated with higher levels of burnout (D'Souza et al., 2011; McLean et al., 2003). They can also interfere with your delivery of the intervention. For example, if you considered it entirely reasonable for someone to have a rule that everyone must be out of bed by 7 A.M. and dressed by 7:15 A.M. on weekends, you might not identify this as a dysfunctional rule that needs to be dealt with in therapy. However, you might identify this as a treatment target if you didn't share the belief. As should be clear, it is not having high standards per se that is the problem; it is the reaction to perceived failure to meet the standard, the all-encompassing way that the standard is pursued, and the importance of achievement to self-evaluation that make perfectionism unhelpful. However, it's important to identify early in therapy which standards may be unusually high or unrealistic and hence predispose the client to perceive him- or herself as a failure or to spend too much time engaging in unimportant tasks.

The Importance of Supervision

Supervision is important regardless of the therapy. Supervision for the treatment of perfectionism can be particularly helpful given the possible effect of the therapist's beliefs on the alliance and the delivery of the intervention. Identification of the domain(s) in which the perfectionism is expressed as well as areas in which perfectionism is absent can all benefit from the eagle eye and observations of the supervisor. Being able to be open with your supervisor about your own standards and reaction to perceived failure as well as any counterproductive behavior you may have will be particularly important. It is often the case that when people have completed their professional training they no longer have a "formal" supervisor of their practice. However, we believe that supervision is very important to ensure good clinical practice. We encourage therapists who do not have any formal supervision arrangements to consider engaging in peer supervision either in pairs or in groups on a regular basis.

Overview of Surveys

Surveys are widely used in CBT for OCD (e.g., Whittal et al., 2010). Based on the pioneering work of Rachman and de Silva (1978), they were originally used to help clients realize that everyone experiences unwanted intrusive thoughts. In the treatment of perfectionism, they are used primarily for information gathering by clients about the standards, beliefs, behaviors, and emotions of other people. Some information may be publically available, but conducting a survey allows clients to gather personally relevant information from people whose opinion they respect or whose opinion is particularly pertinent. The fear of failure and concern over mistakes that are so characteristic of perfectionism are personal values held by our clients, but it is unrealistic to think our clients are not influenced at all by other people. Having information about how successful people with high standards who are not crippled by perfectionism manage to achieve their goals without the adverse consequences of dysfunctional perfectionism can be extremely helpful. Such surveys can also help "set the bar" for striving and achievement.

> Chen was a conscientious man who always went out of his way to help other people. He never said no to anything that was asked of him, no matter how long it took. His partner found this frustrating but also admired him for it. The trouble was, Chen took a very long to complete all the tasks due to his high standards and fear of letting himself and others down. He found that he was helping other people before work in the morning and after work most nights. He couldn't relax if he felt that someone was waiting for him to do something, and he also sometimes woke in the night thinking of ways he could improve the handiwork he was doing for others. He was exhausted and his mood was low. He never felt he was doing enough, or that the work he did was of a sufficient standard. In treatment, it was agreed that it would be important to find out how much morally good people did for others, what they did, how long they spent helping others, whether they had additional ideas of how they could help others, and, if so, what action they took in response to those ideas. Chen also wanted to know their emotional response to helping others, as Chen felt he should feel better than he did

from helping others (and his emotional response indicated to him that he really hadn't tried hard enough).

Chen and the therapist identified six people whom both agreed were moral people. It was agreed that conducting the survey with people Chen did not feel were moral would be of little use. The criteria for inclusion in the survey were that they did not cheat on their partners, did not lie, did help others, and were generally considerate. Chen asked them the following questions via e-mail, telling them it was to help his son with an assignment on morals and values. This can be useful sometimes when clients are concerned about directly asking others their survey questions.

Survey Questions
1. How often do you do "good" for others?
2. What morally good actions do you perform for others?
3. How long do you spend helping others?
4. Do you have ideas for how you could help others? If so, what actions do you take in response to those ideas?
5. How do you feel after you have helped others?

The results of the survey surprised Chen. None of the respondents spent even half as much time helping others as Chen, none thought of ways they could help once the task was finished, and most of them felt that they had not received sufficient thanks when they helped people and were disinclined to help others again. They generally felt relief when the task was finished.

Together Chen and the therapist discussed the results, leading Chen to conclude that he could be a moral person by helping others to a reasonable extent, and that he did not have to drive himself into the ground with exhaustion helping everyone at all times of the day and night in order to view himself as meeting his standards.

Constructing a Survey

No two surveys are exactly alike. The surveys you and your clients collaboratively construct will vary depending on the areas in which the perfectionism is being expressed. Typical questions concern the frequency or duration of a behavior, and anywhere between three and eight questions are optimal. Examples of beliefs that are particularly amenable to information gathered from surveys include the following (see also Handout 9.2 in Appendix 2).

• *Belief*: "I make more mistakes than other people at work." This survey would be given to people who are successful in the client's workplace.

Survey Questions
1. How many mistakes have you made at work in the past month?
2. Can you give examples of the mistakes you have made at work?

3. Do you think others at work make similar mistakes?
4. What is your opinion of others who make mistakes at work?

Typically answers to survey questions like this involve a range of responses, but clients often discover that they are not making more mistakes than others and that they are making similar mistakes to others in their workplace.

- *Belief*: "I am more prone to make serious mistakes compared to others at work." This survey would be given to people who are successful in the client's workplace.

   Survey Questions
   1. How many mistakes have you made at work in the past year?
   2. How many of these mistakes were serious?
   3. What examples do you have of serious mistakes you have made at work?
   4. What were the negative consequences of your serious mistakes?
   5. What is the worst consequence you have ever had due to serious mistakes?

Again, typically clients find their mistakes are not more serious than those of others. In fact, usual responses include mistakes that clients view as being more serious than their own, and they are surprised by the information that others are making more serious mistakes than they are.

- *Belief*: "I should be available for work calls all times of the day and night even when I'm on vacation." This survey could be given to people in the client's workplace and others whom the client respects.

   Survey Questions
   1. How often do you take your work phone with you on vacation?
   2. What do you think of people who do take their work phone with them on vacation?
   3. What do you think of people who do not take their work phone with them on vacation?
   4. Do you answer your work phone at night and on weekends?
   5. What do you think of people who do answer their work phone at night and on weekends?
   6. What do you think of people who do not answer their work phone at night and on weekends?

There are usually a range of responses to this type of survey. Some people might answer calls on their work phone after business hours. However, clients are usually surprised to find that the majority do not, and that generally others have a negative view of those who do answer calls after hours, stating, for example, that they cannot switch off or do not have a balanced life.

- *Belief*: "I am a failure because I didn't get that job." This survey could be given to friends and others whom the client respects.

Survey Questions
1. Have you ever not gotten a job that you interviewed for?
2. If so, what did you think of yourself for not getting the job?
3. What do you think of others who do not get jobs they have applied for?
4. Do you think someone is a failure if they do not get a job they apply for?

Typical responses to a survey like this involve the respondents indicating that they have not always been successful at getting jobs in the past, and they do not think of others as a failure for not getting a job. They also point out that the job might not have been a good fit for the person's skill set, or might have already been filled by an internal applicant at the workplace so that no external applicant could have really competed fairly.

- *Belief*: "The way to better myself is to constantly keep striving." This survey could be given to others that the client respects at work and to friends.

Survey Questions
1. Do you think that successful people have time off and rest time away from work?
2. Do you think successful people strive all of the time and don't let themselves have time off?
3. Do you think it is important to constantly push yourself in order to keep achieving?
4. Have you had any examples in your life where constantly striving resulted in you being less successful?

Clients are often surprised by responses to a survey like this, as they find responses usually indicate others think rest time is important. Respondents also have many examples of how constantly striving leads to poorer performance, for example staying up all night to prepare for a presentation resulting in a poorer presentation than getting adequate sleep the night before.

- *Belief*: "Successful people do not read trashy magazines." This survey could be given to anyone that the client perceives as being successful either at work or among friends.

Survey Questions

1. Do you read gossip magazines?
2. What do you think of others who read gossip magazines?
3. Do you think reading magazines is a waste of time?

Clients usually report they are astonished at results to this type of survey when they find that numerous people they perceive as being successful do indeed read what they perceive as "trashy" magazines, and that some do not view it as a waste of time but rather instead as "downtime" in which they can relax.

The key to constructing a survey is to ensure that it has personal relevance and meaning, so that the information gathered has high evidential value. Surveys are mostly written, but we have used images in the past for a client who was interested in how others rated various examples of how messy other people's houses are. Feel free to be creative and work with your clients to find the most useful form of survey for them. Sometimes you might find that clients do not want to engage in surveys as they are concerned about directly questioning others or worried that others might know the survey is about their beliefs. In that case, you can work creatively with the client to think of a plausible "reason" why the client could ask the survey questions. For example, one client, Rodrigo, who was a teacher, decided he would tell his friends and colleagues that the survey questions were a part of gathering information for use in an assignment for his students. We have also found it useful for clients who use social networking to put questions out via sites such as Facebook, where they can often get a quick response from friends as the medium lends itself to short questions and responses from others in what feels like an acceptable forum for clients.

What to Do with the Information from Surveys

Collecting the Responses

The survey responses should be the first item on the agenda (or the second item, right after reviewing the client's monitoring if that has also been set as homework). Having the responses laid out in front of you on the table so you can work through them together can be particularly helpful.

Drawing Conclusions

Going through the responses together, your goal is to help your client reach conclusions about where other people set the standard, or the impact of the survey on your client's beliefs. You may want to create a summary table or graph to make the information that you've collected as clear as possible. It is likely there will be a range of responses, and discussing this variability can help the client recognize that there is no "right" and "wrong."

The "Reality Check"

Many clinicians are concerned about doing surveys in case the responses are unhelpful. For example, if you ask someone with social anxiety to give a talk and ask the audience what they thought, you might be concerned that the response of the audience would be negative and countertherapeutic. If you have chosen a reasonable audience (as opposed to an audience comprised of people who are particularly negative and critical), then the reaction of the audience will provide useful information. With perfectionism, the fear is that the survey might show that successful people do work to the exclusion of other interests, and that they do base their self-worth on striving and achievement. CBT is about finding out about the reality, and if this is the reality of the respondents who have been asked to complete the survey, then that too can be a subject for discussion. It is rare for the reality check, however unpalatable at times, to be unhelpful therapeutically. Most often, information about the reality enables clients to think about their own standards and beliefs about mistakes, failure, and self-evaluation. Such information will help you and your client to formulate alternative beliefs to the perfectionistic ones.

Following Up Alternative Beliefs

Surveys, like monitoring and psychoeducation, will help the client formulate alternative beliefs. It is highly unlikely that formulation of alternative beliefs will be sufficient for cognitive or behavioral change. Following up the generation of alternative beliefs with behavioral experiments (see Chapter 12) is the key to facilitating a new and more benign perspective in the long term.

Surveys can produce helpful information about where to "set the bar" for standards and for gathering critical information about success and failure. Each survey is idiosyncratic and discussion of the meaning of the results in detail is a priority for the therapy session. Surveys can help facilitate the generation of an alternative belief that should then be further evaluated using some of the cognitive strategies and behavioral experiments described in the next chapters.

CHAPTER 10

Thinking Errors

I n treating clients with perfectionism we employ strategies to help change
their unhelpful beliefs. Which cognitive biases are most salient in perfectionism, and what are the best ways of addressing them? In our clinical
experience, we have found a number of particular thinking styles that are
common in perfectionism. In this chapter we briefly review introduction of
thought records and discuss how to identify and challenge thinking errors
that are common in perfectionism.

Understanding the Link between Thoughts and Feelings

The first step in guiding clients to challenge their negative thinking is helping them to become aware of the impact thinking has on their emotional
states. Don't assume a client has emotional labels and is able to distinguish
between emotional states. It can be useful to provide clients with a list of
feeling states to enable them to more readily access labels for their emotions. A brief list of common emotional states is provided in Table 10.1.

One of the most useful ways to introduce the idea that thoughts impact
on feelings is to use an illustrative vignette and Socratic dialogue. There
are many vignettes that are commonly used by cognitive therapists, and we
provide a few in Table 10.2.

The examples in Table 10.2 are commonly used in cognitive therapy
to introduce the link between thoughts and feelings by prompting clients

TABLE 10.1. Brief List of Emotions

Angry	Sad	Anxious	Frustrated	Happy	Joyful
Nervous	Depressed	Scared	Excited	Irritated	Ashamed

TABLE 10.2. Examples of Illustrative Vignettes for Introducing the Link between Thoughts and Feelings

1. It is 10 P.M. and two neighbors hear a loud bang outside their houses. One neighbor feels angry, while the other neighbor feels scared. They have both heard the same noise, so what accounts for them feeling differently?

2. Two women arrive home to a bunch of flowers from their husbands with an attached note that says "I love you." One woman immediately feels worried, whereas the other one immediately feels happy. What accounts for the difference in their feelings?

3. A teenage boy is walking through a shopping center and brushes past a display stand full of toilet paper. He accidentally knocks it over, and the toilet paper rolls fall everywhere. A few people stop and stare and a child laughs and points at him. The teenager might feel either angry or embarrassed. If he felt angry, what might he be thinking? If he felt embarrassed, what might he be thinking? What accounts for the difference in how the boy might feel in the situation?

4. A woman is walking through a shopping center and notices her close friend walk past. She looks up, smiles at the friend, and stops to say hello, but the friend looks straight past her and just keep walking. She might feel a range of emotions in the situation. If she were to feel angry, what might she be thinking? If she were to feel anxious, what might she be thinking? If she felt sad, what might she be thinking? If she had no change in her emotional state, what might she be thinking? So what accounts for the different ways someone might feel in that sort of situation?

---

to generate possible thoughts that the characters in each vignette might be experiencing. For example, in the first scenario (the noise at 10 P.M.), the person who felt angry might have thought, "I can't believe the neighbor's cat is making noise again," whereas the neighbor who felt scared might have thought, "That could be someone trying to break in."

After introducing the link between thoughts and feelings, the therapist typically moves on to introduce the "ABC thought diary," shown in Figure 10.1 (see also Handout 10.1 in Appendix 2). Here, the therapist introduces the idea of an activating event, the emotional state that went along with it, and the accompanying beliefs. In the case example of Tim, presented in the next section, the therapist and client examine Tim's reactions to his worry about an upcoming presentation he had to deliver at work. Rather than the therapist stating the link between thoughts and feelings in a didactic manner (e.g., "Can you see how your thoughts made you feel anxious?"), it is more useful to ask a Socratic question, such as "What do you think it was that was leading you to feel anxious about the presentation?" Here the therapist guides the client in understanding that it is his thoughts in the situation that influence his feelings.

It is also useful at this stage to introduce the notion of unhelpful thinking styles so that the client is able to understand the particular styles of thinking he or she uses most often. You can provide a list of unhelpful

A—Activating event	B—Beliefs (rate 0–100%)	C—Consequences (emotions—rate 0–100%)
Work Monday morning at work thinking about upcoming presentation	I am going to do a bad job on the presentation (90%)—predictive thinking My company will not win the bid and it will be my fault (85%)—predictive thinking, personalization I feel anxious, so I know I am going to give a bad talk (90%)—emotional reasoning	Anxious—90%

FIGURE 10.1. Example of an ABC thought diary.

thinking styles (see Handout 10.2 in Appendix 2) and ask the client to think about which ones are particularly relevant to his or her thinking, paying attention to the styles that are most common in perfectionism.

Common Thinking Styles in Perfectionism

Of course, many clinicians will be familiar with cognitive biases and thinking errors in cognitive therapy, but how do these present in perfectionism? Once we identify them, we can devise ways of changing them in order to unlock the vicious cognitive cycles that maintain perfectionism.

The cases of Amira and Tim provide examples of some of the common thinking styles in perfectionism. Clients often present with many of the thinking styles that we will discuss in the chapter. As these biased styles of thinking overlap substantially, it is not unusual for specific perfectionistic thoughts to fit more than one category of perfectionistic thinking.

Amira was an international-level athlete who had done well in her 10 km running event, where she held the record for the fastest time for Great Britain. However, Amira reported that she never felt happy with her performance. She said that even though she had won races, including a world championship, it didn't really count, as it was not an Olympic record or medal. She constantly thought, "I should try harder as I am such a failure as an athlete and a person." She reported that she often found herself thinking about how she was letting her family and her coach down by not having won a medal at the Olympics, and when her fellow athletes praised her for her achievements (e.g., her world championship), she thought they were just trying to be nice to her, as they knew she still had not reached her main goal of an Olympic record and gold medal performance. Until she got there, Amira was adamant that she would remain a failure.

Tim was a successful engineer but spent many hours checking over his reports before sending them to clients and was worried about making mistakes in his correspondence with them. He often felt like he was failing at work, and worried a great deal over making mistakes. Tim had recently been promoted to a senior role in his company for his excellent work. Despite regular praise from his boss for doing a good job, Tim was constantly worrying about his performance at work, as he based so much of his sense of self on how well he did in his career.

Selective Attention (Noticing the Negative, Discounting the Positive)

One of the most common thinking styles you will encounter in clients with perfectionism is selective attention, where they habitually notice the negative aspects of their performance. This can be seen in the example of Tim. No matter how insignificant the perceived flaw was (e.g., one spelling error in an e-mail), he discounted the positive aspects of his performance (he had just received a promotion and praise for his excellent work). Because of this style of thinking, Tim often concluded he was a failure, even though others would disagree. However, for many of our clients, anything less than perfect performance is perceived as "failure." Appendix 2 includes a sample handout that can be used to illustrate selective attention with clients (Handout 10.3). When discussing the impact of selective attention, it can also be useful to use an analogy.

The "prejudice metaphor" suggested by Padesky (1990) can be useful to illustrate the impact of selective attention, to help clients see that they confirm their negative core beliefs about themselves, such as "failure," by attending to negative information. The idea behind this technique as outlined by Padesky (1990) is to illustrate to the client through the use of Socratic questioning and a hypothetical example that holding a negative core belief about oneself is like holding a prejudice against oneself. The aim is to get the client to think of someone they know who has a prejudice that they do not agree with, for example, a family member who has a prejudice based on an area such as race or gender. Then the therapist asks the client how they think that person with the prejudice reacts to information that confirms their prejudice (i.e., when they hear a news story that fits with their views it confirms their beliefs) and how they react when they are faced with information that contradicts their prejudice (i.e., they discount this information). The therapist then asks the client what lesson they would take from this discussion, leading to the idea that if one holds a strong belief then this influences the way they process new information in a way that reinforces prejudice. Next, the therapist can ask the client how easy it would be to change that person's prejudice, leading to the idea that it would be difficult to change as new information is distorted to confirm the prejudice, and then the therapist can ask the client what would need to happen for the person to change their prejudice, and discuss the idea that they might need someone to help look for evidence that contradicts the prejudice. Once this has occurred the therapist can ask the client how this example of a prejudice relates to their core beliefs, and how they can go about together starting to view new information in an objective way rather than in their previous manner of being biased in the processing of information like having a prejudice against oneself.

We can also see the thinking style of selective attention in the case of Amira, who discounted the importance of her national record as a runner because it was not an Olympic record. It is common for clients to describe this resetting of standards when they research their goals, saying, "It was not that hard" or "Anyone could have done it." Generally, even when the person recognizes that he or she has met a goal, the self-imposed pressure to try harder next time will still be strong (e.g., "If I can achieve this goal, it must have been a bit easy, so I should try harder and do better next time"). In fact, we have evidence from qualitative research that clients with perfectionism do exactly that, and reset their standards higher after achieving their goals (Egan et al., 2013). The problem is that this discounting of success and resetting goals higher leaves clients in a no-win situation of feeling never good enough about their performance.

Strategies that are useful for challenging this thinking style include completing thought records, recording diaries of positive achievements, and conducting experiments to broaden attention. We'll introduce some of these techniques here but also get into these in more detail in the next chapter. It can also be useful to think of the types of Socratic questions that identify and challenge these particularly salient thinking styles in perfectionism. Examples of what these questions might look like in practice are provided in Table 10.3.

Double Standards

It is common to see our clients with perfectionism holding one set of unrelenting and difficult-to-achieve standards that they apply to themselves, and a more lenient set of standards for others. For example, Tim thought it was okay (though not great) for others to make spelling errors in their e-mails, but absolutely unacceptable for him. While Amira thought of her teammates who had not won Olympic medals as still successful, it was unacceptable for her not to win one. Double standards such as these maintain perfectionism because they lead clients to expect more of themselves than of other people, which in turn leads to self-criticism.

TABLE 10.3. Examples of Socratic Questions to Identify and Challenge Selective Attention

Identifying selective attention

- "When you think about your performance, what do you tend to focus on?"
- "How much do you notice mistakes in performance? Do you notice successes?"
- "How do you react to positive aspects of performance?"
- "How do you feel when you meet a goal or standard? Do you feel satisfied? Not satisfied? How long does that last?"
- "Do you discount your goals when you meet them as being too easy, or that anyone could have done that?"
- "After you meet your goals, do you set the goals for next time higher, lower or the same?"

Challenging selective attention

- "What does focusing in on your mistakes and discounting your successes do to your mood?"
- "What is the impact of focusing on your flaws and discounting the positive aspects of your performance on how much you base your sense of self-worth on achievement?"
- "If you constantly set your goals higher even after you have done well and discount your achievements by saying "it was no big deal," how will you feel satisfied with your performance?"
- "What effect do you think it has on other people when you brush off meeting your goals as no big deal?"
- "If you constantly followed a friend around as a "critical judge" and pointed out everything he or she did wrong, and never commented on what your friend did well, what do you think would start to happen to your friend's mood and self-esteem? What would the judge actually need to do instead in order for your friend of feel like a success?"

Thought records can be useful in challenging double standards. Handout 10.4 in Appendix 2 is an example of a handout that can be used with clients to illustrate double standards. In addition, you can use Socratic questions to help guide the client toward understanding the impact of double standards. Useful sample questions can be seen in Table 10.4.

Another useful technique that can work with double standards is asking the client to do a survey of others' standards (see Chapter 9 for details on how to do surveys). Often clients are surprised to find that other people also hold higher standards for others than they hold for themselves.

Overgeneralizing

Clients with perfectionism commonly overgeneralize from one mistake or flaw in performance to conclude that they are failures overall. Overgeneralizing is pervasive, and when you ask a client with perfectionism to record thoughts, many examples of overgeneralizing may arise in which even the

**TABLE 10.4. Examples of Socratic Questions to Identify
and Challenge Double Standards**

Identifying double standards

- "Do you have one set of rules for yourself, and another set of rules for other people?"
- "Are the rules for yourself harder than your rules for others?"

Challenging double standards

- "Is it fair to have harsher rules for yourself that are different from your rules for everyone else?"
- "What is the impact when someone holds a set of standards for himself that is different from the standards he holds for other people?"
- "What does it do to you go always give yourself these hard standards to meet but think it is okay for others not to meet them?"
- "What would you say to a friend who had a harder set of rules for herself than for other people?"
- "How does it follow that you need to have harder rules for yourself than for other people?"
- "What does holding double standards do to your self-esteem and mood?"

smallest mistakes or errors are perceived by the client as complete failures. This thinking style often goes along with labeling and self-critical thinking in general, whereby clients berate themselves over mistakes (e.g., "I am a screw-up," "I am a failure as a person," "I am useless," "I hate myself"). Overgeneralizing is destructive as it leads clients into intense cycles of defeating self-criticism and continually reinforces the idea of self-worth being based on achievement.

In the cases introduced above, we can clearly see examples of overgeneralizing. Amira saw herself as an overall failure for not having won an Olympic medal. Tim concluded that he was a failure due to small errors he made at work. It can be helpful to use Handout 10.5 in Appendix 2 when discussing overgeneralizing with your client. Useful strategies to combat overgeneralizing can include thought diaries with Socratic questioning to help clients understand both the impact of overgeneralizing on their sense of self and emotional state, and to help them broaden their view of what a "failure as a person" actually is, versus how they apply this definition to themselves. You can help your client to see that there are many aspects that determine someone's worth. Taking an objective view, we can clearly see that making spelling errors in e-mails does not mean Tim is a failure as a person, and that Amira is incredibly successful despite not having won an Olympic gold medal. Useful Socratic questions can focus on asking clients to consider more generally what the universal definition of "failure as a person" is and whether that definition fits them (see Table 10.5).

TABLE 10.5. Examples of Socratic Questions to Identify and Challenge Overgeneralizing

Identifying overgeneralizing

- "What do you think of yourself as a person overall when you make even a small mistake?"
- "What happens to your self-esteem when your performance has not met your standards?"

Challenging overgeneralizing

- "How does it follow that someone's worth as a person can be judged on one instance of not meeting a goal or making a mistake?"
- "What is the universal definition that people in society would hold of a 'failure'? How do you compare to that definition? In what ways are you similar or different?"
- "What do most people judge as important in making up a person's worth?"
- "How is it that making a small mistake or error (e.g., a spelling mistake in an e-mail) can reflect on a person's worth overall?"
- "What does overgeneralizing from one small mistake to mean you are a failure as a person do to your self-esteem and mood?"

"Should" and "Must" Statements

"Should" statements are also common in clients with perfectionism. For example, Tim was always saying to himself, "I should not make any mistakes at work," and Amira thought, "I should have run a better time." As with the thinking style of overgeneralizing, clients with perfectionism may say "should" and "must" to themselves hundreds of times a day, using these types of statements like a whip as a way to motivate themselves and guard against poor performance. This style is what Albert Ellis referred to as "musturbation," which he argued lies at the core of emotional disturbance (Ellis, 1997). In the cognitive-behavioral model of perfectionism, standards are operationalized by clients as rigid rules. One of the central tenets of Ellis's rational-emotive behavior therapy (REBT) was to challenge these insistent demands that clients place on themselves, as they have such destructive emotional consequences.

Cognitive techniques can be useful to combat "should" statements. First, Handout 10.6 in Appendix 2 can be used in session with clients to help you discuss the role of this thinking style in maintaining their perfectionism. It can then be useful to have clients do some simple monitoring of the use of "should" and "must" statements. For example, you might ask clients to keep a simple count of how many times they say "should" to themselves in a day. A fun way of doing this that may appeal to some clients is to put a coin in a jar each time they realize they have said "should" to themselves, and then count up how much money they "owe" at the end of the day. Clients will usually have some fun with this type of exercise, and it can be useful to highlight how habitual this style of pressuring themselves has become. It can also be useful to give some general examples of "should" statements in perfectionism as a way of normalizing how common they are, but also as a way to discuss the impact such statements can have on a person. Examples of common "should" statements can be seen in Table 10.6.

As discussed with the other prominent thinking styles, using some Socratic questions to help clients think about the impact of "should" statements can be a useful way to start helping them change this habitual pattern of self-pressure. Some examples of the types of questions that could be used when engaging in cognitive strategies with clients can be seen in Table 10.7.

The types of Socratic dialogue shown in Table 10.7 can help clients think about trying to become more flexible in their thinking, and replacing "should" and "must" statements with less dichotomous statements, such as "I would prefer . . ." or "I would like to . . ." This type of questioning can sometimes lead naturally into discussion of strategies that are covered later in the chapter regarding rigidity, rules, and extreme standards. It may also lead to discussion of the "coach analogy" (see Chapter 13), regarding the impact of "should" statements on self-criticism: which coach would get a better performance out of someone, the coach who is constantly berating the player or the coach who is encouraging? These techniques can be interwoven in different stages of therapy, as we outlined in Chapter 6. Basically, we want our clients to come away with an understanding that saying "should" to themselves constantly actually leads to worse performance, as they will often feel anxious and engage in self-criticism, and may be more likely to procrastinate. In contrast, if they take a more moderate and flexible approach to what they would like to achieve, then they are more likely to be able to perform and achieve their goals.

TABLE 10.6. Examples of "Should" Statements in Perfectionism

"I should always push myself to achieve."

"I should always do things thoroughly."

"I should never waste time."

"I should always be productive."

"I should always be trying to better myself."

"I should leave as little time as possible for tasks so I don't waste time, even if I am late."

"I should work harder."

"I should try to be the best."

Note. Adapted from Shafran, Egan, and Wade (2010). Copyright 2010 by Constable & Robinson. Adapted by permission.

TABLE 10.7. Examples of Socratic Questions to Identify and Challenge "Should" Statements in Perfectionism

Identifying "should" statements

- "What do you say to yourself to really get yourself going when you think you have to get something done?"
- "What runs through your mind when you think of the 'to do' list that you have to get through?"
- "How often do you say 'should' and 'must' to yourself when you are thinking of everything you have to do?"

Challenging should statements

- "How does saying 'should' to yourself constantly make you feel? In what way does it impact on your sense of self?"
- "If a friend wanted to engage in exercise more, how would she feel if she said to herself, 'I should exercise 7 days a week'? What would it do to her sense of pressure on herself? Now consider if she said to herself, 'I would like to engage in exercise more regularly, if I can.' Which one do you think would make her feel more stressed? Which statement would lead her to be more likely to engage in exercise?"

General Thinking Styles That May Present in Perfectionism

As we discussed earlier, some of the central thinking styles in perfectionism include dichotomous thinking, selective attention, "should" statements, overgeneralizing, and double standards. However, other well-known cognitive biases may also be present at times in clients with elevated perfectionism. Consider again the case of Tim.

Tim recalled recently having to do a presentation to win a job for his company. He stated that he became very nervous before the presentation, thinking he would do a bad job. Tim reported that he felt like he had failed at the talk. At the start of the presentation he stumbled over his words a little and said "um" too much for the first 5 minutes. But for the rest of the presentation he felt less anxious, and everyone received it well. Even his boss told him he had done a good job. Tim felt that because he had stumbled over his speech at the start everyone would think he was a "loser" and "incompetent fool," and that his company would probably not get the job because of him. He said that despite everyone saying he had done a good job, he knew that they were just trying to be nice. He could tell they didn't like his talk, he said, because some people looked out the window while he spoke, suggesting they were bored. Also, they didn't ask as many questions about his talk as they had when his colleague had presented a similar talk to another client group. Tim said he felt miserable after the talk and ruminated about it all night. He felt like a "complete failure."

Catastrophizing

Catastrophizing is a familiar thinking style associated with "what if?" statements that lead clients to blow things out of proportion, imagine the worst-case scenario, and therefore feel anxious. Catastrophizing about the consequences of failure is a common way in which this thinking style manifests in perfectionism. In the earlier example, Tim was catastrophizing that what he perceived to be a bad presentation would result in his company losing a job with a potential client. It can be useful to ask standard "downward-arrow" questions, which can often reveal progressively more catastrophic scenarios that the client imagines may occur. An example of how this questioning unfolded in Tim's case can be seen in Table 10.8.

Of course, when the therapist questioned Tim about this example, she found that the likelihood of his losing his job even if his company did not get the deal was slim. Tim stated that it was common for potential clients to go with other companies, and that he had never seen anyone lose his or her job over it. However, despite knowing this logically, Tim said he had times of "panic" where he would engage in catastrophic thinking that he "might be the first one" to lose his or her job over poor performance. Note that the questions asked by the therapist to gain access to Tim's thoughts about the presentation were aimed not only at verbal thoughts, but also at images. Working with imagery is an important and often underutilized component of cognitive therapy (Hackmann, Bennett-Levy, & Holmes, 2011; see Chapters 13 and 16 for further information on imagery).

TABLE 10.8. Using Downward-Arrow Questions to Explore Catastrophic Thinking

THERAPIST: What did you imagine would happen as a result of your presentation?

TIM: That my company would lose the job with the client.

THERAPIST: And if that happened, what would be the worst thing about that?

TIM: Well, it would be really bad, as it is a multimillion-dollar deal we stand to lose, so I might lose my job if we did not land the deal.

THERAPIST: And if that were true, what do you think would be the worst outcome of that?

TIM: Well, I might not be able to find another job, and then my family and I would be out on the street. It's pretty scary thinking about that!

THERAPIST: That does sound scary, and when you are thinking about this, do you have a picture or an image in your mind's eye about these scary outcomes?

TIM: Yeah, the same one I get all of the time. I imagine standing in the street in the cold and dark with nowhere to go and my wife and kids looking up at me. I feel like a failure, totally responsible for what happened, and such a loser.

Emotional Reasoning

Clients often base their views of a situation on their feelings rather than on facts. Recall that Tim engaged in emotional reasoning before his talk, thinking, "I feel anxious, therefore I know I am going to give a bad talk." Standard evidence testing questions can be used to address this thinking style—for example, "What evidence do you have that stumbling over some words at the start of the presentation means the whole presentation was bad?" Socratic questions (such as "Can you think of any examples of people you know who have appeared slightly anxious in a talk but still have given a good presentation?") can also be useful.

Labeling

Labeling is associated with self-critical thinking, and is common in perfectionism. It often occurs when clients feel that they have failed to meet their standards or goals and includes negative self-labels such as *failure, loser, screw-up, useless,* and *idiot.* We saw this when Tim labeled himself as a failure over his presentation. In addition to the cognitive therapy techniques discussed in this chapter, strategies covered in Chapter 13 to combat self-criticism can be useful to reduce this pervasive style of negative self-talk. It is also useful to ask Socratic questions (e.g., "What effect does it have to constantly call yourself a 'loser' and a 'failure'?" and "What does calling yourself a failure do to your sense of self being based on achievement?"). Socratic questioning helps to highlight for the client the impact of this negative self-talk in keeping the cycle of perfectionism going by continually reinforcing the idea of self-worth based on achievement, and the client's tendency to strive toward standards in order to "make up" for perceived deficiencies and failures.

Personalization

The client who personalizes assumes full responsibility for events and outcomes in which responsibility is actually shared, without taking into account all of the factors that contribute to the outcome. In the case of Tim, he was personalizing that it would be 100% his responsibility if his company did not win the deal. He failed to recognize that success required a team effort, that he was only one person among seven colleagues who were working on the project, and that many people had input into the final decision, which was outside of his control. It can also be useful to challenge personalization by drawing a "responsibility pie chart," which therapists routinely use in cognitive therapy for OCD, following the work of Salkovskis (1999). This strategy involves having the therapist draw a circle on the whiteboard and ask the client to consider all of the potential contributing factors responsible for a given situation for which the client has assumed responsibility. The client estimates the degree to which each factor is responsible for the situation, and the therapist draws that portion of the pie chart to reflect the degree of responsibility. The client's responsibility is left until last, after all other factors have been considered and drawn on the chart. Thinking back to the earlier case, Tim assumed the success of his company's bid was entirely dependent on his performance during his presentation. Figure 10.2 includes an example of how a responsibility pie chart might be used to challenge this belief. The first pie chart represents Tim's feeling that he was completely responsible for the outcome. After the therapist asked him about other possible contributing factors, he recognized there were numerous other factors that were also important, and it was not possible for him to be 100% responsible for the outcome.

1. Tim's initial assessment, that he alone was responsible for the company's losing the bid.

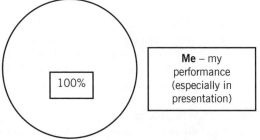

2. Consideration of all factors that are responsible for whether the company wins the bid.

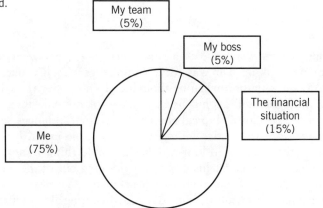

FIGURE 10.2. Example of a pie chart to combat personalization and overresponsibility cognitions in perfectionism.

As shown in Figure 10.2, when he considered all of the factors that might contribute to the outcome, Tim was able to recognize that he was not in fact wholly responsible for it. Although the therapist questioned whether Tim was really still 75% responsible, and whether his colleagues did not actually hold more responsibility, Tim was adamant that as team leader, he was ultimately responsible for the majority of the outcome. It is useful here for the therapist not to become engaged in a debate with the client, as arguing with the client can contribute to rigidity regarding what is "right" or "wrong," as seen in the troubleshooting box below.

Troubleshooting: The Impact of Cognitive Rigidity on CBT of Perfectionism

Inevitably at some point in working with your client with on perfectionism, the very problem he or she is struggling with regarding dichotomous thinking and cognitive flexibility will affect the therapy itself. It is important for you not to become engaged in an intellectual debate with your clients regarding what is "right" or "wrong" in terms of their beliefs, or to become frustrated if your clients are having difficulty shifting to a more flexible way of thinking. It can be useful for you to remind yourself that this is the very issue for which your client is presenting for therapy, and to "roll" with what you may perceive as resistance to viewing things in a different way. If the therapy session starts to turn into a debate, you should consider changing course, and instead of considering evidence for and against a belief, examine the impact of the client's thoughts or thought process (see metacognitive strategies), or design a behavioral experiment to test the cognition that the client is having difficulty taking a different perspective on.

Mind Reading

Mind reading occurs when clients assume they can guess what others around them are thinking. Tim was mind reading regarding his colleagues' reactions to his presentation when he thought, "I know they thought the presentation was bad and boring because some of my colleagues were staring out of the window." Typical cognitive therapy techniques such as evidence testing and perspective taking are likely to be useful here. For example, Tim's therapist asked him whether he could think of any other factors that might account for his colleagues' looking out of the window (e.g., they were worried about their own workloads; they were thinking about problems in their own lives; they were daydreaming about what they were going to do after work). The point here is for the therapist to help clients recognize that they are only guessing when they assume they know what others think, and usually in a very unhelpful way. Rather, the only way that anyone can ever know what other people are really thinking is to ask them.

Predictive Thinking

Clients with perfectionism typically form negative predictions regarding how they are going to perform with respect to meeting one of their standards. This can be seen in Tim, who had a strong negative prediction that he was going to do a bad job of his presentation, and then another negative prediction that his company would not win the bid. In addition to standard cognitive therapy techniques discussed in this chapter, it is important to engage in testing negative predictions that clients hold using behavioral experiments, as outlined in the next chapter. Behavioral experiments are perhaps the most powerful and effective way to arrive at change in cognition, and there are recent data to support the idea that behavioral experiments have some advantages over thought records when changing negative thinking (McManus, van Doorn, & Yiend, 2012). As reviewed in Chapter 12, behavioral experiments appear to bridge the gap between the client's rational perspective regarding the situation and the emotions that often lead the client to take a different, more negative perspective.

Dichotomous Thinking and Perfectionism

Dichotomous ("all-or-nothing") thinking is one of the most relevant thinking styles for maintaining perfectionism. In their cognitive-behavioral model of clinical perfectionism, Shafran et al. (2002) proposed that dichotomous thinking played a central role in the maintenance of perfectionism: clients with perfectionism judged whether they had met their standards and rules in a dichotomous manner. In the earlier example, Tim was engaged in dichotomous thinking regarding his performance in public speaking. He felt that because he had made mistakes early on, the entire talk was ruined and a complete failure. Tim viewed his performance in an all-or-nothing manner. Similarly, Amira had a rule that anything less than an Olympic record was a failure; hence, she was judging her performance as an athlete in a dichotomous manner.

Research evidence has demonstrated that dichotomous thinking is a predictor of perfectionism (Burns & Fedewa, 2005), and, in particular, that it can account for differences between positive and negative aspects of perfectionism (Egan et al., 2007). Consider the example of Mei.

Mei was a student in her final year of studying to become a teacher. She had always been a good student and received honors throughout her schooling. However, during the final year, Mei received the lowest mark of her college career, just scraping through the course. She recounted that she had had a lot of stress that semester, as she had just broken up with her long-term boyfriend and also had to take on a new job to support herself. When Mei received her grade, she felt shocked and thought to herself, "You complete failure." She had a dichotomous rule set that she should always get high grades, and because this grade was lower, she felt she was a failure. Mei said this resulted in a bout of intense self-criticism, and in working long hours into the night for all of her courses to get even better grades than she usually received. She stated that because of the failure she now wanted an A in every class to prove to herself that she was not a failure.

Dichotomous thinking has a central role in the maintenance of perfectionism. People with perfectionism commonly judge their rules and standards in a dichotomous way. This leads to a continual cycle of perfectionism: individuals judge that they have not met their standard, resulting in intense self-criticism and thinking that they need to try harder next time. As discussed earlier, even when they do judge that they have met a standard, they see it as "no big deal" and set the bar even higher next time. Hence, dichotomous thinking maintains the dependence of self-worth on achievement. Strategies that are useful for reducing dichotomous thinking include behavioral experiments (covered in Chapter 12) as well as challenging dichotomous thinking through continua, replacing rules with guidelines, and various other cognitive strategies discussed in the next chapter.

CHAPTER 11

Cognitive Strategies

In the previous chapter we introduced the ABC thought diary and techniques to identify and challenge thinking errors in perfectionism. Once this groundwork has been laid, the focus can move to further challenging of the unhelpful thoughts that maintain perfectionism. In Chapter 10 we also examined a number of cognitive strategies, including Socratic dialogue and pie charts, to challenge common thinking styles in perfectionism. In this chapter we consider additional cognitive therapy techniques for challenging cognitive biases in perfectionism (such as dichotomous thinking), including metacognitive approaches. The section on thought diaries is relatively brief, as these are standard techniques that most therapists are aware of, and they are covered in detail in other texts (e.g., Beck, 2011).

Examining Evidence and Perspective Shifting

After introducing the basic ABC thought diary, you can introduce the notion of challenging thinking by adding a "disputation" column to the thought diary. Although asking general evidence-testing questions such as those in Figure 11.1 (e.g., "What would a friend say?" or "Is there another way of viewing this thought?") may have its place, particularly for clients when they are completing thought diaries outside of the sessions, using a range of Socratic questions based on the particular situation the client is discussing is more useful. It is useful to remind you about stylistic aspects of cognitive therapy that we believe lead to more effective belief change. We have already given several examples of the types of Socratic questions that can be used to challenge particular thinking styles in the previous chapter. In our experience, therapists (particularly beginning therapists) sometimes feel unsure about the types of Socratic questions they should ask. While a discussion of how to do Socratic questioning is outside of the scope of this

A—Activating event	B—Beliefs (rate 0–100%)	C— Consequences (rate 0–100%)	D— Disputation	E—Evaluate outcome
What was the event, situation, thought, image, or memory?	What went through my mind? What does it say about me as a person? Am I using unhelpful thinking styles?	What was I feeling?	What would a friend say? Is there another way of viewing this thought?	How do I feel now?
At home Monday night lying in bed thinking about presentation that I gave in the afternoon	I said "um" a lot and stumbled over my words at the start, so the whole presentation was ruined (90%) (noticing the negative, discounting the positive, dichotomous thinking) I screwed up the presentation; I am such a failure; what a loser (90%) (overgeneralizing, labeling) I should be able to do a better job of presentations by this point in my career (80%) (shoulds) I may lose my job (60%) (catastrophizing) I know the audience was bored as some people were looking out of the window (80%) (mind reading)	Anxious (90%)	Just because I stumbled over a few words does not mean the whole thing was ruined; I was more confident after the start. No one said the presentation was bad. Just because someone says "um" a lot in the first 5 minutes of a presentation does mean he is a failure as a person. I would like to not be anxious about presentations, but telling myself I should be doing better at them just makes me more anxious. There is no evidence I will lose my job. I don't know they were bored, they were probably thinking about other things.	Anxious (45%)

FIGURE 11.1. Example of completed thought diary.

TABLE 11.1. Examples of Socratic Questions to Challenge Beliefs

- "How does it follow that stumbling over a few words at the start of your presentation means the whole thing was ruined?"
- "Can you think of any examples of colleagues whom you admire but who say 'um' in presentations? Do you think they give good presentations?"
- "How does society in general define what is a 'failure' as a person? In what way does saying 'um' in presentations fit, or not fit, with that view?"
- "Can you think of any examples of colleagues who have lost their jobs over poor presentations or not getting deals?"
- "What reasons might account for people looking out of the window during your presentation other than your thought that they must be bored?"

chapter, and this topic is covered elsewhere (e.g., Kennerley, 2012), the idea is for the cognitive therapist to ask a question that is likely to help the client start to think differently about the belief, which will help to shift the client's perspective on the belief. An example of a completed thought diary for Tim, whom we introduced in a case example in Chapter 10, can be seen in Figure 11.1 (see also Handout 11.1 in Appendix 2).

If the therapist had only asked evidence-testing questions regarding Tim's situation, generating some good challenges to Tim's beliefs as seen in Figure 11.1, there may have been some decrease in anxiety, but it is unlikely that this level of challenging would lead to Tim "feeling" that the disputation was true, and it is possible that Tim's perfectionistic beliefs would remain unchanged. Instead, the therapist is best advised to ask a range of Socratic questions, such as those in Table 11.1.

Core Beliefs

The most typical core beliefs (schemas) that clients with perfectionism hold are around worthlessness and incompetence, and they can usually readily access core cognitions regarding being "not good enough." To get to the core belief level, you can use the "downward-arrow" technique. Consider the types of beliefs in the thought diary example in Figure 11.1. In this example, the therapist asked a range of "chaining" questions to identify the core, such as "What was the worst thing about that?" and "If that were true, then what would that mean about you?" and "What does that say about you as a person?" until the therapist and client arrived at the core belief of "not good enough/worthless." To help the client challenge these core beliefs, it can be useful for the therapist to first introduce a diary such as the one used in Figure 11.2 (see also Handout 11.2 in Appendix 2).

To help the client complete the diary, the therapist shows the client how to gather evidence that does not fit with his or her negative core belief.

Core belief: *I am not good enough, I am a failure/worthless.*

Evidence that shows this belief is not true:

1. *I recently received a promotion.*
2. *My boss gives me regular positive feedback.*
3. *I have a loving family—my wife and kids think I am good enough!*
4. *I have lots of friends—they regularly call and invite me to play sports with them.*

Helpful new core belief: *I am good enough; I am more than just my work; I am a good husband, father, and friend.*

FIGURE 11.2. Core belief diary 1.

It was helpful for the therapist to help Tim see that he was more than just his achievements at work (which in fact were good anyway, but he was overlooking this), and this helped to broaden his view of himself to include other areas of his life and roles such as a father, husband, and friend. This level of challenging core beliefs can also move nicely into changing self-evaluation based on achievement, which we cover in Chapter 13.

While it can be useful to have a client complete diaries such as the one in Figure 11.2 (see also Handout 11.2 in Appendix 2) outside of sessions to gather evidence for new core beliefs, it is important to also test core beliefs using behavioral experiments to get a more "believable" change in the core belief. That is, clients often report that when they change beliefs through thought diaries they can understand on an "intellectual" level that the new beliefs make sense but do not "feel" that they are believable. Behavioral experiments can help to bridge the intellectual understanding and the feeling that a new belief makes sense. In this way, behavioral experiments are often more effective in changing core beliefs than diaries alone. An example of a core belief that was used for Tim can be seen in Figure 11.3 (see also Handout 11.3 in Appendix 2). The therapist asked Tim how he thought he might know whether the core belief was true, and together they discussed the idea of using a behavioral experiment to test the core belief.

Testing out core beliefs using behavioral experiments can be one of the most effective ways to change core beliefs and develop more helpful new beliefs. Behavioral experiments are covered in detail in the next chapter.

Specific Techniques to Challenge Selective Attention

In addition to standard thought diaries, specific forms can be used to help clients notice the positive aspects of performance. As discussed earlier,

---

Core belief: I am not good enough; I am a failure/worthless.

Experiment: Ask my boss for honest feedback on my presentation style.

Prediction: If I ask my boss for feedback, he will say I was really anxious, that he was disappointed, and that I need to try and learn some skills in public speaking.

Outcome: My boss said it was excellent, even when I directly asked him if he thought I looked anxious and said "um" too much. He laughed and said he did not notice me saying "um" at all, and that he says "um" much more than I do. He was surprised that I might be concerned about my presentation, and said that I am known as one of the best presenters in the company.

Helpful new core belief: I am okay at my job, and a good enough person; my work does not equal my worth.

FIGURE 11.3. Core belief diary 2.

when we considered the impact of selective attention, it can be useful to use Socratic dialogue along the lines of "What do you think would happen to someone if they constantly had a judge walking beside them commenting on everything they did wrong, no matter how small, and ignoring anything that they were doing well in?" Here you attempt to get the client to recognize being stuck in a habitual pattern of scrutinizing his or her own performance, noticing all the negative aspects and minimizing any successes. You can use an analogy to illustrate selective attention, for example, asking the client if he or she has ever had the experience of buying a new car and then suddenly noticing many more cars on the road that are the same as the new one. Here you help the client see that by focusing attention on something, he or she will be more likely to notice it. The example of the "moonwalking bear" in the next chapter can also be used to illustrate the effects of selective attention.

Completing specific diaries (both in the session and for homework) can be useful in helping clients broaden their attention in situations where they engage in selective attention and help them to see positive aspects of a situation that they have overlooked. It can be useful to have clients think about simple ways to broaden attention, for example by focusing on a conversation they are having, or colors they can see in a room. Handout 11.4 in Appendix 2 can be used to help clients broaden their attention. A sample of this handout completed for Tim can be seen in Figure 11.4.

It is useful to encourage clients to practice broadening their attention *at the times* they engage in selective attention. It is also helpful if you point out examples of selective attention in session to demonstrate to the client the impact of focusing of attention. Another strategy that can be useful

Situation	Noticing the negative thoughts (rate 0–100%)	Ways to broaden my attention in the situation	Outcome
Work	The fact that I said "um" a lot in my presentation means it was a complete failure (90%)	1. I am ignoring the fact that the content of the presentation was good and feedback was positive from the client 2. I can focus on questions and notice details around me (e.g., what color shirts is everyone wearing?)	When I consider the evidence, the presentation was a success overall. Focusing on conversation and colors broadens my attention.

FIGURE 11.4. Noticing the negative and broadening attention. Adapted from Shafran, Egan, and Wade (2010). Copyright 2010 by Constable & Robinson. Adapted by permission.

for combating selective attention is to encourage the client to record *actual* evidence of performance in situations using Handout 11.5 in Appendix 2. This can help break the habit of noticing negative aspects of performance and ignoring positive ones. An example of this handout completed for Tim can be seen in Figure 11.5.

Many people with perfectionism believe that in order to be a success, they must not make any mistakes. They operate on the rule "If I make a mistake, I am a failure as a person," an example of overgeneralization.

Area	Positive evidence	Lack of negative evidence
Work	Boss commented that I did a good job on my presentation	No one criticized the presentation
Parenting	My children are happy to see me when I get home from work	My kids have never said they hate me like my friend Simon's kids have said to him
Social	People approached me to talk	No one said I looked anxious or that I was boring

FIGURE 11.5. Diary of positive comments and lack of negative comments. Adapted from Shafran, Egan, and Wade (2010). Copyright 2010 by Constable & Robinson. Adapted by permission.

One strategy for tackling this type of assumption is the use of orthogonal continua, as described by Padesky (1994). As with standard continua to challenge dichotomous thinking as covered in the next section, orthogonal continua provide a measure of change. The technique is also an important tool for changing beliefs. In Figure 11.6 we illustrate how this method can be adapted to tackle beliefs that typically occur in perfectionism. First, together with the client, draw the correct horizontal and vertical axes. In the case of the belief "If I make a mistake, I am a failure as a person," the horizontal axis has "complete failure as a person" at one end and "complete success as a person" at the other end. The anchor at the top of the vertical axis is "lots of mistakes" and at the bottom it is "no mistakes."

An example of how to use orthogonal continua is shown below with Pete, a perfectionist who felt highly negative about himself.

THERAPIST: Pete, looking at the grid, where would you put yourself?

PETE: Well, I am a complete failure as a person, but I don't make huge numbers of mistakes because I check so much and I am so careful. I guess I would put myself on the horizontal line near the end, "complete failure as a person."

THERAPIST: Okay, now let's take someone who you regard as highly successful. Who might that be?

PETE: I guess someone like the adventurer and entrepreneur Richard Branson. He's a complete success as a person and never makes mistakes.

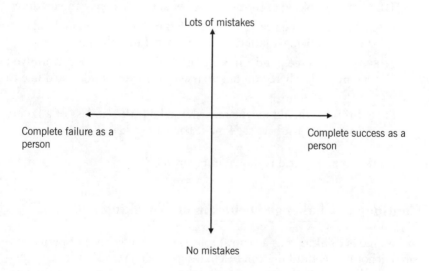

FIGURE 11.6. Orthogonal continua.

THERAPIST: None? What about the air balloon ventures that failed and he had to be rescued?

PETE: Oh, yeah. And he did have some failed businesses, but he's still a success as a person.

THERAPIST: Can you put him on the grid?

PETE: Okay.

THERAPIST: Where would you put the president?

PETE: Well, he's made a lot of mistakes and is obviously a successful person!

THERAPIST: Can you put him on?

PETE: Okay.

THERAPIST: Do you know someone who has made few mistakes and yet you would consider a failure as a person?

PETE: My friend Joe. He's just a bit . . . you know . . . nothing. Nothing bad but nothing good. A nothing person. I would put him in the bottom left quadrant.

THERAPIST: Anyone you know who has made lots of mistakes and you might think is a failure as a person?

PETE: Does it have to be real?

THERAPIST: No

PETE: Okay, then. Bili from *Nights of Our Lives*, the soap opera on television. I would put him there.

THERAPIST: Looking at the grid now, what conclusions can you draw?

PETE: That there is quite as strong a relationship between making mistakes and being a failure as a person as I first thought.

THERAPIST: I agree. And thinking of all those other people, are you happy with where you put yourself or do you think you'd like to move yourself?

PETE: I think I should maybe move myself a little—to less of a failure as a person just because I make some mistakes.

Pete's completed grid is shown in Figure 11.7.

Continua to Challenge Dichotomous Thinking

Dichotomous thinking has a central role in the maintenance of perfectionism. Dichotomous thinking can be challenged using standard thought diaries as outlined earlier, or behavioral experiments (see Chapter 12). However, another cognitive technique to shift this thinking style is the use of

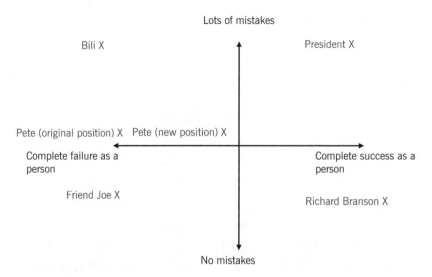

FIGURE 11.7. Example of completed orthogonal continua.

continua. The idea behind this technique is to facilitate flexible thinking by helping clients see that their performance rarely falls into the "all" or "nothing" categories, and that seeing things in shades of gray is both more accurate and more helpful. Your role is to identify the client's dichotomous belief and help the client to identify where on a continuum (or continuous line) his or her performance belongs (see also Handout 11.6 in Appendix 2). In the case of Tim, the therapist used continua to help him realize that his performance in speaking was not a "complete failure" as seen in Figure 11.8.

As illustrated in this example, continua can help clients who view their performance in a dichotomous way to gain flexibility. In this example, Tim was able to recognize that actually he was more of a success at work than he was a failure, and that there were no examples of when he had "completely" failed in his work.

Techniques to Challenge Rigidity in Thinking

As we discussed in Chapter 7, a key issue in perfectionism is that clients set multiple, rigid, and demanding rules and standards that they must meet. For example, Tim's overall goal was to do well at work, and he set rigid rules that he should never making spelling mistakes in e-mails and should never stumble over his words when delivering presentations. Amira had a rigid rule that she should run each race faster than her last, to help her meet her overall goal of winning Olympic gold.

1. Identify the all-or-nothing thought
2. Specify the categories on the continuum
3. Think of examples of evidence along the continuum
4. Reflect

1. What is my all-or-nothing thought?

My presentation was so bad; I am a complete failure at my job.

2. Specify the all-or-nothing categories on the continuum.

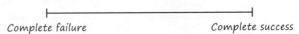

Complete failure   *Complete success*

3. Examples of evidence that falls at various points along the continuum in the thought/ behavior:

Stumbled over my words in the presentation.

Colleague sent me an e-mail thanking me for the hard work I had put into her project.

Boss recently said I did a good job on a report.

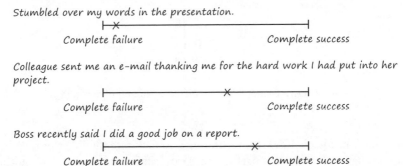

4. What I learned from the continua:

When I consider examples of evidence that falls along different points on the continuum, there are shades of gray in my performance at work. I am neither a "complete failure" nor a "complete success." I am somewhere in between.

FIGURE 11.8. Example of continuum to challenge dichotomous thinking. Adapted from Shafran, Egan, and Wade (2010). Copyright 2010 by Constable & Robinson. Adapted by permission.

It is useful to discuss the impact of rigid rules with clients using a phrase coined by Christopher Fairburn (2013): "Rules break, guidelines bend." An example can be useful in introducing this idea. You can ask the client what effect a rigid rule such as "I must never eat chocolate" might have on the likelihood that an individual will actually eat chocolate. You can help the client recognize that setting such rigid rules is likely to be unhelpful because breaking the rule even once might lead individuals to eat more chocolate than if they had a more moderate "guideline" along the lines of "I have a general guideline to eat healthily and not to eat chocolate every day, but it's okay to eat it occasionally." It is useful to explore with clients their rules for their performance, and for other aspects of their lives. You can ask the client to generate all of the "should" and "musts" they say to themselves. Clients may be surprised to learn that they expect themselves to meet numerous rules during the day. An example of what this would look like in the case of Tim can be seen in Figure 11.9.

After generating such a list, it can be useful to ask the client, "Do you ever get time off from the prison of rules you impose on yourself?" Usually the client will answer "no," and it can be helpful here to introduce the idea that "even prisoners get time off for good behavior!" You should help the client see that the imposition of such rigid rules is unhelpful, and that it is more useful to think about guidelines for behavior. It is also helpful at this point to think of the client engaging in behavioral experiments to text this flexibility, for example, doing something less than perfectly (see Chapter 12 for details).

Brush my teeth twice a day	Do not make spelling errors in e-mails	Exercise five times per week
Comb my hair before going out	Make sure my reports are perfect	Never drink alcohol
Make sure my shirt is perfectly ironed before going to work	Get back to e-mails on the same day that they are sent	Read my children bedtime stories every night
Flush the toilet after using it	Order my work shirts by color in the wardrobe	Phone my mother once a week
Clean my bike once a week	Return phone calls within 24 hours	Keep track of my clients' business cards by having them neatly ordered
Always phone friends back within a few hours of their calling me	Back up my computer with a memory stick	Ensure my wife's car is always in good order
Always respond to requests from my boss immediately	Do better at work than others in my team	Don't eat high-fat foods
Do something to improve my performance at work every day	Never waste time	Mow the lawn once a week to ensure the yard looks good
Read books that will further my career and not waste time reading the paper	Ensure my car is thoroughly clean each week	Always listen to every word my children say in order to be a good dad
Eat five fruits or vegetables per day	File my papers each day before going home	Do something productive each day

FIGURE 11.9. Example of rules identified for performance and behavior.

Another useful way of challenging dichotomous, rigid, rule-based thinking is to help the client to *accept* less-than-perfect performance. For example, you can ask the client to think back to the pros and cons of perfectionism already identified near the start of treatment and consider whether living by such rigid rules and guidelines actually costs more than what he or she gets out of it. You can emphasize the value of sometimes accepting the possibility of not being completely happy with one's performance, and how the negative impact of living by such rigid rules is sometimes worse than being not completely satisfied with how something has turned out. Through this discussion, clients can learn to accept that their performance is not always going be perfect, and that it can be useful to accept a performance they are not entirely happy with in order to lead a more balanced life overall. For further discussion of acceptance-based strategies, see Chapter 13.

Mindfulness-Based Approaches to Challenging Perfectionism

Following from some of these "acceptance"-based ideas, mindfulness-based approaches can be used to help clients adopt a different perspective toward their perfectionistic beliefs. A discussion of mindfulness-based therapy is outside the scope of this chapter, and we refer the reader to one of the many comprehensive texts on the topic (e.g., Segal, Williams, & Teasdale, 2013). There are also self-help books available on mindfulness that may prove useful (e.g., Somov, 2010; Williams, Teasdale, Segal, & Kabat-Zinn, 2007). At a minimum, it is useful to encourage clients to disengage from self-critical and perfectionistic thoughts (e.g., "I am a failure," "I am not good enough") and view them as just thoughts, rather than facts (Segal et al., 2013).

Mindfulness-based cognitive therapy (MBCT; Segal et al., 2013) can help clients to get distance from their thoughts. Rather than getting caught up in their perfectionistic thinking, they can be taught to take a step back, observe, and label their thoughts (e.g., "I have had a thought arise that I am not good enough"). This process is sometimes referred to as "decentering." You can also discuss with clients the idea of resisting the tendency to engage with these thoughts by "tuning them out" in the same way that one might turn down the volume on a radio. Other useful metaphors in the MBCT literature include seeing perfectionistic thoughts as an old, repetitive music DVD, and making the decision not to "play" the DVD or to turn the volume by stepping back, observing the thoughts, labeling the thoughts, and disengaging from them.

CHAPTER 12

Behavioral Experiments

Overview and Definition

Have you ever experienced a client saying "yes but" in response to a cognitive-behavioral formulation, or when gathering of evidence for and against a particular belief? We have! Many of our clients know rationally that nothing dreadful will happen if they don't engage in a particular behavior such as checking, and they know rationally that hours spent finding the "right word" or "perfect Christmas card" are not helpful. They are likely to be aware that procrastination and avoidance can be unhelpful to them. They know they *should* think differently, and they *should* behave in a different way, and this may be their motivation for treatment. However, despite knowing rationally that they should try to behave in a different way, they remain fearful of the cognitive, emotional, and behavioral consequences of doing so. They are stuck. Behavioral experiments are one of the most powerful treatment techniques used to help close the gap between our clients' heads and their hearts. They test the validity of clients' negative automatic thoughts and conditional beliefs in a controlled, contained way that manages risk. For clients with perfectionism, any identification and cognitive evaluation of thoughts or beliefs is routinely followed by a behavioral experiment.

Behavioral experiments have always been given prominence in cognitive-behavioral interventions, and were first described by Beck and colleagues in their seminal treatment manual of CBT for depression (Beck, Rush, Shaw, & Emery, 1979). They can be defined as "planned experiential activities, based on experimentation or observation, which that are undertaken by patients in or between cognitive therapy sessions" (Bennett-Levy et al., 2004, p. 8). Behavioral experiments are derived directly from the cognitive-behavioral formulation (see Chapter 7) and are also used to test the formulation. For example, it may be central to the cognitive-behavioral formulation that the client has lots of rules, and when these are broken the client reacts with self-criticism, which leads to lowered mood. A behavioral experiment could be used to see what happens when that client does break a rule, in terms of self-criticism and mood. Such an experiment brings the cognitive-behavioral formulation to life, helps with engagement, and also tests the validity of the client's beliefs about the helpfulness of rules.

One of the main purposes of behavioral experiments is to gather new personally relevant evidence to test clients' beliefs about their own and others' emotional, cognitive, and behavioral responses. They are also used to test beliefs about how the world works. Such beliefs may be part of the maintenance of perfectionism, and such information is used as a powerful way to challenge existing beliefs. For example, Grieg (who is described in more detail later in the chapter) believed that to be successful, you needed to always be "on the go" and lived by the motto "The devil finds work for idle hands." Grieg was never "idle," but was exhausted. Therapy included a series of behavioral experiments observing the "idleness" of moral people and the consequences of some relaxation/idle time for him. Such consequences included the impact on his self-evaluation and the worry that he thought would be associated with "idleness."

It is not only existing beliefs that can be challenged using behavioral experiments. One of the most common lay myths about cognitive therapy is that it is about "positive thinking." It is not. It is about realistic, balanced, and flexible thinking. The therapist's role is to help the client find out how the world really works and to help the client construct a realistic view of the world that will stand up to scrutiny and future tests. This can be hard. It may be the case that clients are right—they are very bad at giving presentations, they do stutter, or their blush is obvious. If this is the case, then they need to know so that they can make changes and acquire the necessary skills to improve (if that is important to them.) If, on the other hand, they only *believe* they are bad but they are actually good, then the intervention is about belief change. Some of the cognitive work described in the previous chapter may have led to the construction of new, more realistic beliefs about how the world works, and behavioral experiments are then used to test such beliefs.

The Value of Behavioral Experiments

We are not alone in strongly advocating the value of behavioral experiments. In their book on cognitive therapy for delusions, voices, and paranoia, Chadwick, Birchwood, and Trower (1996) write, "Beliefs rarely change as a result of intellectual challenge, but only through engaging emotions and behaving in new ways that produce evidence that confirms new beliefs" (p. 37). For the treatment of anxiety disorders, Wells (1997) clearly argues that "behavioral strategies offer the most powerful means to cognitive change in cognitive therapy" (p. 78). And Padesky and Greenberger's (1995) classic cognitive therapy treatment manual for managing mood problems has the same perspective: "The best way to increase the believability of your alternative or balanced thoughts is to try them out in your day-to-day life" (p. 113).

In a nutshell, the best way to acquire (and retain) information is not by talking about thoughts but through personal experience. You can be told that the oven is hot, but it is only when you burn yourself as a child that you fully understand the significance of this remark and don't go near a hot oven again. You can be told that you won't drown if you take your armbands off and try to swim in the way you've been practicing, but it is only by trying that this becomes clear. Learning from experience is arguably the most powerful method to help our clients obtain a different perspective (Kolb, 1984), and this is the reason the "evidential value" of behavioral experiments is so high. In a study by McManus and colleagues at Oxford University (McManus et al., 2011), 91 people took part in a study to compare the efficacy of one session using thought records, one session of behavioral experiments, and a control intervention. The results showed that while both thought records and behavioral experiments were better than the control condition at changing beliefs, anxiety, behavior, and symptoms, the target belief changed earlier and generalized to beliefs about others as well as the self more with the use of behavioral experiments than with thought records. When behavioral experiments and thought records are used in conjunction with each other, the therapeutic outcome is likely to be even better.

Purposes of Behavioral Experiments

The main purposes of behavioral experiments are to test and elaborate the formulation, to examine the validity of unhelpful beliefs, and to construct and gather evidence for newer, more realistic beliefs (Bennett-Levy et al., 2004). Clients typically grasp this idea right away, and discussion about their own personal experiences reaching a new perspective on a situation can be helpful. For example, have they ever had an experience in which they found something out (i.e., "gathered new information") that changed their mind about a particular situation or person (e.g., "whether a friend was trustworthy")? Paul Salkovskis developed a "builder's apprentice analogy" that we have adapted and often use with clients (Stott, Mansell, Salkovskis, Lavender, & Cartwright-Hatton, 2010) to illustrate this point.

THE BUILDER'S APPRENTICE

Joe, 16, was about to start his first day as a builder's apprentice. He was nervous and eager to please his new bosses and do well. When he came to work promptly at 9:00 A.M., the builders decided to play a trick on him. They told him they had a very important job to do. They asked him to hold up the wall that was just being built. It was about 10 bricks high and 2 bricks wide. Joe thought this was a bit of an odd request, but he was eager to please his new bosses, and he had been told this task was very important. He dreaded the consequences of not doing what he had been asked. What if the wall fell down? What would his bosses think of him for even questioning them?

So Joe held up the wall while the builders sniggered to themselves in private. At about 11:30 A.M., a passerby asked him what he was doing. Joe explained. The guy laughed, told him he was being taken for an idiot, and of course Joe could let go of the wall without anything happening. Although what the passerby said made sense, Joe simply couldn't take the risk. It was his first job, his first day at work, and he couldn't let anyone down.

By lunchtime, Joe's arms ached, he needed to use the restroom, and he was hungry and thirsty. His boss, who was enjoying Joe's predicament, told him that he was doing really well, he was really pleased with him, and could he please just keep going a bit longer? Joe nodded and responded, "Of course." By 4:00 P.M., Joe was completely miserable, terrified to let go of the wall, and unable to continue any longer.

We then ask our clients the following questions:

"What would happen if Joe let go of the wall?" (Response: "Nothing.")

"How can Joe find that out for himself?" (Response: "He has to let go.")

"Why wasn't the passerby's comment enough?" (Response: "He has to find out for himself.").

"What is the similarity with your situation?" (Response: "I have to find out what happens if I 'let go.'")

Behavioral experiments can be used to address negative automatic thoughts, dysfunctional assumptions, or core beliefs. What is fundamental to the success of the experiment is that it is appropriate to the stage of the intervention. Behavioral experiments can be done in the session, and in fact one should be in order to give clients the experience and support of doing one before trying an experiment on their own. It is optimal for behavioral experiments to be conducted when you are seeing clients twice weekly, which is the frequency we recommend for the first six sessions. The reason for this is that it can be tough for the client to do these experiments, and knowing that he or she will be seeing the therapist in only a couple of days can make the experiment seem more manageable and less of a risk than if the next session were a week away. If an experiment is set for homework, it is at the top of the agenda for discussion at the subsequent therapy appointment. If you are unable to see clients twice weekly for the first 3 weeks, or if the experiment is being conducted when your sessions are weekly, then you may want to schedule a brief telephone call or e-mail exchange to check on the progress of the experiment.

Clients may have concerns about the behavioral experiment as it is likely to involve some perceived risk. Being aware of this and empathic to the courage it takes to engage in such experiments is vitally important. It is also crucial that you give the client a clear rationale for the experiment. This means the rationale needs to be clear to you so that it can be communicated clearly to the client to allow a full collaborative discussion. Discussion of the rationale for the experiment should not be rushed and squeezed into the last 5 minutes of the session because it was on the agenda. It is better to leave it to the next session so that you and the client are crystal clear that the purpose of the experiment is to evaluate a specific cognition/prediction that can be understood in terms of the formulation, and that the design of the experiment is appropriate for such an evaluation.

What also becomes clear from the above analogy is that in order to gather new information, the client, like Joe, will have to take some sort of risk. Your job as therapist is to ensure the risk taken is manageable, and that the prospective usefulness of the information gathered helps give the client the motivation to risk doing the experiment.

General Guidelines

The exact behavioral experiment to be devised will depend on the thought or belief to be tested. There is no "right" behavioral experiment—there are many possibilities, all equally valid, to help your clients test their beliefs. It is important that you be flexible about the behavioral experiment, open to change, and willing to set aside your own cognitive biases. For example, many therapists remember the time that a client did not conduct a behavioral experiment as opposed to all the clients that did do them successfully. Some search for the "perfect" behavioral experiment or stick rigidly to their ideas rather than being open to collaboration. Being aware of such tendencies is fundamental to ensuring the experiment is flexible and developed collaboratively with the client.

Perhaps the beliefs that are most easily tested concern specific, observable outcomes that would result from a particular behavior. For example, a client might predict that a friend will refuse if the client asks him or her to come over and watch a video. Another client might fear that if an assignment is done in 10 hours instead of 12, he or she will fail the assignment. Both of these beliefs can be tested in a straightforward manner. If a client has a belief concerning what other people may think (rather than do) in response to his or her actions, this is harder to test and it requires operationalizing. An example of a behavioral experiment can be seen in the case of Grieg.

> Grieg believed if he was "idle" he would be perceived as "lazy" by his course instructors. He tested this in a behavioral experiment in which he did not take notes for 20 minutes of his 2-hour class. Grieg predicted that the instructor would (1) notice his idleness, (2) be insulted by his idleness, and (3) think worse of Grieg for such insolence. Grieg also had a number of predictions about his own emotional and cognitive reactions to the 20 minutes of "idleness." He thought he would be unable to concentrate at all on the content of the lecture, and that he would think badly of himself as a result of being idle for 20 minutes. A fundamental component of behavioral experiments is eliciting specific predictions, so it was agreed that Grieg would be able to establish whether the instructor noticed his idleness and (if he noticed) how he viewed it only by asking him afterwards. It was agreed that after the lecture Grieg would go up to the lecturer and apologize for failing to take notes for 20 minutes. If the lecturer said, "I didn't notice" or looked surprised, then Grieg would know that he had not noticed. If Grieg concluded that the instructor had noticed, it was agreed that Grieg would then say he hoped the instructor had not been insulted or thought worse of Grieg for not taking notes, but Grieg was trying to concentrate on the content of the lecture by listening harder. Specific predictions and ratings were also made about his own responses to the experiment.

The general principles for designing and setting up a behavioral experiment include the following:

1. Make sure the rationale is clear and explicit for both you and the client.
2. Be clear about the belief to be tested—try where possible to also test the alternative or more helpful belief that the client is less convinced about.
3. Ensure that behavioral experiments are set up in a systematic way.
4. Design the experiment such that it does not involve too great a perceived risk for the client, and that it yields useful information to test the belief.
5. Design the experiment collaboratively and ensure that it is the focus of the session, rather than rushing through it at the end of the session. Consider whether the experiment can be simplified (don't try to do too much in one go) or altered to yield more information (or more meaningful information) to help change the client's belief.
6. Ensure the experiment or associated predictions are SMARTER— that is, specific, measurable, achievable, realistic, and time-limited. The experiment should provide results that have a clear bearing on the validity of the assumption (e.g., if the assumption is correct, then X will happen, but if an alternative perspective is correct, then it won't).

7. Design and personalize the materials that will be required to record the outcome of the experiment.
8. Ideally, conduct a behavioral experiment in session so that the client can have some experience of what it requires and how it works.
9. Ensure that you anticipate any difficulties and work together to resolve them. Being specific about when and where the experiment will be conducted can be helpful in ensuring that it does take place.
10. Clients are usually correct if they predict they will experience some discomfort and worry, and this should be discussed as part of setting up the experiment. However, it is extremely unusual for the catastrophic prediction to be accurate (e.g., "I will faint"; "I will make a fool of myself"; "I will collapse and no one will help me"; "people will reject me"). It is also important to emphasize that such experiments cannot "go wrong" because the outcome of any behavioral experiment will provide valuable data to discuss in the next session. (See further discussion later in this chapter about fears that behavioral experiments will "go wrong.")
11. Make the review of the experiment your priority in the next session, which ideally will take place soon after the experiment rather than several days later. Consider adding an extra session to review the experiment, even if it is just by phone. Emphasize how impressed you are that the client successfully conducted the behavioral experiment, took a chance, and did something differently. This should be recognized as a significant and worthwhile achievement to be valued by the client.

Bennett-Levy and colleagues (2004) describe different types of behavioral experiments, including surveys, which we discuss separately (see Chapter 9). Experiments can be observational (i.e., the client does "hypothesis testing" by observing other people). There is rarely one definitive behavioral experiment, just as there is rarely one definitive cognitive method. Instead it is likely you will use a series and sequence of different types of experiments to gather information about the way the self, others, and the world works. Such experiments will test existing beliefs and help generate alternative perspectives that can themselves be subsequently tested. For clients with perfectionism, we have a particular liking for "contrast" experiments in which clients compare how they have always behaved (e.g., spending a long time on cleaning) with a new way of behaving (e.g., spending a reduced amount of time on cleaning). It can be extremely powerful to make the same predictions for the original and new way of behaving and contrast the experience of doing the same behavior (cleaning) in different ways. If there is a longer time between therapy sessions, we also ask clients to repeat the experiment. For example, on Monday and Wednesday they could be cleaning in the original way, and on Tuesday and Thursday the new way. We then suggest that they review the results of the experiment to decide which way of cleaning works better for them and their lives, bearing in mind their treatment goals, for Friday, Saturday, and Sunday, or until the next appointment. The way we discuss this with clients is that manipulating (e.g., increasing or decreasing) the behaviors associated with their perfectionism and contrasting the consequences is a great way to gather personally relevant, important information about which way of behaving works best for the client. This information gives clients real choices about the way they want to live their lives.

Specific Guidelines

We recommend the following specific steps for the design of the behavioral experiment.

- Step 1: Consider the formulation. Collaboratively identify a key belief/thought/behavior/process that keeps the client stuck in the vicious cycle of perfectionism. Ask the client to rate how much he or she endorses that belief (0–100%).
- Step 2: Collaboratively brainstorm ideas for an experiment to test the thought/belief/behavior/process. Ensure the experiment is not likely to be too challenging, and that it will likely yield useful and meaningful information. Be specific about when and where the experiment will be conducted.
- Step 3: Elicit multiple specific predictions about the outcome of the experiment and devise a method to record the outcome.
- Step 4: Anticipate problems and brainstorm solutions.
- Step 5: Conduct the behavioral experiment.
- Step 6: Review the experiment, including the predictions; rerate belief in the target belief and draw conclusions.

As an example, the steps for another of Grieg's behavioral experiments are described below.

Step 1: Consider the formulation.

Grieg's key beliefs: The devil makes work for idle hands. In other words, I must always be busy, and it is wrong not to be busy. I could not tolerate being idle. Belief rating: 100%

Step 2: Collaboratively brainstorm ideas for an experiment to test the thought/ belief/behavior/process.

"Idle" was defined as "not being engaged in some productive activity." The therapist suggested that Grieg relax by watching trashy TV or reading a trashy magazine.

Grieg's disdain for this suggestion was obvious. Grieg suggested relaxing by reading a novel on quantum physics. The therapist considered that this would be "productive" and not fall within the definition of "idle." It was agreed that sitting in a café and reading a newspaper, which was viewed as "idle" and would only take 20 minutes, was all the idleness Grieg felt he could tolerate.

Step 3: Elicit multiple specific predictions about the outcome of the experiment and devise a method to record the outcome.

Grieg predicted that (1) he would feel acutely uncomfortable sitting in a café reading a newspaper (100%); (2) he would feel so uncomfortable that after about 15 minutes he would have to leave (60%); (3) he would judge himself as immoral for engaging in idleness for 20 minutes (100% certainty that he would judge himself as immoral; immorality level— 80% in recognition that he was not stealing or harming others, which would be 100%).

Step 4: Anticipate problems and brainstorm solutions.

Grieg couldn't do the experiment in a local café, as he did not want local people to think of him as idle. On the other hand, he wasn't prepared to travel a long distance to find a different café because that would take up too much time and not be productive. It was agreed he would do the experiment in a café near where the therapy appointment took place, and time it so that it was just before an appointment.

Step 5: Conduct the behavioral experiment.

Grieg did the experiment. Owing to the bus schedule, Grieg ended up spending 27 minutes in the café rather than the agreed 20 minutes.

Step 6: Review the experiment and draw conclusions.

Something very unusual happened during the experiment, which Grieg was concerned would invalidate the experiment. After about 10 minutes, a father and young child asked Grieg if they could share his table, as the café was crowded and it was lunchtime. They became engaged in conversation as the father apologized for the child's various misdemeanors. Grieg found the interaction pleasant but felt it hadn't been a proper test, as he hadn't been idle but instead had been chatting and had helped clean up a spill. The therapist considered the experiment to still "count" as it was what actually tended to happen in life—even when you are "idle," distractions arise and conversations and interactions occur. Grieg agreed and the results were reviewed. Grieg reported he had felt uncomfortable at first (100%), but this decreased rapidly to about 50% after 5 minutes and disappeared when the father and young child joined him. He didn't leave, and much to his surprise, he did not judge himself as immoral because (1) he was doing something for therapy and (2) the café was so crowded with people that it just seemed "normal." He had enjoyed it. It was agreed to try the experiment again, in a café closer to home, at a less busy time. His rating for his original belief was reduced from 100% to 50%.

Grieg's experiment led to the generation of an alternative belief that "it is okay to be idle sometimes." He did not endorse this belief very highly when it was first generated (10%), so another experiment was developed in which he tested that more positive alternative belief by allowing himself to have 10–20 minutes of idleness per day or 2 hours of "idleness" a week. He worked out that this was less than 2% of his day (assuming that he was awake for 14 hours a day), for a total of 840 minutes, and so was tolerable. At the end of this experiment, his endorsement of the alternative belief that "it is okay to be idle sometimes" was 95%.

Behavioral Experiment Record Sheets

It can be helpful to use a behavioral experiment record sheet such as Handout 12.1 in Appendix 2. A completed record for Grieg is shown below in Figure 12.1, based on Grieg's original café experiment described earlier. An alternative behavioral experiment record sheet is also provided in Figure 12.2, where the prediction is specified before the experiment. This alternative record sheet can be a useful simplified sheet for use with clients.

Comparison between Exposure and Behavioral Experiments

Behavioral experiments typically involve exposure to feared stimuli and situations, but they are not the same as exposure. The differences are shown in Table 12.1.

It is rare for a client to ask for an elaboration on the differences between exposure and behavioral experiments, but it is common for therapists to get confused. The two are conceptually and practically different. Exposure is systematically graded, and although behavioral experiments are not, no competent therapist would suggest an experiment that is too difficult to conduct. In a client group that is sensitive to perceived failure, procrastination, and avoidance, it is critical that the experiment be agreed upon collaboratively and be manageable.

Client Concerns about Behavioral Experiments

If someone asked you to risk your life, or that of a loved one, you would be reluctant and fearful to do so. For many of our clients, that is what it seems as though the therapist is asking them to do. Clients with perfectionism

---

Belief to be tested (Rate degree of belief (0–100%): *I could not tolerate being idle* *(100%).*

Is there an alternative belief? (Rate degree of belief 0–100% if applicable): *I might not like being idle but I can tolerate it (0%).*

Experiment that will test the belief (specify what you will do in detail including when, where, and how).
Go to a café and be idle for 20 minutes (i.e., read the newspaper and have a drink).

Specify the prediction precisely (specify behaviors and rate intensity of beliefs and emotions): Feel 100% uncomfortable (I am 100% sure of this).
I will leave (60%) because I will feel so uncomfortable.
I will judge myself as immoral (100%)—level of immorality 80%.

What problems might occur, and how will you overcome them? *I might chicken out. I will tell myself that I am being idle for good reason and that I do really need to try to change.*

Experiment—what did you actually do?
I did the experiment as we agreed and went to a café with a newspaper.

Results—what happened? *Did the experiment but Peter and Flynn shared the table after 10 minutes, which made it much better but I am not sure it counts.*

Rerate the predictions made: What can you conclude?
I was right—I was 100% uncomfortable but it did get a bit easier (50%) quite quickly and was fine when Peter and Flynn arrived. I didn't feel at all immoral— the café was completely packed and actually it made me feel normal for once.

Rerate the belief you were testing and the alternative belief (if you had one): *I could not tolerate being idle (75%).*

Reflection (including plans for any follow-up experiments): *I am not sure this counts because I am not sure I was really idle. It was not as bad as I thought, and I feel strangely proud of myself for doing something others do. Peter and Flynn made it a really good time but perhaps this means I cheated. I think I should do this again properly.*

Revised belief/behavior: *Going to a café, reading a paper, and having a chat is probably idle, and it is probably okay sometimes. I didn't feel as bad as I thought I would for very long, I didn't leave, and I feel normal. I believe this 50%.*

FIGURE 12.1. An example of a completed behavioral experiment record sheet for Grieg's idleness experiment.

Situation	Predictions	Experiment	Outcome	What I learned
	What I think will actually happen. How much I believe it will, 0–100%. What will happen to my anxiety? How much do I believe this, 0–100%.	What I can do to test my fears. How can I find out what will happen to my anxiety?	What actually happened? Were any of my predictions correct?	What do I make of the experiment? How much do I believe my initial predictions will happen in the future, 0–100%? How can I test this further?

FIGURE 12.2. Alternative behavioral experiment record sheet.

TABLE 12.1. A Comparison of Behavioral Experiments and Exposure

	Behavioral experiment	Exposure
Primary purpose	Test validity of beliefs	Decrease anxiety
Frequency	Typically once	Typically repeated
Systematically graded?	No	Yes
Duration	Usually brief	Usually prolonged
Anxiety	Not necessarily evoked	Evoked
Okay to leave situation when anxious?	Almost always	Many therapists believe that clients must stay in the situation for exposure to be effective
Need to focus on anxiety?	No	Believed to be beneficial

have a fear of failure because failure is so very personally meaningful and significant to them. When the therapist suggests an experiment that could result in perceived failure of the task (and consequently as a person), it can provoke enormous anxiety. For clients who believe it is right and moral to strive for perfection, the threat of such experiments is that the client may end up immoral, slovenly, average, and "bad." Each client is different, so the concerns will be different. It is important for you to take a significant amount of time eliciting these concerns, empathizing with them, and finding an experiment that will be useful in testing beliefs but is also manageable for the client. Doing the first behavioral experiment in session helps with some of the concerns. When reviewing the outcome of the experiment, it is important not only to evaluate the impact of the experiment on the validity of the beliefs, but also to reflect on the client's concerns about the process of doing such experiments.

Therapist Concerns about Behavioral Experiments

Therapists have a number of concerns about behavioral experiments and typically they involve worries about the experiments "going wrong" in some way. Therapists mostly seem concerned that the client's predictions will be valid. In Grieg's case, the therapist might worry that Grieg can't tolerate idleness, that it is so aversive that he will leave, and regard himself as entirely immoral. While this would not help in forming an alternative belief to the original one, what it does reveal is that Grieg's appraisal of the situation is accurate and realistic. What then? The answer is that this is important information for the therapist to know, and it needs to be fed into the formulation. If Grieg cannot tolerate idleness, then the therapist may wish to help him focus more on what idleness means to him and help him build up a tolerance to idleness. It may mean that the experiment was "too much, too soon" and it is necessary to go back a step to understand better the origins of those beliefs and the factors that are maintaining them before going ahead with change at that particular stage of therapy.

An important part of the treatment of perfectionism is acceptance (see Chapter 11). On their self-evaluation clients are encouraged to accept the reality of their standards and the cost of striving to achieve goals. Therapists may also require a bit of acceptance with regard to the therapy session. You will not design the perfect behavioral experiment, and it may be the case that the results of the experiment are not in keeping with your formulation or with what you regard to be most therapeutic. However, in science, the most important findings are the surprising and unpredictable ones and the same is true of therapy. Knowing how the world works for your clients is the only way to understand where, when, and to make the changes needed to improve their quality of life and help them meet their goals. The most important characteristic of the therapist in setting up behavioral experiments is not omniscience (knowing the outcome) but having an intense curiosity to see what will happen and what information this will yield about how the client can best interact with the world.

Therapists are often wary about behavioral experiments that involve other people's reactions. They seem less controllable and therefore "higher risk." Since we live in a social world where other people's reactions are likely to influence the standards clients have for themselves as well as their reaction to perceived failure and its impact on self-evaluation, behavioral experiments will undoubtedly need to involve others at some time. It is important to operationalize how you will obtain information about what others may think (e.g., by observing their reactions or by going up and asking them, as was the case with Grieg's course instructor). If the experiment "goes wrong" and the person your client asked to watch television refused the invitation, that is important information to have and reflect upon. Was your client as devastated as he or she predicted? How did your client feel about having at least taken the first step and asked someone over? If it was all dreadful and the client regretted ever taking that step, then that is important to know in considering how your client wants to live life in the future. No information is "bad" or "wrong." Your hypotheses about maintaining factors and your predictions may be "wrong," but they will still yield essential information to help your clients on the road to recovery.

Having said all the above, it is obviously important to be sensible in designing and implementing behavioral experiments. It is not sensible to ask someone with a heart condition to engage in strenuous exercise to "see what happens" or to test the belief that such exercise will lead to a heart attack (unless, of course, you happen to have particular medical expertise in this area). It is not sensible to ask elite athletes to make changes to their training without the requisite expertise. The experiments should be contained within your area of expertise and should focus on facilitating belief and behavioral change.

Troubleshooting Problems in Behavioral Experiments

It may be tempting to set up an early behavioral experiment involving "making a mistake." Clients may believe that making a mistake will lead to awful consequences, such as an inability to cope and concentrate. Although you may want to test out this belief early in therapy by having the client purposely make a mistake (e.g., write a postcard with a spelling error in it), we recommend delaying until later in therapy and ensuring that these experiments are conducted in an appropriate context. Clients who have spent a great deal of their lives preventing themselves from making such mistakes and whose self-evaluation is dependent on being precise and flawless can react to such a suggested experiment negatively, with responses such as "Why would you make a mistake on purpose?" "What is the point of such an experiment?" "A deliberate mistake isn't like a real mistake anyway because it doesn't reflect on me." A similar reaction may occur from suggesting experiments in which clients do something badly—the purpose needs to be clear and the timing needs to be considered carefully. Such experiments are best done in conjunction with the cognitive work and methods for adjusting self-evaluation rather than in isolation.

While experiments cannot "go wrong," it is worth considering how to maximize their impact and troubleshoot any difficulties. The most common problem is that the therapist and client underestimate the amount of perceived risk the client is taking, and when it comes to it, the client cannot engage in the experiment. It is worth emphasizing that this is not a "failure" on your client's part, but a source of information about the perceived level of risk and meaning to the client. Using that information to devise a more acceptable, realistic behavioral experiment is what should follow, and if it can be done immediately with the therapist's encouragement in session, then so much the better. It is an advantage in the treatment of perfectionism that a "mistake" in therapy (i.e., underestimating the perceived difficulty of the experiment) is particularly helpful therapeutically. Instead of self-flagellation for the experiment being too difficult, together you reflected on the experiment, generated a hypothesis as to why it was tricky, and came up with a more realistic experiment that could be done. And perhaps it was even better that it was done together in session!

How Behavioral Experiments Link to Engagement, Formulation, and Cognitive Challenges

The most competent therapy that we have observed by others is when it hardly looks like any therapy is happening at all. There is an agenda and goals, and therapy techniques are being implemented, but the session is more like a conversation. It flows naturally. Behavioral experiments should not be seen as a "technique" that is used independently of other issues such as engagement, alliance, developing a formulation, or using thought records. It is a tool that can be seen to have all of these aspects. When you develop a behavioral experiment and discuss the merits of doing it, it is likely that the conversation will include a discussion about how the best way to facilitate change is to start by changing behavior. Making such changes will help with the therapeutic alliance, and it will certainly inform the formulation. Cognitive biases that may not have been apparent in verbal discussion may come to the fore when conducting such an experiment. Integrating behavioral experiments in a seamless way will impact positively on all aspects of therapy.

Your Own Experiment

It would be hypocritical to have spent the first half of this chapter extolling the virtues of learning by doing and then continue without asking you to conduct an experiment. You may believe what you have just read, and you may even remember it (which would be good going). But there is only one way to really consolidate the learning, and that is by doing your own experiment.

Either in supervision or on own, take time out to think about a behavioral experiment to test a belief you may hold about yourself, others, or the world. If such a belief were in the domain of standards, self-evaluation, rules, self-criticism, or other aspects relevant to perfectionism, that would be even better. If you now do the experiment using the record sheet presented earlier, we suggest that will really help consolidate the information in the chapter so far. Clearly, it is not linked to a formulation and you are not in therapy, but it will nevertheless enable you to contrast theory with practice and become familiar with the record sheet that you will use with your clients. When we are running workshops on how to do CBT for perfectionism, attendees will often try to conduct their own behavioral experiments by making a mistake on purpose during the lunch break. For example, a therapist who has high standards regarding her appearance will go to the bathroom and take off some of her makeup before joining the lunch line, or one with high standards for his social behavior will purposely stumble over a couple of words when speaking to a colleague.

Specific Experiments

As is clear from Chapter 7, people with perfectionism engage in various performance-related behaviors to prevent mistakes and perceived failure, and they also respond to perceived failure to meet standards with counterproductive behavior. Performance-related behavior and counterproductive behavior are often the same for a particular client. Although no two clients are the same, typical behaviors include trying to find the "right word," checking work repeatedly, making multiple lists, avoidance, procrastination, and overpacking "just in case" something is needed. Specific experiments involving these behaviors are described below, each with an associated example and completed worksheet. Some come directly from experiments described in psychological research and others were developed from our clinical practice. Both the research literature and clinical practice are helpful sources of inspiration in devising such experiments.

Repeated Checking

The treatment of compulsive checking in OCD has been advanced by a cognitive theory of checking (Rachman, 2002), and robust experimental findings from independent research groups have demonstrated that repeated checking in a relevant domain decreases confidence in memory. In treatment, this is most easily described as "checking causes memory distrust" (see Radomsky, Shafran, Coughtrey, & Rachman, 2010, for further information, including a video illustration of a behavioral experiment if you are accessing the article online). There is no reason to expect that repeated performance checking or counterproductive checking in response to perceived failure in perfectionism is any different from the repeated checking that characterizes OCD and other disorders.

You may wish to describe these research findings when providing psychoeducation at the beginning of therapy, or it may be better to provide this specific piece of psychoeducation (or at least to revisit it) when you discuss the rationale for a behavioral experiment to help decrease checking behavior.

Many clients respond with scepticism to this information. The reason that people check is to improve their performance and to decrease their worry and anxiety about their performance for the next time. Such skepticism is most welcome as it is fertile ground for a behavioral experiment. A typical experiment to address this scepticism is to contrast the impact of repeatedly checking something highly salient (as clients usually do) on a given occasion, with the impact of checking just once. Clients often predict that when they check repeatedly they will be reasonably certain they have not made a mistake, they will only feel moderately anxious for a short time, and their worry will not be excessive throughout the day and so will not interfere with important tasks that require full concentration. Clients predict that if they were only to check their performance once, they would be very unsure whether there was a mistake, that it would certainly be considered suboptimal in terms of quality, and they would feel highly anxious and worried immediately and for a long time afterward.

We quantify their predictions using a scale of 0–100 for severity/intensity and specifying the duration of predicted anxiety. In keeping with the general principles described earlier, we like to ask clients to do this experiment twice, so that they have more data points from which to draw conclusions. Depending on the client, we suggest that therapists give the clients a choice as to whether they wish to continue checking once or if they prefer to check repeatedly until the next appointment. It would be important to know if clients find that checking repeatedly does not impact their memory or cause anxiety, and whether it is much better than checking once. However, if they find (as is almost always the case) that checking increases uncertainty and anxiety, then they are likely to choose to check only once. When we review the experiment, we discuss the amount of time the client will gain by checking once as well as the obvious other advantages such as increased confidence in memory and anxiety reduction. We agree on a pleasurable activity that the client can do during this newfound time. An example can be seen in the case of Joachim.

> Joachim was a 32-year-old man who worked as a management consultant in New York in a highly pressured, well-paid job. He believed he had achieved his position through hard work and dedication as well as having some natural ability. By nature he was a competitive, determined, and ambitious man. He came to therapy in a state of extreme distress as he had only been given a rating of 4 out of 5 on his performance review. Such a rating influenced his salary but that was not of concern. Joachim was told that the reason he had not been given 5 out of 5 (as on all his previous reviews) was that his peers had commented that he was "slow," overly persnickety, and overly critical when they failed to live up to what his peers perceived to be unrealistic standards. Joachim told the therapist that at first he had been outraged by these comments, which he felt were grossly unfair, but upon reflection he thought they had a point. He wanted 5 out of 5 on his next review and so had come to therapy to see if he could reduce his concern for detail and perfection.
>
> During the course of therapy, it emerged that Joachim not only checked his own e-mails to ensure they were error free, but he also asked his subordinates to send him important e-mails they were going to send to clients so that Joachim could ensure they were error free as well. He also had an unpopular habit of correcting typing errors in other people's e-mails and returning them to the sender. He knew this was unpopular, but he also described the need to do this to make things right and said that all e-mail traffic that passed through his e-mail account was "clean." Checking his own and other people's e-mails was time-consuming, and Joachim often did this at home late at night. He said it could take him up to an hour as he

checked and rechecked the same e-mail more than once to make absolutely sure he did not make a mistake. Joachim predicted that if he did not do this, he would be unable to sleep, sure there would be a mistake, and highly anxious. He agreed to a behavioral experiment using an e-mail that the therapist would send him. On one occasion he agreed to check it for mistakes just once (the therapist promised there would be a few on purpose) and on other occasion he agreed to check it repeatedly. He predicted that he would miss mistakes if he checked just once, he would be highly agitated, and he would want to check again. He thought he would do a better job if he was able to check repeatedly, and that he would be less agitated, with very little desire to check again. As you can see from the behavioral experiment record sheet below, the reality was that when Joachim checked repeatedly, he was less sure he had checked properly and more agitated and anxious than when he checked once and went straight to bed, where, to his great surprise, he fell asleep. Reflecting on this experiment, Joachim agreed that repeated checking was not helping his performance—he had corrected the e-mail perfectly when he checked once, just as when he checked multiple times—and that it was distressing, time-consuming, and kept him up late. He agreed to repeat the experiment using e-mails from work as the subsequent homework assignment. Joachim's record sheet is shown in Figure 12.3, together with examples that test beliefs about multitasking and list making. Feel free to make each record sheet slightly different to personalize it for the client; such adaptations are recommended providing that the essential principles of the steps remain the same. Flexibility is for therapists as well as clients!

Completed record sheets for client experiments related to multitasking and list making are provided, respectively, in Figures 12.4 and 12.5. Please note that the record sheets for both examples have been altered slightly to illustrate how these forms can be adapted for the individual client.

Avoidance and Procrastination

Avoidance is the hallmark of anxiety disorders, and procrastination the hallmark of perfectionism. As we will describe in Chapter 14, people with perfectionism procrastinate for a variety of reasons. Some procrastinate because the scale of the task ahead of them is daunting, as it must be completed to the highest possible standard and is therefore time-consuming. Others procrastinate to leave themselves too little time to complete a task so that performance on the task cannot be considered to be a true reflection of their ability. Understanding the reason for avoidance, procrastination, and indeed all the behaviors that characterize perfectionism is critically important to understanding what the appropriate intervention should be. Behavioral experiments to decrease avoidance often resemble exposure so bearing in mind the key distinct purpose of an experiment compared to exposure can be helpful in designing an experiment with a clear purpose.

Belief to be tested (rate degree of belief 0–100%):

I need to check over and over to make myself sure that I haven't missed any mistakes and so that I can go to sleep at night. (Belief: 98%)

Is there an alternative belief? (rate degree of belief 0–100% if applicable):

I prefer to check, but I would eventually fall asleep if I didn't. (Belief: 2%)

Experiment that will test the belief (specify what you will do in detail including when, where, and how): *Check repeatedly vs. check once, and see how sure I am that I haven't missed any mistakes, how upset I get, and whether I sleep.*

Specify the prediction precisely (specify behaviors and rate intensity of beliefs and emotions):

When I check [the therapist's] e-mail over and over, I will be 100% sure I have picked up all the mistakes, I will not want to go back and check (100%). My anxiety will be 0 (100%) and I will go straight to sleep (100%).

When I check [the therapist's] e-mail once, I will be totally UNSURE I have picked up the mistakes (100%), I will want to go back and check (100%), I will be 100% anxious, and I will not sleep all night (so I will do this on a Friday so it won't affect my work the next day).

What problems might occur, and how will you overcome them?

I could get stuck checking and not be able to only check once. If that happens, I will ask Maggie (my friend) to help me.

Experiment—what did you actually do? *As above. When I checked over and over, it took 45 minutes for an e-mail of 10 lines.*

Results—what happened?

When I checked the e-mail over and over, I was only 90% sure I picked up all the mistakes. I began to doubt if I had checked properly. I did want to go back and check, and my anxiety was about 10%. It took me 30 minutes to go to sleep.

When I checked once, I was surprised, but I was 100% sure I picked up all the mistakes. I didn't want to go back and check at all and was only about 10% anxious (the same as when I checked over and over). It took me the same amount of time to go to sleep (30 minutes) and I went for a run the next day.

Rerate the predictions made: What can you conclude? *See above for predictions. I conclude checking once wasn't as bad as I thought.*

Rerate the belief you were testing and the alternative belief (if you had one):

RE: Belief—I need to check over and over to make myself sure that I haven't missed any mistakes and so that I can go to sleep at night. (Belief: 40%)

(continued)

FIGURE 12.3. Sample record sheet for Joachim's behavioral experiment.

RE: Alternative belief—I prefer to check but I would eventually fall asleep if I didn't (Belief: 60%)—depends on what I am checking though!

Reflection (including plans for any follow-up experiments): I was surprised that when I checked once it wasn't nearly as bad as I thought. In fact, it was slightly better than when I checked over and over. If there is no difference in picking up mistakes when I check once and when I check lots of times, what am I doing it for?! Follow-up experiment is to do it again with something more important.

Revised belief/behavior: I could never not check at all but checking once is okay rather than over and over.

FIGURE 12.3. *(continued)*

Behavioral experiments to decrease procrastination can be very helpful as clients know rationally that "putting things off" is unhelpful and that the tasks just "hang over them." However, it is only when they have the experience of doing a task with less procrastination that the true extent of the disadvantages become clear and that they begin to have confidence that they can indeed do tasks without significant delay. They learn that they are capable of enduring real tests of their performance and they can be pleasantly surprised by the results.

If you and your client have a good relationship and access to the Internet, you may want to look up "Procrastination" (*www.youtube.com/ watch?v=4P785j15Tzk*) on YouTube for a brief and humorous look at the nature and futility of procrastination.

Procrastination in clients with perfectionism is illustrated in the case of Sonal.

Sonal was a 40-year-old, highly glamorous assistant professor of biology at Harvard University. She had not been granted tenure and was producing work far too infrequently for her to be considered for promotion. She had an annual contract that was constantly subject to renewal. She felt if her contract was not renewed, it would have rendered her life meaningless, and no other job would carry with it the status as the one at Harvard. She had conducted lots of experiments with interesting results but had not been able to send off the papers she had written to journals for fear of rejection. Without such publications she could not secure funding and this is why her contract was reviewed annually. At night, Sonal would reread the articles she had written, making tiny changes here and there. She told herself they were not good enough to send off and they would be rejected. She said that such a rejection would "be the end of me."

An example of Sonal's behavioral experiment to overcome perfectionism is shown below in Figure 12.6.

Belief: Multitasking is efficient and the only way I will manage all the many tasks I have to do (95%).

Experiment that will test the belief:

Multitask the chores one night; do the chores sequentially the next night. Repeat the experiment and choose which one works better for me.

Specify the prediction precisely (specify behaviors and rate intensity of beliefs and emotions):

I will get more done when I multitask, without any loss of efficiency (100%).

I will finish earlier when I multitask than when I do things one by one (50%).

My stress level will be 80% when I do things sequentially and 60% when I multitask (I am quite a stress person!).

Experiment—what did you actually do?

Multitask night: 6:00 P.M. Ran the bath, put on supper, put clothes away, turned off bath, chased kids to get in bath (!!) (They never come when I call them!) Finished making supper, got them out the bath, had supper, told them to brush their teeth when I cleared up, put kids to bed, got Zoe out of bed because her face was dirty from supper as she hadn't cleaned it when brushing her teeth and also she hadn't done her teeth properly as usual. Finished chores and sat down to X Factor at 9:00 P.M. and grabbed something to eat for myself in front of the TV. Not bad!

Sequence night: 6:00 P.M. Ran bath, turned off bath, got kids to go into bath by bringing them (no yelling), washed them myself. Let them play while I put clothes away. Made supper and tidied up as I went along (I had time as I was actually in the kitchen). Bit later than usual so I ate with the kids. Tidied up and then washed kids' faces (especially Zoe's), made sure they went to the toilet again, and I brushed their teeth, which made me feel better. Finished chores and sat down to X Factor at 9:00 P.M. I had already eaten.

Results—what happened?

I got the same amount done when I did the tasks all together as when I did them sequentially. Funnily enough, I felt I did things better when I did them sequentially, I was calmer, and there was less yelling. I finished at the same time but my stress level was about 80% when I multitasked and only 60% when I did them sequentially.

Reflection (including plans for any follow-up experiments): I prefer doing things sequentially—there is no loss of efficiency and I feel less stressed. My original belief that multitasking is efficient and the only way I will manage all the many tasks I have to do is now 60%.

Revised belief/behavior: Less multitasking! I can manage the tasks without trying to do them all at the same time—doesn't increase my efficiency.

FIGURE 12.4. Example of a behavioral experiment to test multitasking.

Belief: *I am stupid; if I don't make lists I will forget what I need to do (75%).*

Experiment that will test the belief: *Don't make a list and see what I forget.*

Specify the prediction precisely (specify behaviors and rate intensity of beliefs and emotions):

I will forget at least 3 items on my "to do" list (which has about 10 items on it). (Belief: 100%)

I will be anxious about forgetting something important (100% sure I will be anxious; anxiety intensity will be 75%).

I will end up rehearsing what I have to do in my head all day and that will distract me from my work (100%).

What problems might occur and how will you overcome them?

I am not sure. If I run into problems, I will just review my notes.

Experiment—what did you actually do? *On Tuesday, I did not make a list.*

Results—what happened?

I did not forget any items on my "to do" list.

I was anxious, but the intensity was about 60% and soon faded to about 10% during the day, although a bit worse when I thought about it at lunch.

I did not rehearse the list in my head because I was actually doing the work—I focused well on my work. This prediction was not true!

Reflection (including plans for any follow-up experiments): *I still like lists, but I surprised myself by not forgetting what I had to do. I am not sure what this experiment says about whether or not I am stupid. I guess I am less forgetful than I thought.*

Revised belief/behavior: *I can remember tasks without making lists (80%). Multitasking is efficient and the only way I will manage all the many tasks I have to do (15%).*

FIGURE 12.5. An example of a behavioral experiment to challenge beliefs about making lists.

Belief to be tested (rate degree of belief 0–100%): *My paper is not ready to send off yet. If I send it off and it is rejected, I will be devastated—unable to eat, work, or sleep again (95%).*

Alternative belief: *It might be okay to send off and I could possibly cope with rejection as other people do (5%).*

Experiment that will test the belief (specify what you will do in detail including when, where, and how):

Send off a paper—maybe the one I think is best and nearly ready. I will send it on Tuesday as it is the first of the month, fresh start. I will drop it in a mailbox so I can't just retrieve it from internal mail when I panic later.

Specify the prediction precisely (specify behaviors and rate intensity of beliefs and emotions):

It will get rejected (95%). I will be devastated (100%). I won't be able to eat for days (100%), or sleep for days (100%) or go to work and face my colleagues (100%).

What problems might occur and how will you overcome them?

I could wimp out. I will remember that I need to make progress and it's an experiment.

Experiment—what did you actually do?

Sent off the paper with a cover letter asking for a rapid editorial opinion about suitability for publication.

Results—what happened?

The editor wrote a nice letter back saying it was "out of scope" for his journal, but he recommended another. I was not devastated at all, and I ate, slept, and worked just fine. My colleagues often have their papers rejected as "out of scope."

Rerate the predictions made: What can you conclude? *It will get rejected (100%—it was rejected). I will be devastated (20%). I won't be able to eat for days (20%), or sleep for days (10%) or go to work and face my colleagues (50%).*

Rerate the belief you were testing and the alternative belief (if you had one):

Original belief—My paper is not ready to send off yet. If I send it off and it is rejected, I will be devastated—unable to eat, work, or sleep again (10%).

Alternative belief—It might be okay to send off and I could possibly cope with rejection as other people do (90%).

(continued)

FIGURE 12.6. Example of a behavioral experiment to challenge procrastination.

Reflection (including plans for any follow-up experiments): *I can't believe I did it! It was rejected as "Out of Scope" but weirdly, I didn't care too much because I SENT IT OFF. I will probably be more upset if it gets rejected from the other journal I have now sent it to but I SENT IT OFF. The journal editor didn't say it was below standard or not ready and he recommended that I send this "interesting" paper to another journal. He thought it was interesting! I feel I have really achieved something by sending it off after so long. I need to do this with other papers, especially ones that are more risky as they are not as good.*

Revised belief/behavior: *I can cope if my papers are rejected.*

FIGURE 12.6. *(continued)*

Other Behavioral Experiments

There are a range of other relevant behavioral experiments for people with perfectionism. Once cognitive work has been done to address "all-or-nothing" thinking and clients are beginning to see the "gray area," it can be extremely useful for them to act "as if" they have a more moderated thinking style even if they don't adhere to it at the time of the experiment. By having the experience of thinking and behaving differently, clients are in a position to discover whether such beliefs and behaviors are helpful and desirable for them. Acting as if the client has flexible guidelines rather than rigid rules will give invaluable and direct insight into the benefits of such flexibility. Being able to operate in a less rigid manner is intrinsically reinforcing as it typically is less stressful and saves time. If the client does have extra time as a result of changing beliefs and behaviors, it is helpful to suggest that the time be filled with pleasurable activities rather than more goal-directed striving.

Experiments that address hypervigilance and selective attention to threat are also helpful. YouTube has an "awareness" test that illustrates the phenomenon of selective attention very well (*www.youtube.com/watch?v=47LCLoidJh4*). In this brief video clip of less than a minute, the viewer is asked to count the number of passes that the basketball team in white makes. The answer is 13 and the viewer is told this but then asked if they saw the "moonwalking bear" that was present in the video. The video is rewound and the moonwalker bear becomes clear. This text then comes up on screen: "It's easy to miss something you're not looking for." Having watched the moonwalking bear on YouTube to illustrate the phenomenon, clients can then be encouraged to spot activities and events that they would usually miss and contrast this to being hypervigilant for success and achievement. Another activity in session to illustrate the role of selective attention is to ask clients how itchy their scalp feels and to rate that. Then ask your clients to take a few moments to concentrate on the itchiness of their head and to close their eyes and focus attention on their scalp. Afterward, ask the client to rerate the itchiness. It usually goes up, illustrating the power of selective attention to internal sensations. It is often helpful for therapists to do the experiments in parallel with clients and, where possible, to go out with clients when conducting an experiment about hypervigilance and selective attention so that two sets of information can be gathered to address beliefs.

Other Behavioral Strategies

Habit Reversal

Behavioral experiments are not the only behavioral interventions that are useful for clients with perfectionism. It may be the case that people with perfectionism are checking or avoiding and engaging in particular behaviors associated with perfectionism out of habit rather than due to any particularly strongly held beliefs. For example, Carol used to check that the corners of the bed were like "hospital corners," and the bed made "properly" a few times a day even though she was alone in the house. She said she did this automatically when she passed the bedroom door rather than from any belief that someone had gotten into the house and messed up the bed.

Habit reversal is a highly effective behavioral intervention to help decrease behaviors such as hair pulling that occur outside awareness. It was developed in the 1970s (Azrin & Nunn, 1973) and has been redeveloped recently by researchers in Canada and the United States (O'Connor et al., 2001; Piacentini & Chang, 2006). It can be used for people with perfectionism whose behaviors are driven by habit.

Habit reversal involves bringing the behavior (such as checking) into awareness. This is done by asking clients to describe in detail each time they carry out the behavior, or by asking others to notice when the person carries it out. The client may use self-monitoring to help identify early warning signs for the behavior and to identify the situations in which such behavior occurs.

The next step to habit reversal is to pair the habitual behavior with an incompatible one. If the behavior is hair pulling and the recording reveals that this is done whenever the client is in the bathroom, then the incompatible behavior is for the client to clench his or her fists prior to going into the bathroom. In the case of checking behavior, the incompatible behavior could be to look elsewhere when passing the bedroom so she doesn't see the bed and find herself checking it without fully realizing what she is doing. Other components of habit reversal may include contingency management, relaxation training, and training to help habit reversal generalize. More in-depth information about habit reversal can be found in treatment manuals for disorders such as Tourette syndrome (e.g., Woods & Miltenberger, 2001).

Graded Exposure

We have discussed the differences between graded exposure and behavioral experiments in Table 12.1 earlier in the chapter. The majority of the chapter has focused on behavioral experiments as we consider this to be the most appropriate and effective cognitive-behavioral intervention to test beliefs and bring about behavioral change. However, graded exposure is the mainstay of the majority of interventions for anxiety disorders and is shown to bring about belief change that is equal to other cognitive-behavioral interventions. If your client is highly anxious and avoiding situations is a primary symptom, it makes sense to incorporate graded exposure into treatment (see Abramowitz, Deacon, & Whiteside, 2011).

CHAPTER 13

Self-Evaluation and Self-Criticism

As we mentioned earlier, clinical perfectionism has been defined as "the overdependence of self-evaluation on the determined pursuit of personally demanding, self-imposed standards in at least one highly salient domain, despite adverse consequences" (Shafran et al., 2002, p. 778). The model of clinical perfectionism considers the overdependence to be a pivotal maintaining factor of perfectionism, along with one of the adverse consequences of perfectionism, namely self-criticism.

When self-worth is judged mainly in terms of the degree to which a person can achieve demanding or rigid standards, it is difficult to move away from the influence of clinical perfectionism. Therefore, one of the important objectives of therapy is to help clients address this overdependence and broaden their scheme for judging self-worth so it is less dependent on achievement and striving. While we have addressed this work indirectly in discussing the therapeutic processes described elsewhere in this book, it is also important to address overdependence directly if it has been identified as part of the personal formulation, and to address its adverse consequences, one of which is self-criticism. If a person with clinical perfectionism achieves a goal, he can criticize himself for not having "set the bar high enough" and thus minimize the achievement ("Anyone could have done it") or disregard it ("It doesn't count"), and thus draw no pleasure from it. As this process continues, inevitably the point will come when he sets the bar so high that the goal is not achievable.

On the other hand, if the goal is not achieved, either because the person tried but failed, or because he or she avoided the goal due to fear of failure or fear of discovery (e.g., "People will know I am no good," "I am a fake"), then self-criticism results or is strengthened. Self-criticism promotes the vicious cycle of clinical perfectionism, in that it weakens self-esteem and self-worth and impels a person even more strongly to prove him- or herself through ever higher levels of achievement. Therefore, another important objective of therapy is to help such a person respond to successes, failure, or avoidance with less self-criticism and a greater focus on self-compassion.

These two objectives of therapy are not quickly achieved, and require a gentle focus over a period of time. We expect to see gradual rather than rapid changes occur. The earlier in treatment these goals are introduced, the better. The assessment procedures discussed in Chapter 5 introduce these issues, and the collaborative formulation should allow for justification of these therapeutic objectives. In this chapter we look at two key strategies for reaching these objectives: *broadening self-evaluation* and *moving from a primarily self-critical stance to a more self-compassionate stance*. In broadening self-evaluation, there are four steps to consider with your client:

1. Compare the original assessment of the impact of performance on self-evaluation to the current situation.
2. Examine the pros and cons of the current situation.
3. Conduct a historical review of the origins and development of the overevaluation.
4. Directly alter the client's scheme for self-evaluation.

Much of our work on self-evaluation is informed by that of Christopher Fairburn and his colleagues in developing a CBT approach for eating disorders (Fairburn, 2008).

Similarly, there are five main steps in moving a client from a primarily self-critical stance to a more self-compassionate stance:

1. The identification of self-criticism and its pervasiveness.
2. Positive beliefs about the usefulness and value of self-criticism.
3. Identification of the costs of self-criticism.
4. Developing a self-compassionate and respectful response.
5. Practicing a new way of responding.

Broadening Self-Evaluation

Compare the Original Assessment of the Impact of Performance on Self-Evaluation to the Current Situation

The initial assessment of self-evaluation was previously outlined in Chapter 7. When starting this work you should help clients in session generate a pie chart that reflects how much each domain of their life influenced their judgment of their self-worth at the time they started therapy. The relative influence of such domains is indicated by how bad clients feel about themselves when things are not going well in that domain. Then the client should be asked to reflect on which of these domains are primarily influenced by achievement and meeting strict goals. These are typically the ones that, when they are not going well, tend to "poison" the other domains of life. An example of such a discussion is presented below in remarks by a therapist to a client called Serafina, along with a pie chart showing her current system of self-evaluation (Figure 13.1) (see also Handout 13.1 in Appendix 2):

> "People who are perfectionistic often demand higher levels of performance than it is actually possible to achieve and judge themselves or others based on their ability to perform to these high levels. Often, they judge themselves almost entirely by whether they meet their rigid, extreme standards. When we first met, you identified that the domain of your life that most impacted on you in this way was your university studies. You felt worthy when you were doing well in this area of your life. However, you generated such high and unobtainable standards that you expected yourself to meet (i.e., that you had to write the perfect assignment in one sitting) that typically you did not feel good about your university studies and therefore you did not feel good about yourself as a person. When this happened the bad effects started to flow over to other parts of your life, such as your friendships. You would avoid seeing friends because you felt that you couldn't be fun enough, and you also didn't want them to know that you were struggling emotionally. At these times you would also become less tolerant of the possibility of making mistakes in your part-time work as an administrative assistant and refuse to adopt new work systems in case they weren't 'right.' Also, eating became more problematic, as you would become more dissatisfied with your appearance and start on a strict dietary regime, and then start binge eating. When we put

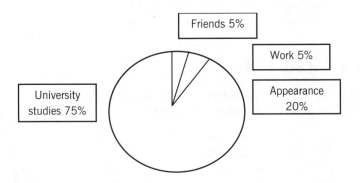

FIGURE 13.1. An initial assessment pie chart generated with Serafina about the domains of life in which performance influenced her self-evaluation.

this in a pie chart showing the domains of your life that you currently use to evaluate yourself and that impact on how worthy you feel as a person, we found that doing well at university studies took up most of the space, followed by appearance, with small slices left for friends and work."

Some people seeking help for perfectionism judge themselves based on their performance in multiple domains. An example of this is shown below with a client called Lauren, along with a pie chart showing her current system of self-evaluation (Figure 13.2):

"When we first met, you identified a number of domains of your life where meeting your rigid standards influenced your judgment about whether you were worthwhile as a person. This included your part-time university studies (getting less than top of the class made you feel bad about yourself), your part-time work as a fitness trainer (you needed to have all your clients keep returning for sessions or you felt like a failure), being a great mother (if you did not organize structured and interactive educational quality time with your 3-year-old daughter every day you felt that you were a bad mother), having a clean and tidy household at the end of each day (you felt that you would not be able to sleep if there was a mess because this would tell you that you were becoming a slack and lazy person), and maintaining the weight you had when you left high school (which has been really difficult, resulting in your feeling like a failure and leading to self-induced vomiting

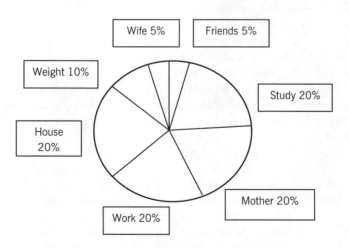

FIGURE 13.2. An initial assessment pie chart generated with Lauren about the domains of life in which performance influenced her self-evaluation.

most days when you feel that you have eaten too much). You felt that your studies, being a great mother and housekeeper, and work had the most impact on your self-evaluation. If things were going according to plan in these domains, then you felt able to enjoy downtime with your husband and friends, but if things were not going well, you would work harder in these domains and sacrifice time with your husband and friends. You also said you haven't done anything for yourself for a long time, such as a getting a massage, doing exercise, or just reading a book. When we put this in a pie chart showing the domains of your life that you currently use to evaluate yourself and the impact on how worthy you feel as a person, we found that performing to your standards as a student, mother, worker, and housekeeper took up most of the space, followed by weight, with small slices left for being a wife and friend."

Up to six sessions may have elapsed since this therapy began, so it is useful to allow the client to reflect on what (if anything) has changed since therapy began. For example, the client may have noticed that self-evaluation is starting to be impacted by domains that are not performance related, that the domains in the pie chart have become less dependent on performance, or that he or she has become interested in pursuing new domains in life that are not performance based. For example, Serafina noticed that she is more grateful for her friends and their support and what this says about her worth as a person, as well as adopting more of an "exploration of ideas rather than getting it right the first time" approach in her studies. Lauren reported that she enjoyed unstructured play time with her daughter on one occasion and noticed that her daughter was more physically affectionate than usual during this time. She has also managed to leave the house "untidied" at the end of the day on two occasions, and was surprised by how much more relaxed her husband was on these occasions, which helped her to reflect that maybe she was better company when less focused on getting things done. This has made her wonder if she and her husband should arrange for babysitting on some occasions so that they could go for walks in the country, something they used to enjoy doing together but have not done for a long time.

As part of clarifying the current system of self-evaluation and exploring some of the disadvantages, it can be useful to employ self-monitoring around this issue for a week. This has the advantage of making clients more fully aware of what currently impacts on their self-evaluation, and, importantly, how adversely this can affect them. The urgency for change can become stronger through this process. A self-monitoring sheet completed by Lauren over a 2-day period is shown in Figure 13.3 (see also Handout 13.2 in Appendix 2).

Day	What area did you use to evaluate yourself?	Record the thoughts that you had about evaluating yourself.	Describe how you felt and rate the intensity of the feelings from 0 (low) to 100 (high).
Mon	Household tidiness	If I don't get this mess tidied up then I am a second-rate person who can't keep her life in control	Angry with daughter and husband for making the mess (75), guilty at feeling angry (80), felt bad for telling off daughter (85)
Mon	Ate 2 slices of bread at lunch when I had only intended to have one	If I can't exercise control over this small area of my life then I am weak and despicable	Guilty (100) Sad that this matters so much to me when I have so many more important things to focus on (80)
Tues	Class assignment— received second-highest mark in class	I am incapable of being the best; there is something wrong with me	Emptiness (85) Frustration (90)
Tues	Mother—tried to engage my daughter in a nature lesson in the garden but she wanted to draw instead	If she can't be provided with a stimulating learning environment at home before starting school, then I am a bad mother	Frustration (90) Anxiety (75) Stress (85)

FIGURE 13.3. Self-monitoring of self-evaluation.

Examine the Pros and Cons of the Current Situation

If there have been some changes since the beginning of therapy, this can provide useful information for a discussion of the pros and cons of allowing self-evaluation to be primarily influenced by achieving rigid (i.e., all-or-nothing) and extreme standards. Start with a discussion about the advantages of the current system for self-evaluation. Often, clients will suggest that focusing so much on achievement allows them to achieve more than others, or at least as much as others. The discussion about the disadvantages of the current situation should explore whether this is always true and whether there have been times when this has in fact made them achieve less than others. In the case of Serafina, she could see clearly that when she felt unable to turn out the perfect piece of university work in one sitting she often delayed handing in the work until the last moment, when she would dash something off or indeed did not hand it in at all. This had caused her to fail one year, so not only was she behind her peers in terms of her progress at school, but her marks were consistently average, and not in the A range to which she aspired. She also felt that life that was leaving her behind, as her strategy meant that she had fewer intimate relationships with others than she had hoped for at this stage of her life, and that failure at university had made her try to compensate with achieving rigid standards in other areas of her life (weight and work), which made her feel more depressed with her life.

In the case of Lauren, she felt that her organized approach to life that used every minute maximally allowed her to keep control of her busy life and that people looked up to her as she got so much more out of life. However, when she looked at the people who mattered in her life (husband, daughter, friends, family), she admitted that her organized approach was sometimes difficult to live with and could cause some exasperation, impacting adversely on the quality of these relationships. Generation of the disadvantages can also be considerably enhanced by consideration of what clients have experienced with the changes they have made so far. In the case of Lauren, she had noted that both her daughter and husband were more relaxed when she was less organized and seemed to enjoy her company more. She also noted that when she had not tidied up at the end of the day, her worst fear (i.e., that the next day would be completely out of control) had not come true.

While some disadvantages of the current situation will be generated by the client, you should take an active role in introducing and exploring possible disadvantages, including:

• Over time has the client been feeling better or worse about him- or herself? Does this relate to the setting of demanding and unrealistic goals that can often be arbitrary or misinformed (as explored previously in the psychoeducation section of Chapter 9), and in fact make no difference in performance or diminish performance? When the client feels worse, does this enhance or diminish performance?

• Is the client living his or her life in the way he or she might want for a child, close relative, or friend? If not, why not?

• Is there something about the ways others live their lives that is not related to achievement and that the client feels he or she is missing out on or has stopped noticing? Have other important areas of life been marginalized or neglected? How has this impacted on the client's development as a person?

• If people judge their self-worth by the attainment of goals that are not always realistic or under their control, then this ensures that their self-esteem will be a victim to circumstance. For example, consider elite athletes who work hard to ensure high-level performance and think about how many times you have heard of injuries or psychological blocks that have occurred and interfered with their ability to attain their goals. If achievement in this one area primarily determines their self-worth, then they have nothing left to feel good about. It is what Christopher Fairburn (2008) refers to as "having all your eggs in one basket" (p. 99), which places self-evaluation continually at risk of being damaged. The more areas of life clients build their self-worth on, the more robust self-worth will be.

Review the Origins and Development of the Overevaluation

It is useful to engage in a thorough historical review of why clients have become sensitized to their performance, thus continually raising standards, instituting rigid rules, and focusing on achievement as a primary way of judging self-worth. The sensitization may have developed for a variety of reasons, and it is not unusual for a train of events to appear relevant. This process should be done collaboratively with the therapist leading the client through the various topics of potential relevance. This can sometimes lead to discussion of events that the client has experienced as quite traumatic or emotionally distressing, and you need to work sensitively and empathically in dealing with these topics. Among the various subjects to cover are the following:

- Family history: family values concerning achievement, family history of clinical perfectionism.
- Personal history: personal history of concerns about performance, family expectations to succeed (family comparisons), pressures to perform to a high standard, critical comments from significant others about performance, benefits that have come from striving to achieve, adverse effects that have arisen, fear of failure, devoting too much time to achievement, avoidance of tests of performance (i.e., procrastination), exposure to unusual pressures to perform in specific environments (e.g., in certain schools or occupations such as professional dance or music).

As part of this discussion, it can be useful to have the client fill out a historical review chart, as shown in Figure 13.4 for Serafina.

When going through the historical review, we are working to help clients value the lessons they have learned (i.e., it is important to achieve, it makes me feel more worthwhile) while strengthening bigger-picture thinking (i.e., achievement is only one of many things that makes me feel better about myself) and cognitive flexibility (i.e., one rule won't fit all situations, all-or-nothing rules just cause more problems than they solve). The primary goal of this historical review is to help clients distance themselves from

Age	Event or circumstance that sensitized me to performance	Thoughts I developed about striving, performance, and perfectionism
5 to 12 years	My older brother was at the top of his class at school, my parents were always comparing my academic performance unfavorably to his.	You have to be the best to be acceptable. Only the top mark is good enough.
13 years	Came out at the top of the class with an A in my essay—when I told my dad he looked at me and asked, "why didn't you get A+?"	I am not good enough;I have to try harder.
14 to 17 years	When I didn't hand things in on time, the teachers would work with me to get the assignment finished.	I am incapable of completing a quality product on my own. I am a fake.
18 years to present	Competition at university, reluctant to have my work and lack of knowledge scrutinized.	If I can't do the best work in the class there is no point in handing it in.

FIGURE 13.4. Historical review of the development of Serafina's sensitization to achievement.

excessive reliance on performance in the present time and, importantly, be able to separate themselves from unhelpful messages and make choices about principles they can use to guide their current life choices. This process can lead to the further generation of pros and cons (especially the latter), when considering if the client has adopted someone else's judgements that he or she no longer needs to live up to or believes in.

Unhelpful thoughts that remain currently active can be discussed and alternative beliefs explored. It may be important in some cases to examine the reinterpretation of past experiences or events from the vantage point of the present. There may also be imagery accompanying some of these historical events that is distressing to the client (e.g., of being teased or ridiculed) and that contributes to current concerns. A body of experimental research has found that imagery has a greater impact on both negative and positive mood than verbal processing (e.g., Holmes & Mathews, 2010; Holmes, Mathews, Dalgleish, & Mackintosh, 2006). In such cases imagery rescripting may be useful (Arntz & Weertman, 1999), as it has been shown to reduce distress associated with past memories and negative affect associated with current imagery (Nilsson, Lundh, & Viborg, 2012). This process and its rationale should be explained fully to clients before it is used with them.

Imagery rescripting involves three phases: reliving, mastering, and compassion. During the reliving phase the client is instructed to imagine the memory at the age that it happened as if it were happening now. The client can describe the event to the therapist in the present tense (e.g., "Suzie is grabbing the test from me and I am shouting at her to give it back. She looks at the mark and then starts shouting in a singsong voice, 'Paul failed his test! Paul failed his test!' Everyone in the playground can hear. I feel humiliated. I just want to sink into the ground"). Mastering involves instructing the client to imagine the same scene as a bystander at his or her current age. Clients are instructed to watch what is happening to their younger self, describe their adult bystander reactions, and suggest how they could help their younger self to feel more secure or to act in a more assertive way (e.g., "I would ask Suzie to come to me, talk to her calmly and firmly about the inappropriateness of her bullying behavior, and take the test from her and return it to the other child. I would ask Suzie to apologize," or "I would instruct the child to ignore such an unpleasant bully, and to walk away and find some other children to play with"). The compassion phase involves the client being asked to relive the memory as his or her younger self with the adult self present and to explore what actions would be necessary for the younger self to feel better (in line with extra nurturing and compassion) and to ask for this. The use of compassion will be explored further later in this chapter.

An example of imagery rescripting using positive imagery can be seen in the case of Tim, whom you may remember from Chapters 10 and 11, who had perfectionism related to his work and a great deal of worry over his presentation and public speaking skills. In the course of addressing cognitive strategies with Tim, the therapist found that he had a specific distressing image related to a memory of being ridiculed as a child by a teacher in front of a class. Tim recalled that he was around 12 years of age and he had to read aloud in front of the class. He remembered that his teacher laughed at him and called him stupid when he mispronounced some words, and he had an image of himself back in the situation feeling very small, shaking and feeling ashamed. The therapist helped Tim to rescript the image by imagining himself back in the situation, standing tall and proud, and speaking clearly. He also imagined speaking back to his teacher and letting him know that he was not stupid, that he would go on to graduate at the top of his class in engineering, have a successful job, and a great family life with a loving wife and children. With the help of his therapist, he finished off the image on a positive note by imagining his teacher becoming small and fading into the background of the image, and he and the other children laughing at the teacher as he faded off into the distance like a deflating balloon. Tim described feeling very positive after this image, as he knew that his teacher was a bully to him and other children, but the upsetting image had stuck with him throughout his life. While further research is required to determine the efficacy of imagery interventions for perfectionism, the incorporation of imagery rescripting may hold promise for reducing the distressing images regarding performance that often accompany perfectionism.

The historical review process can also lead the client to generate some further disadvantages of overevaluating oneself based on achievement (e.g., "I am focusing on just one aspect of me and not the whole person," "I am ignoring or dismissing all the effort that I put into various tasks," "I bully myself to get things done in a certain way and it makes me feel bad"). As further pros and cons are generated, they should be added to the client's list. One way of making more salient the idea that reinterpretation of past experiences or events can provide benefit from the vantage point of the present is to complete another historical review, this time with events that support the alternative perspective: "Being worthwhile as a person is about more than striving and achievement."

Directly Alter the Client's Scheme for Self-Evaluation

To reduce the overevaluation of striving and achievement, the emphasis of the work with clients is to help them base some of their self-worth on areas of life that are independent of achievement, and that are based on who they are and their intrinsic worth as a person. To this end, it is important to help the client work on three related goals: (1) expand the current domains that contribute to the client's scheme for self-evaluation that are not performance based, (2) introduce new domains in life that are not performance based, and (3) decrease the extent to which performance impacts on self-evaluation in the domains that have most influence on self-worth. This latter goal is partly addressed in the second half of this chapter and also addressed in Chapters 10–12. In this section we discuss working on the first two goals with the client. The hope is that if clients are engaged in a broader range of activities and interests that are not reliant on performance, then these will assume more importance in the client's life, thereby displacing achievement as the primary factor in their scheme for self-evaluation.

It is useful to ask the clients to draw an alternative pie chart that shows more emphasis on multiple life domains (e.g., family, work, friends, home, school, relationships, role as father, mother, daughter, or son, sports, community participation, spirituality) that are less reliant on achievement, and that resembles something they would like to see happen in their lives within a 6-month period. To do this, you help clients identify activities and interests they might like to become more engaged in, especially ones of an interpersonal nature that are independent of achievement. Discussing areas they used to enjoy but have given up is also an important aspect of this discussion. As can be seen in the case presented below, the formation of this alternative pie chart is interwoven with behavioral experiments and further revision of the pie chart in light of these experiences.

After exploring these issues, Serafina felt that she would like to shrink the importance of university studies to 50% rather than the current 75% of the pie. As part of this discussion, she reasoned that her university studies would have an important impact on her future life options, but she also recognized that she wasn't learning very much given her avoidance of feedback, and she felt that she would like to be more open to getting feedback so she could enjoy the process of learning and broadening her perspectives. A behavioral experiment was set up in which Serafina agreed to attend the statistics tutorial that she had been avoiding, to ask one question of the instructor, and observe his reaction and the degree to which this helped her learning. She was pleasantly surprised—the instructor had commented that it was a good question and answered it enthusiastically and at length, and other students later commented to Serafina that they had been wondering about the same issue. She also felt that her understanding of the issue had progressed considerably, and she felt less alone in her studies.

The discussion then moved on to any activities that Serafina had once enjoyed but had been dropped. Serafina immediately offered that horseback riding had been a very enjoyable activity for her, not so much because of the achievement but because she enjoyed the freedom and sensation of riding and was very fond of animals. While this particular option was too expensive for Serafina to return to, she was asked to think about any voluntary activities involving animals that she would be interested in pursuing. Over a few weeks, Serafina contacted a local animal shelter (for cats and dogs) and started doing a few hours of volunteer work each week, which was enjoyable to her and made her feel good about herself because she felt that the activity made a real difference in the animals' quality of life.

Serafina also mentioned that she used to attend a church youth group when she was a teenager but had ceased attending when she started university. She was interested in attending a different church as she felt that she would like to keep exploring the role of God and spirituality in her life, even though she was not sure about what her beliefs were. Over the course of therapy, Serafina attended two or three different churches and had not yet made up her mind as to whether this would be a long-term feature in her life, but she enjoyed thinking and reading about the issues as she felt that this broadened her perspective about herself and life.

Finally, when looking at some domains that had small sections in her pie chart (friends, work, and appearance), Serafina thought that it would be useful to broaden her focus on friends and her part-time work as a personal trainer. She recognized that she needed to maintain ongoing quality contact with friends despite how she was feeling, and that at times her friends really appreciated her sharing her problems with them. They felt that she was treating them as a true friend, and this also gave them the opportunity to share some of their issues with her. At work, Serafina experimented with trying out new systems and evaluating how useful this was for work efficiency. When returning to the revised pie chart, Serafina felt that 50% for university studies was too much and reassigned allocations as shown in Figure 13.5.

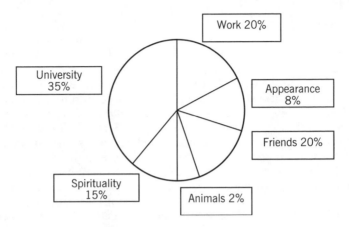

FIGURE 13.5. Serafina's revised pie chart of the domains contributing to self-evaluation.

You should strongly encourage clients to engage in a broad range of activities that are not reliant on achievement for self-evaluation and thus do not reinforce clients' tendencies to evaluate themselves based on achievement—therapists should avoid falling into the trap of encouraging clients to take part in activities they do not enjoy or are not good at. Such activities are not relevant to broadening the scheme for self-evaluation as they are not valued, and they can also negatively affect the therapeutic relationship. If you think it would be useful for a client to have the experience of engaging in activities he or she is not good at, this should be done in the context of challenging beliefs with a behavioral experiment. In order to help the client engage in a broad range of activities, ask them to complete a pie chart with a focus on self-evaluation using the new domains or non-performance-based domains. An example of how this was used for Serafina is shown in Figure 13.6.

Troubleshooting: What to Do When Clients Are in Environments That Emphasize Perfectionism

Workshop participants commonly want to know what to do about the person who has "perfectionism imposed upon them" in a certain domain. A case example is a professional ballet dancer who, despite a history of having anorexia nervosa from which she had recovered, was required to be below a weight that she could maintain without disordered eating to stay in the dance company. While all avenues should be explored for trying to resolve this situation, realistically there are some pressures that are unable to be negotiated around. In this case the difficult questions have to be asked. Does this domain need to be removed from your life? Can it be transformed to another domain that is less destructive (e.g., becoming a teacher of dance, joining a dance company that specializes in a style of dance that requires athleticism rather than a specific shape or weight)? A full understanding of the advantages and disadvantages of retaining this domain needs to be explored, as do the disadvantages and advantages of transforming or removing it. Then it can be useful to "collapse time"—look at what life would look like across different domains (e.g., work, health, emotions, intimate relationships, friendships, finances, relationships with significant others, hobbies, community involvement) in 5 years' time if this domain were retained, and if it were transformed/removed.

Day	What area did you use to evaluate yourself?	Record the thoughts that you had about evaluating yourself.	Describe how you felt and rate the intensity of the feelings from 0 (low) to 100 (high).
Mon	Friends—met Sarah for coffee at university	It is great to have such a loyal friend as Sarah—she is interested in me and cares about me and enjoys my company.	Happiness (50) Content (60)
Tues	2 hours of volunteering at the animal shelter	The people here really appreciate the gift of my time and the dogs love my company—they don't care what I have or haven't done.	Happiness (80) Feeling at peace (30)
Wed	3 hours of class at university	When I ask questions, usually someone else has the same question, which means that I am being (1) brave for asking and (2) wise enough to know what we need to know more about.	Less lonely (65) Competent (40) Courageous (80) A bit stupid (20)

FIGURE 13.6. Broadening self-evaluation worksheet completed by Serafina.

Moving from Self-Criticism to Self-Compassion

Identify Self-Criticism and Its Pervasiveness

The self-critical voice may have become so established in the client's life that he or she has difficulty actually identifying it or seeing it as something that can be changed. It can be useful to assess self-criticism using the *Dysfunctional Attitude Scale* (DAS; Weissman & Beck, 1978), where many of the items are similar to those of the concern over mistakes (CM) scale from the FMPS (Frost et al., 1990). Examples of items are: "If I don't set the highest standards for myself, I am likely to end up a second-rate person" and "If I am to be a worthwhile person, I must be truly outstanding in at least one major respect." Assessment of self-critical perfectionism (Clara, Cox, & Enns, 2007) shows that this factor is also indicated by the socially prescribed perfectionism (SPP) subscale from the HMPS (Hewitt & Flett, 1991b) and the self-criticism subscale from the *Depressive Experiences Questionnaire* (Blatt, D'Afflitti, & Quinlan, 1976).

The nature of self-critical self-commentary should also be discussed with the client to aid in identification of this type of thinking. Self-criticism is, by nature, like an internal critic or bully—a voice in one's head that continually points out faults. One of the hallmarks of the critical voice is that it makes personal judgments (e.g., "you are a complete failure") and indulges in name-calling (e.g., "you are . . . bad, a fake, hopeless, a loser, useless, a failure"). In addition, you can return to the self-monitoring first introduced in Handout 13.2 and help the client identify which were the self-critical thoughts, and to what degree these thoughts have more adverse consequences than other types of thoughts.

Identifying self-critical assumptions can also be useful in session using the downward-arrow technique. Situations that have arisen over therapy that provoked strong negative feelings can be discussed with the client, and common underlying assumptions explored. For example, in the case of Gina, a 16-year-old student with type 1 diabetes, three situations were explored with the downward-arrow technique as shown in Figure 13.7 (see also Handout 13.3 in Appendix 2). As can be seen, Gina was experiencing intense self-loathing and her self-critical thoughts always drew her to the conclusion that she was useless and worthless across a variety of situations—the worksheet helped identify this as a particular "tag" for her self-critical voice.

Explore Beliefs about the Usefulness of Self-Criticism

A client is likely to argue that without self-criticism, he or she would become lazy, ordinary, or second rate. Clients often see self-criticism as a

Situation 1: Asked to babysit for a new family	Situation 2: Exam due tomorrow	Situation 3: Used insulin as prescribed
Feeling: anxious	**Feeling:** anxious	**Feeling:** guilty and anxious
Thought: They won't like me and I won't do a good job.	**Thought:** I haven't studied enough; I am going to fail.	**Thought:** I shouldn't do that again.
First question: What does it mean if this happens?	**First question:** What does it mean if this happens?	**First question:** What does it mean if this happens?
Answer: It will all go badly and they won't want me back again.	**Answer:** I am going to look stupid.	**Answer:** That is just what you deserve.
Second question: If that was true, what would that mean about you?	**Second question:** If that was true, what would that mean about you?	**Second question:** If that was true, what would that mean about you?
Answer: I'm not likeable and I am useless.	**Answer:** I am incapable and don't deserve to do well.	**Answer:** I am disgusting, unlovable, and undeserving.
Third question: What is the "if . . . then . . ." statement?	**Third question:** What is the "if . . . then . . ." statement?	**Third question:** What is the "if . . . then . . ." statement?
Answer: If people don't like me, then it just proves I am pathetic and unlikable. If I don't do a good job, then I am useless.	**Answer:** Unless I do well, I am stupid and useless and undeserving.	**Answer:** If I don't take care of myself, then that is treating myself as worthless, which is what I am.

FIGURE 13.7. The downward-arrow technique examining assumptions involving self-criticism.

motivation to work hard, stay on task, and achieve more. They say that it "keeps them on their toes." Self-criticism may be viewed as a good sign, or an indicator that an individual is committed to self-improvement and has an open mind. There may be a belief that being less critical will lead to smugness, self-indulgence, boasting, and becoming big-headed. This style of thinking has been around for centuries, as typified by the quote from Catherine of Siena (1347–1380) first provided in Chapter 3 and repeated here, indicating that the road to growth is through self-criticism: "Make a supreme effort to root out self-love from your heart and to plant in its place this holy self-hatred. This is the royal road by which we turn our backs on mediocrity, and which leads us without fail to the summit of perfection."

It is important to differentiate between constructive criticism/feedback and self-criticism. Discuss with the client that setting goals and standards to achieve is a normal part of life, and that growth is obtained through receiving and adapting in response to feedback. However self-criticism involves becoming very critical of *yourself as a person and your value as a person* when you don't meet your personal standards. Making this point can be aided by the use of the parable shown in the box "Which Coach Would You Choose?" The example uses basketball but it is likely to be most helpful if you can choose an activity or sport that has most relevance for your client.

WHICH COACH WOULD YOU CHOOSE?

Imagine that as a parent you took your daughter along to coaching sessions to teach her to play basketball. It has always been your child's dream to play basketball well, so she is really excited and determined to try hard in the lessons. Now imagine that your daughter has lessons under three different coaches: Coach Moe, Coach Larry, and Coach Curly.

Coach Moe does not say anything every time your child bounces and throws the ball. However, when she drops the ball or misses a catch, Coach Moe calls her names, such as a "wimp," "pathetic," and "useless." He says that unless your daughter can play faultlessly, she will be considered as an inferior person and blackballed by the team.

Coach Larry is quite a different type of person, and welcomes everyone to the team. Regardless of performance on the court, he praises every player lavishly, only gives them feedback on what they do well, and ignores any problems with their basketball technique.

Coach Curly is different again. He does not tell your daughter off every time she drops the ball but rather encourages her and says she is doing well when she catches the ball, and says things like "It is okay to make mistakes because it helps us to learn how to do it better." He takes time with each player at the end of the game to emphasize what he or she did well and what needs to be improved. He gives each player specific skills to work on over the week to facilitate performance.

Now, which coach would you choose to teach your child? Why? Importantly, which coach do you think would get a better performance out of your child—Coach Moe, Coach Larry, or Coach Curly?

Adapted from Hoffman and Otto (2008). Copyright 2008 by Routledge. Adapted by permission.

Troubleshooting: Self-Criticism

When discussing beliefs about the usefulness of self-criticism, you may notice that the client starts to criticize himself for using self-criticism! As part of discussing the pros and cons of self-criticism, it is important to use validation, discussed in Chapter 8. You can communicate to the client that these current responses make sense within his current and past life experiences. It may be that the client was raised under the "spare the rod and spoil the child" philosophy, where faults were highlighted and achievements downplayed, and he has adopted this system for himself, but needs to practice cognitive flexibility to decide when it makes sense to apply this rule. This offers you a chance in the therapy session to work through rigid and unhelpful rules with the client.

Identify the Costs of Self-Criticism

Although clients should first be invited to speculate on the costs of self-criticism in their own lives, they may find it difficult to step outside their current framework to do this. Therefore, you should also provide psychoeducation on the costs of self-criticism. In her book *Overcoming Low Self-Esteem*, Melanie Fennell (1999) lists a number of the costs of self-criticism. Two of these are highlighted below.

Self-Criticism Paralyzes You, Blocks Your Learning, and Makes You Feel Bad

This idea can be explored using a number of behavioral experiments. Fennell suggests two such experiments, the first involving having the client look at a list of critical words (e.g., *incompetent, ugly, unlikable, pathetic, worthless, useless*) for a few minutes and noting what happens to his or her mood using "before" and "after" ratings. The second is using imagery to focus on a person the client knows and perceives as being talented and self-confident, and imagining that this person is followed around for weeks by a self-critical imp who is always calling him or her names, pointing out mistakes, criticizing performance, and ignoring any achievements. What does the client think will happen over time in the face of this unrelenting barrage? How does the client think the person might feel? What might happen to the individual's confidence and ability to cope and succeed in life?

Another behavioral experiment that can be powerful (in either a group or individual therapy context) involves a version of the game Twenty Questions. In a group context, one person is sent outside and the group agrees on an object. The person is brought back in to ask questions that can only have a "yes" or "no" answer in order to guess the object. Unbeknownst to the person who has the task of guessing, on the first occasion the group is instructed to be empathic, encouraging, and constructive (e.g., "not quite, but it was a good guess: you're getting closer"), and on the second occasion the group is instructed to be critical (e.g., "that is a stupid suggestion; don't be so useless; this is taking a really long time"). Ask the person to reflect on the difference between these two situations in terms of feelings that were triggered, the ability to think clearly, and the ability to come up with the solution. The group can also reflect on how this felt for them and what they noticed about the person's ability to provide an answer. Typically the person takes a lot longer to guess the answer under the second condition, and the implications for the impact of self-criticism can then be discussed. This discussion can be linked in with the psychoeducation about self-criticism provided in Chapter 9.

Self-Criticism Is Unfair and Ignores the Realities

The nature of self-criticism is that it unilaterally judges the person for a specific mistake or weakness with respect to a specific area or task. It also ignores legitimate and important reasons why mistakes were made (e.g., being tired or preoccupied with another issue, not having all the information required to make an informed decision). The client can be asked to judge how fair this is by imagining doing this to another person. It can also be useful to discuss how consistent self-criticism is with the values that the client holds to be important in terms of how others should be treated. Some commonly held values are shown in Figure 13.8 , but clients should

Acceptance: To accept my friends no matter what they do	Caring: To be caring toward others	Compassion: To feel concern for others
Courtesy: To be polite and considerate to others	Forgiveness: To be forgiving of others	Generosity: To give people the benefit of the doubt
Helpfulness: To be helpful to others	Hope: To keep believing in my friends	Fun: To have fun with friends and share a sense of humor with them
Justice: To treat my friends fairly	Service: To be of service to others	Respect: To treat my friends with respect and not put them down

FIGURE 13.8. Values that guide how others should be treated. Adapted from Shafran, Egan, and Wade (2010). Copyright 2010 by Constable & Robinson. Adapted by permission.

generate their own values and assess how self-criticism measures up against each one of these (see also Handout 13.4 in Appendix 2).

After these discussions, clients can be invited to summarize the issues discussed and discovered as a written "impact statement," such as is used in cognitive processing therapy with people who have experienced a traumatic event (Resick & Schnicke, 1996). This entails writing their thoughts about why self-criticism developed in their life, the impact it has had on themselves and others, and the ways the event involved has influenced their beliefs about themselves, others, and the world. It is helpful if the client can read this impact statement out loud in session, and the content and meaning can be further discussed, focusing on potential "stuck points" that interfere with moving from a self-critical stance to a more self-compassionate one.

Develop a Self-Compassionate and Respectful Response

When introducing the client to the alternative to self-criticism, the idea of self-compassion can be explored. Self-compassion is a construct that can be used by the client to guide the development of new responses. While various definitions of self-compassion exist, Kristen Neff (2003) refers to a three-dimensional definition, where each positive facet has a companion negative facet, a structure supported in studies of teenagers and young adults (Neff, 2003; Raes, Pommier, Neff, & Van Gucht, 2011). The first dimension is self-kindness, or treating oneself kindly and tolerating perceived inadequacies, coupled with self-judgment, an intolerance for perceived inadequacies. The second dimension is a common sense of humanity, or seeing suffering as a unifying aspect of the human experience, coupled with isolation, or a sense of being alone with one's suffering or inadequacies. The third dimension is mindfulness, acknowledging internal affective states in a nonjudgmental fashion, coupled with overidentification with these affective states.

Self-compassion has been shown to buffer people against negative emotionality after adverse life events (Leary, Tate, Adams, Allen, & Hancock, 2007) and mediates the relationship between MBCT and reductions in depressive symptoms (Kuyken et al., 2010). Self-compassion has been found to buffer against negative self-evaluation in people who have low self-esteem (Leary et al., 2007) and is more strongly related than mindfulness to lower levels of psychopathology and higher levels of well-being (Van Dam, Sheppard, Forsyth, & Earleywine, 2011). It is positively associated with mastery goals (which involve the aim of improving one's own performance), and negatively associated with performance goals (which reflect the pursuit of outperforming others), as well as being associated with fewer avoidance-oriented strategies in the face of perceived academic failure (Neff, Hsieh, & Dejitterat, 2005).

To help clients develop some self-compassionate responses that they can road test, we suggest working with the client in session to generate a range of responses that are written down and "ranked" by the client with respect to how helpful the responses are likely to be (e.g., from most helpful to least helpful). Techniques for generating these self-compassionate responses include formulating responses from an "arm's length" view, therapeutic letter writing from the view of a compassionate other, asking key questions to generate alternatives, using an ideal image of compassion, using surveys, and cultivating a stance of acceptance.

Formulating Responses from an "Arm's Length" View

First return to the self-monitoring that has been done over the course of therapy to date and generate self-compassionate responses from the view of self-kindness, common humanity, and mindfulness. Use Socratic questioning and avoid placing words in the client's mouth. It is highly likely that clients will have great difficulty generating alternative responses, so helping them to take an "arm's length" approach may be helpful (e.g., "what would you say if a close friend was expressing the same self-critical thought" or

Self-critical thought	Exercising self-kindness	Exercising common humanity	Exercising mindfulness
If people don't like me, then it just proves I am pathetic and unlikable.	Not everyone will like me, but I have people who love me.	No one is completely unlikable.	This critical voice just focuses on the bad and doesn't look at the whole picture—the good and the not-so-good bits about me.
Unless I do well at studying, then I am stupid and useless and undeserving.	Not doing well at studying doesn't make me a bad person.	Everyone fails something at some stage, and they aren't lesser people because of it—in fact, failure can promote growth.	The times when I don't do well need to be viewed as part of the total picture of what I have achieved to date.
If I don't take care of myself, then that is treating me as worthless, which is what I am.	Focus on my positive aspects instead of the negative.	I am allowed to feel well—it is a basic human right like being able to breathe.	Thoughts are not always true—I don't need to listen to the critic.

FIGURE 13.9. Generating self-compassionate responses.

"what might someone who cares about you say in response to your critical thought?"). Alternatively, return to the values that the client rated as being most important, and ask how these values would look if applied to the client him- or herself. In Figure 13.9 (see also Handout 13.5 in Appendix 2), we look at the types of responses generated by Gina in response to the self-critical thoughts identified in Figure 13.7. Gina found this work quite difficult and was rather dismissive of the potential usefulness of these responses because "she didn't believe them; they were just made up." She was asked to write down some of the key self-compassionate phrases on a small piece of cardboard, carry it around with her for the next week, and read them regularly. When she returned for her next appointment, she said that she was surprised at how much the responses had helped her mood and how they "seemed a lot less stupid" than they had the week before.

Therapeutic Letter Writing from the Point of View of a Compassionate Other

This approach has previously been adopted in work with eating disorders (Schmidt, Bone, Hems, Lessem, & Treasure, 2002). A specific situation or event is chosen to write about, and four short letters are written about it. The first is from the perspective of the client and describes what happened, how the individual felt about it, and the self-critical thoughts that were associated with it. The second is written from the perspective of a close friend who describes the event and its interpretation in a kind and loving manner. The third letter is written by someone the client knows and respects who describes the situation in a manner that is balanced and fair toward the client. Finally, a letter is written by someone who is perceived as being compassionate and wise (e.g., the Dalai Lama or Mother Teresa), and whose view of the incident has the focus of a world view that is kind, loving, and honest.

There are some important principles to emphasize for this type of writing (Wade & Schmidt, 2009):

1. Writing should go for no longer than 20 minutes at one sitting (so for the exercise described above, around 5 minutes should be allocated per letter).
2. Potential topics should be discussed with the therapist beforehand so that any upsetting subject matter can be set up in a safe way.
3. The same basic content or information should be included in each perspective—it is changing perspectives and trying to see it from another person's point of view that is important.
4. There should be no gaps in time between writing the different perspectives—the writing should flow immediately from one perspective to the next.

Troubleshooting: Overcoming Obstacles to Therapeutic Writing

Be sure to explore potential obstacles to therapeutic writing. Clients struggling with perfectionism may find it difficult to write something because of concerns about negative judgment. Discuss the rationale and practicalities of writing with the client, with a brief explanation of the scientific basis of expressive writing (which indicates it can help alleviate low mood and improve health outcomes, e.g., Sexton & Pennebaker, 2009). We tell clients they are not expected to produce A-quality essays and that the more open and honest with themselves they can be, the more useful the exercise will be. Clients are asked to write continuously and spontaneously in order to minimize internal censorship, and we encourage them to engage with the task fully.

Using Key Questions to Generate Alternatives

Melanie Fennell (1999) provides a list of questions to identify cognitive biases in self-critical thinking (p. 115) that can be helpful for the client to address, including: "What is the evidence?," "What alternative perspectives are there?," "What is the effect of thinking about myself in this way?," and "What are my biases in thinking about myself?" (e.g., "Am I condemning myself as a person on the basis of a single event?" "Am I blaming myself for things that are really not my fault?").

Using an Ideal Image of Compassion

This technique comes from Paul Gilbert's compassionate mind training (Gilbert & Irons, 2005). Clients are invited to spend time visualizing the age, appearance, facial expression, postures, and inner emotions of their ideal compassionate image. Clients are asked to record these characteristics in a written format, and then imagine that a self-compassionate part of themselves could be thought of as a person. They are then asked to slowly visualize themselves becoming that person. This exercise is followed up by a letter-writing exercise from the perspective of this self-compassionate person, recognizing their own positive qualities, achievements (no matter how small), the challenges they have faced, the skills and talents they have developed, and the aspects of their personality that have helped them thus far and are appreciated by others.

Surveys

As outlined in Chapter 9, surveys are a flexible tool and are set up individually with the client. You should work with the client to devise a survey that examines what others say to themselves when they face an experience of failure or disappointment in the achievement of goals. Those surveyed should include people who are respected by the client or who are perceived as being high achievers.

Cultivating a Stance of Acceptance

Metacognitive acceptance plays a significant role within the broader practice of mindfulness and denotes the ability to experience thoughts, feelings, and physical sensations without making judgments or evaluations and without the need to avoid, change, or control them (Baer, 2003). A relationship exists between the use of acceptance techniques and decreased negative mood (Singer & Dobson, 2007, 2009). In terms of its application to self-critical thoughts, the client can be instructed as follows:

> "Notice the critical thoughts and voice—observe what they look like— and then you can let them go. One way of doing this is to think of these thoughts as if they were projected on the screen at the cinema. You sit, watching the screen, waiting for thoughts or images to arise. When they do you pay attention to them so long as they are there 'on the screen' and then let them go as they pass away."

These techniques have been further outlined in work related to MBCT (Segal et al., 2013).

This approach may not be for everyone. Our own research on body dissatisfaction shows that while acceptance works well to decrease negative affect, it was only used by around two-thirds of the people studied, whereas the remainder used cognitive reappraisal, positive thinking or reassurance, avoidance, problem solving, or overthinking despite receiving detailed instructions about the use of acceptance strategies (Atkinson & Wade, 2012). Nonengagement with acceptance strategies was not a random event but rather was predicted by higher levels of negative affect, emotion regulation difficulties, and avoidant coping. However, some clients prefer this approach to generating alternative thoughts. For example, Gina experienced especially strong feelings of self-loathing, and found it helpful to write the following responses to the self-critical voice in her self-monitoring: "Thoughts are just thoughts. They are not always right and I don't have to listen to them."

Practice a New Way of Responding

An important tool that supports the development and maintenance of a self-compassionate way of responding is the use of self-monitoring. As suggested in Chapter 9, real-time monitoring can help clients distance themselves from their self-critical thoughts and become observers of these thoughts rather than accepting them without question. While clients may well argue that they wish to avoid focusing on such upsetting thoughts, they should be reminded that it is only by confronting these thoughts that they can put different responses into place. The monitoring also includes the generation of a self-compassionate response, and reminders to take a stance of acceptance, thus making these new styles of responding more habitual and automatic over time. The self-monitoring form can be devised with the client for his or her specific needs, but headings we have used previously on such forms include "Triggering Events," "Self-Critical Thoughts," "Feelings," "What Does the Self-Compassionate Voice Say?," "What Skills Can I Practice?," and "What Happens to My Feelings When I Respond This Way?"

CHAPTER 14

Procrastination and Time Management

One of the fundamental problems we see in our clients with clinical perfectionism is poor time management. For example, they may try to fit too much into their schedules due to achievement striving, so that they are always rushing, running late, and never allowing time for rest or relaxation. Or, they may have periods of procrastination in which they ruminate and put off tasks that need to be done, often due to worry over not doing them well enough. Typically clients with clinical perfectionism swing between periods of continual work toward achievement of goals and times of procrastination and avoidance. Such swings are consistent with the dichotomous thinking styles that we discussed previously. Even when a person procrastinates over starting a task, he or she rarely engages in pleasant or enjoyable activities. Often clients have the belief that doing things they enjoy is a "waste of time," and that all time should be spent being productive and achieving progress toward their goals. When they procrastinate, instead of using that time to engage in a pleasant activity, they often engage in rumination and self-criticism over their standards and will not "allow" themselves to do something enjoyable. They believe they have not been productive enough, and so have not "earned it." In this chapter we look at ways that you can help your clients understand the impact of perfectionism on their time management, and ways they approach the idea of leisure time. The aim is to guide your clients toward the idea of balance in life, in which they can try to achieve some of their goals but balance this with time for rest and relaxation.

Techniques to Overcome Procrastination

When we ask clients in our research studies what they found to be the most useful aspects of treatment, among the most cited strategies were those used to combat procrastination (Steele et al., 2013). This is not surprising given that procrastination is a common behavior we see in the majority of our clients with clinical perfectionism. It is associated with a high degree of distress and can be one of the main reasons why someone presents for treatment for perfectionism. Given that our clients value using their time well and achieving their goals, times when they are being unproductive and putting off tasks lead to a lot of distress.

Clients often put off doing tasks due to their high standards. Many times they report that they put off doing a task due to worry about failing or not doing it well. Other common reasons for engaging in procrastination include thinking it will take too long to complete the task well, an inability to leave a task partway through (meaning the task will take up too much time), and concern about feeling overwhelmed while trying to complete the task perfectly. Clients may also report preferring to leave the task until the last minute so they have an excuse if it is not done well. We see this in the case of Claudia.

> Claudia reported that she often left writing reports until the night before they were due, as she knew that completing them to her standard required a great deal of work, and that she would not be able to find time during her busy work day to devote hours to the reports. However she also reported that she left them until the night before so that if she had negative feedback on her reports, she could blame it on not having had enough time to do them. She said that receiving negative feedback on a report written the night before it was due would be much worse than receiving negative feedback on a report she had started earlier. If she worked hard on a report and still received negative feedback, this would be a confirmation that she was not good enough at her job.

The belief that leaving things to the last minute protects one from self-criticism is self-defeating and counterproductive and keeps the unhelpful cycle of procrastination and perfectionism going. In the case of Claudia, this pattern is likely to lead to poorer performance due to the lack of time available. People with clinical perfectionism often become locked in vicious cycles of perfectionism and procrastination, and as therapists we need to help our clients to both understand how this is maintained and learn strategies to combat these unhelpful patterns.

Identifying Areas of Procrastination

A first step in addressing procrastination is to encourage clients to think about the domains in which their perfectionism leads to procrastination. At this stage in treatment the domains of the client's perfectionism will likely have been identified by the therapist and client ; however, sometimes it can be useful to encourage clients to think about areas in which they procrastinate, using the handout in Figure 14.1 (see also Handout 14.1 in Appendix 2).

Socratic dialogue can be useful at this stage to help clients become more aware of their patterns of procrastination. For example, do they procrastinate across many domains or only some areas of striving? Are there other domains in which they procrastinate of which they were previously unaware? Self-monitoring of procrastination and the predictions that drive procrastination can also be useful. In the case described earlier, Claudia's procrastination stemmed from her prediction that she would not write reports well and that she would receive negative feedback from her boss. An example of a completed self-monitoring form for Claudia can be seen in Figure 14.2 (see also Handout 14.2 in Appendix 2).

Perfectionism area/ behavior	Example	My procrastination behavior
Eating/shape/weight	Delay trying on clothes	_____
Social performance	Put off phoning a friend	_____
Organization	Delay writing to-do lists	_____
House cleanliness, neatness	Delay starting cleaning	_____
Appearance	Delay ironing clothes	_____
Artistic performance	Postpone new painting	_____
Musical performance	Postpone violin practice	_____
Athletic performance	Put off training	_____
Academic performance	Ask for extension	_____
Work performance	Delay starting report	_____
Intimate relationships	Put off asking for a date	_____
Parenting	Delaying choice of school	_____
Health, fitness	Put off going for a walk	_____
Entertaining	Delay cooking for party	_____
Other perfectionism areas:		_____
_____	_____	_____
_____	_____	_____
_____	_____	_____
_____	_____	_____

FIGURE 14.1. In which areas of my life do I procrastinate? Adapted from Shafran, Egan, and Wade (2010). Copyright by Constable & Robinson. Adapted by permission.

Perfectionism area and situation	Perfectionist prediction	Procrastination behavior	Feelings (rate 0–100%)
Work At work thinking about writing reports	I will not be able to write the report to an excellent standard (90%). My boss is not going to be happy with my work (85%).	Read e-mails all day instead of doing report Thought about how my boss has corrected some areas of my reports before Delayed writing report until the night before it was due	Anxious (90%)

FIGURE 14.2. Self-monitoring procrastination. Adapted from Shafran, Egan, and Wade (2010). Copyright by Constable & Robinson. Adapted by permission.

This type of worksheet, in which clients monitor their perfectionistic predictions that lead to procrastination, can then be used in treatment to help clients identify the vicious cycle between perfectionistic beliefs and procrastination behavior.

Another strategy that can be useful in helping clients recognize their patterns of procrastination is to encourage them to think more broadly about procrastination and to develop some perspective on how others engage in procrastination through watching the YouTube clip "Procrastination" in Lev Yilmaz's *Tales of Mere Existence* (discussed previously in Chapter 12). This is a short, lighthearted clip of someone engaging in procrastination and shows a typical pattern of putting off work by getting distracted by other nonrelevant tasks. Short clips such as these are often amusing to clients but also can help to provide a more objective perspective when thinking about their own procrastination, thereby providing motivation to change, and to avoid being stuck in the vicious cycle portrayed in the clip.

Troubleshooting the Impact of Procrastination on Therapy

It is useful to note that procrastination is an issue that may interfere with clients completing homework and engaging in self-monitoring. Address this potential problem directly when assigning self-monitoring for procrastination. Strategies that may help clients engage in self-monitoring include reminders to complete the self-monitoring at the time the behavior occurs, keep self-monitoring worksheets in a prominent position, or set reminders to do self-monitoring (e.g., smartphone alerts). However, if it is clear that the client has difficulty engaging in homework or completing worksheets, you can use this problem in session as an example to illustrate the issue of procrastination. You and the client may choose to complete a self-monitoring form in session, focused on completing worksheets and homework in therapy. This strategy can help clients identify beliefs that contribute to procrastination and help to address issues in homework compliance that may interfere with treatment progress.

Conducting a "Vicious Cycle" Formulation of the Link between Perfectionism and Procrastination

One of the most important steps in addressing procrastination is helping your client understand the reciprocal relationship between procrastination and perfectionism. By this point in treatment, you will have worked with the client to develop a collaborative formulation that includes the possible role of procrastination in keeping perfectionism going. However, it is useful at this point to elaborate on this through use of Socratic dialogue following up on earlier discussions, or worksheets identifying perfectionistic predictions arising in the context of procrastination. Using these identified beliefs, you can expand from one of these examples and ask the client what the impact of procrastination was on perfectionistic predictions and the tendency to evaluate oneself based on achievement. Note this line of inquiry in the following dialogue from the case of Claudia.

> THERAPIST: Claudia, you had predicted that you would not write your reports well, so you left them until the night before. What effect do you think procrastinating had on your belief that you don't write reports well?
>
> CLAUDIA: Well, it probably made it worse because when I write reports late at night I am really tired, and I tend to make silly mistakes, especially when I am rushed. That probably feeds into my ideas that I am no good at doing reports.
>
> THERAPIST: Okay, so it seems that procrastination actually increases your predictions that you won't do well, and sometimes that may be based on the reality of leaving it to the last minute and actually making a few mistakes. What effect does that have on this problem of basing your self-worth on how well you are doing at work?
>
> CLAUDIA: Well, I suppose it makes it worse again, as I always feel like I am not doing well, which makes me think I have to try harder next time. But I get so caught up in worrying about doing a good job that I just keep putting it off and leaving it to the last minute.

THERAPIST: Yes, it certainly sounds like that is the case. Claudia, I wonder if there is a cycle going on here where you base your sense of worth on your work achievements, which leads you to worry about doing a good job, putting your work off. Then, after you procrastinate, you worry even further about doing a good job and get self-critical about having procrastinated, leading you to put off your work even more.

You can make this point clear by drawing a figure illustrating the cycle between predictions and procrastination. Such a figure can help clients understand that the more they procrastinate, the stronger their perfectionistic predictions become, and the more likely they are to procrastinate again, which in turn further increases perfectionism. Overcoming this vicious cycle requires helping clients understand how perfectionistic predictions and self-evaluation based on achievement increase due to procrastination, and then challenging the associated thoughts and behavior. Sometimes it can be helpful at this stage to use other examples to illustrate the vicious loop between perfectionism and procrastination, as seen in Figure 14.3 (see also Handout 14.3 in Appendix 2).

How Procrastination Is Maintained by Increasing Beliefs in Perfectionistic Predictions

Having the client read the examples in Figure 14.3 will help to highlight the vicious cycle that links procrastination and perfectionism, and will also reinforce the idea that procrastination is often maintained because it increases how much clients believe in their perfectionist predictions, which makes it more likely they will keep procrastinating. You can then use this knowledge as leverage to help clients see they need to change both their predictions and their behavior to combat procrastination, and that decreasing procrastination will help to decrease perfectionism (because of the strong reciprocal link between the two).

How Procrastination Is Maintained by Increasing Self-Evaluation Based on Achievement

In the earlier sample dialogue, the therapist helped Claudia see that procrastination reinforced her view that self-worth should be based on achievement, and that the more this view is reinforced, the more likely Claudia is to worry about meeting her standards and to procrastinate. In discussing the vicious loop, use both the vicious cycle diagram of procrastination and the collaborative formulation diagram (Chapter 7, this volume), with the goal of helping the client see how procrastination leads to the perception that one is failing at tasks and is therefore a failure as a person. A useful

Example	Perfectionism area	Perfectionistic prediction	Procrastination behaviors	How procrastination keeps going by increasing belief in predictions
Taj	Work	I will not be able to write reports to an excellent standard.	Delay writing reports. Write detailed lists to delay doing reports. Stare at clock thinking about reports. Line up business cards.	The more Taj procrastinated, the less time he had to do reports, thus not doing them to the standard he would like, which increased his belief in his prediction he would not do reports to an excellent standard, and made him more likely to procrastinate again.
Anil	Cleaning	I will not be able to get every room perfectly neat and tidy, so I might as well not start cleaning.	Put off cleaning until house became very messy.	The more Anil put off cleaning, the more he believed his prediction that he would not be his standard, and this made him keep procrastinating.
Clare	Study	I will never be able to write a good assignment.	Sleeping in. Staring at computer trying to think of ideas. Not handing assignment in.	The more Clare put off working on her assignment, the more she believed her prediction that she would not write a good assignment, and the more she continued to procrastinate.
Matias	Work and social life	If I do not leave things to the last minute, I will get so caught up in checking they are perfect that I will not get anything done.	Put off sending in job application and then made the mistake of forgetting stamp on envelope.	The more Matias procrastinated, the more likely he was to make small mistakes due to rushing, which increased his belief that he needed to check for a long time and made him more likely to procrastinate.
My example				

FIGURE 14.3. Understanding how procrastination is maintained by increasing belief in perfectionistic predictions. Adapted from Shafran, Egan, and Wade (2010). Copyright by Constable & Robinson. Adapted by permission.

technique that can be used at this point is Socratic questioning with the client—for example:

> "So given we know that procrastination leads you to continue thinking you are a failure and only good enough if you are achieving, if you were able to break this pattern of procrastination, what do you think that would do to your sense of self-worth?"

With this line of questioning, clients can learn to see that reducing procrastination can have a big impact in decreasing the problem of viewing self-worth as a function of achievement which, as discussed throughout this book, is a fundamental problem in clinical perfectionism. This type of questioning can then lead nicely to the use of motivational strategies.

Motivational Enhancement Techniques for Procrastination

Standard motivational enhancement techniques can help the client understand the negative consequences of procrastination, and how changing procrastination may be helpful. Established strategies of considering benefits and costs can be used to help clients examine the negative consequences of procrastination. Once you and the client derive a list of the benefits and costs of procrastination, you can help the client to consider the negative consequences of procrastination by elaborating on the costs and generating more detailed information regarding impact. You can also enhance motivation by challenging some of the perceived benefits of procrastination (e.g., the belief that putting off a task will reduce anxiety). It is useful to highlight and contrast short-term versus long-term consequences and validate some of the perceived benefits of procrastination. For example, you can acknowledge that in the short term individuals may experience some anxiety relief from putting off a task, but then ask what impact procrastination has had on the client's anxiety over the long term. Help the client to understand that relief following procrastination is short-lived, and that procrastination often leads to an increase in anxiety as tasks build up, triggering thoughts such as "I should be doing those tasks," which in turn increase anxiety further. One take-home message from this discussion is that procrastination has no real benefits, or if there are benefits (such as a slight reduction in anxiety at the time), they are short-lived. In the long term procrastination costs the client a lot more in increased stress and pressure.

Another take-home message from the consideration of benefits and costs is the negative impact procrastination has on actual task performance, the thing that people with perfectionism care so much about. For example, you can help clients see that allowing tasks to build up can lead to high anxiety, which may impact on their performance once they do start the task. It can be useful here also to remind them about the Yerkes–Dodson curve (see the section on psychoeducation in Chapter 9), illustrating how some anxiety can help performance but too much can impede it. It is also useful to elaborate on the impact of procrastination on the time available to complete required tasks. For example, if a person puts off doing a task for so long that there is limited time left to complete it (as in the case of Claudia), then the individual may in fact end up completing it in a less satisfactory way than if there had been more time to spend on the task. This point can often be tricky, as clients may explain that they "work better under pressure" and that it has always been their strategy to leave things to the last minute. To address this issue it is useful to propose behavioral experiments such as those discussed below.

Cognitive Strategies to Overcome Procrastination

Behavioral experiments can be helpful to combat procrastination and associated beliefs (e.g., the belief that leaving tasks until the last minute results in better performance). Strategies for setting up behavioral experiments were covered in Chapter 12. To illustrate how behavioral experiments can be used to challenge procrastination-related beliefs, consider the example of Tyler, a university student who presented for treatment of problems with anxiety and procrastination. Tyler often left his assignments until the night before they were due as he believed he worked best under pressure. Tyler's therapist suggested that he complete two behavioral experiments—one in which he had adequate time to complete an assignment and another where he completed the assignment at the last minute. Tyler was asked to rate how well he completed the task, how much anxiety he experienced, and any other observations that were relevant, as seen in Figure 14.4 (see also Handout 14.4 in Appendix 2).

This type of experiment can be useful to help clients understand the negative impact procrastination can have on performance and realize that procrastination often results in the very consequence they worry about (i.e., performing more poorly) and that reducing procrastination can lead to improved performance. A similar experiment could be used in the case of Claudia, who predicted that her boss would give her negative feedback about her reports. Claudia might be asked to rate the degree of negative feedback she might receive for a report completed the night before versus one prepared earlier, and examine whether reports prepared earlier are really more likely to receive negative feedback than those prepared at the last minute.

Thought diaries can also be used to combat procrastination. Clients often have a range of unhelpful thinking styles regarding procrastination, as illustrated by predictions described in the earlier cases of Tyler (e.g., "I will do better if I leave it to the last minute," "I will feel anxious if I start it early") and Claudia (e.g., "My boss will give me negative feedback

Belief to be tested (rate degree of belief 0–100%): *I work best under pressure; procrastinating and leaving assignments to the last minute helps me to do better (85%).*

Alternative belief to be tested (rate degree of belief 0–100%): *Procrastinating and leaving tasks to the last minute actually makes me do worse (15%).*

Experiment that will test the belief (specify what you will do in detail including when, where, and how):

1. Start an assignment 1 week before it is due; hand it in a day early.

2. Start an assignment 1 day before it is due; hand it in 5 minutes before the deadline.

Rate the following and compare your notes for experiment 1 versus 2:

How anxious did you feel? (0–100). How good was your performance? (0–100). What was the result? Which one led to a better performance?

Prediction: *If I start assignments earlier I will feel overwhelmed and anxious and do a poorer job, as I work better under pressure.*

Specify the prediction (specify behaviors and rate intensity of beliefs and emotions):

I will not produce a good assignment if I start it a week before instead of the night before (90%), I will feel anxious for the whole week (80%).

What problems might occur and how will you overcome them?

I might not be able to do the experiment on an important assignment—I may have to do it on one that I care less about.

Experiment—what did you actually do?:

I did the experiment that I planned.

Results—what happened? *I got a slightly better mark for the assignment that I started early, I felt more anxious when I started it the night before.*

Rerate the predictions made: What can you conclude? Rerate the belief you tested, as well as the alternative, if you had one.

Predictions: *I will not produce a good assignment if I start it a week before it is due instead of the night before (60%); I will feel anxious for the whole week (10%). I can conclude that my predictions did not come true—I did produce a good assignment and was less anxious than when I did it the night before.*

Alternative belief to be tested (rate degree of belief 0–100%): *Procrastinating and leaving tasks to the last minute actually makes me do worse (75%).*

(continued)

FIGURE 14.4. Behavioral experiment to overcome procrastination.

Reflection including plans for any follow-up experiments: *It is not helpful to leave things to the last minute. I actually worked better when I had more time and felt less pressured. I need to do it with a different type of assignment, however, to really change my beliefs.*

Revised belief: *Leaving things to the last minute is stressful and makes me get poorer marks; I can do better if I start things earlier and I will try and hand things in with a day to spare.*

FIGURE 14.4. *(continued)*

about my reports"). Standard thought records can be used to challenge these ideas, though behavioral experiments are likely to be a more effective way to demonstrate to clients that some of their predictions may be unfounded.

One benefit of thought records is to generate reminders or "coping statements" that a client can later use to dispute procrastination-related thoughts. Consider the following example in Figure 14.5. This type of thought record may help the therapist to derive with Claudia a flash card of helpful reminders regarding her procrastination that she can keep handy (e.g., pinned up near her desk, or as a screen saver on her computer).

Other types of helpful reminders that clients have often found to be useful are illustrated in Table 14.1 (see also Handout 14.5 in Appendix 2).

Behavioral Techniques to Overcome Procrastination

One of the most common reasons provided for procrastination is a lack of motivation to start on the task, and a belief that it is best to wait until one feels motivated to begin. Of course this belief is unhelpful, as motivation tends to increase after one gets started. This "waiting for motivation" trap (Shafran et al., 2010) can be identified by the therapist, followed by the introduction of Socratic questioning, in which the therapist asks a series of questions regarding how the client believes that motivation will happen, and whether the client has had the experience of feeling unmotivated followed by suddenly feeling motivated to do something. It is also useful to ask whether the client has had the experience of becoming motivated after starting a task. An example that can be useful for this discussion is exercise, for which the belief that one must feel motivated before starting exercise stops an individual from exercising. On the other hand, as anyone who has ever exercised knows, motivation typically begins after the initiation of exercise, and continues to increase as an individual exercises more regularly. This idea can be illustrated by the therapist using a whiteboard, as seen in Figures 14.6 and 14.7.

A—Activating event	B—Beliefs (rate 0–100%)	C— Consequences (rate 0–100%)	D— Disputation	E—Evaluate outcome
What was the event, situation, thought, image, or memory?	What went through my mind? What does it say about me as a person? Am I using unhelpful thinking styles?	What was I feeling?	What would a friend say? Is there another way of viewing this thought?	How do I feel now?
Staring at computer, thinking about report	I never write good reports (90%) (predictive thinking) My boss will think I have done a bad job and criticize my reports; I am stupid (80%) (mind reading, predictive thinking, labeling)	Anxious (90%)	I have received good feedback from my boss before on my reports. I won't know if my boss will say I did a bad job until I hand it in; he has never said that I am stupid; he has praised me before.	Anxious (50%)

FIGURE 14.5. Sample thought record to challenge procrastination.

You can introduce some humor here with an analogy, such as "waiting around for the motivation bus." Consider a person sitting around waiting for the motivation bus to arrive, but waiting for an express bus at a stop that is only served by a local bus. Such a person is going to be waiting at the bus stop for a long time, and is unlikely to get where he or she needs to go. On the other hand, if the individual gets up and starts walking in the right direction toward the correct bus stop (a metaphor for taking action) or getting on the local bus and riding a few stops until getting to the express bus stop, there is a much better chance of achieving what the person wants to achieve and to feel more motivated to continue.

TABLE 14.1. Helpful Reminders for Procrastination

"I feel better once I start something."

"I feel less anxious once I get going with a task I am putting off."

"If I put it off I will feel worse."

"Getting started with a task makes me feel more confident to keep going."

"I am not a failure because of procrastinating; if I make a small start I will feel better."

"Procrastination makes me feel anxious, so it's best to not put things off."

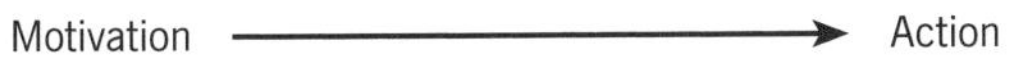

Motivation ⟶ Action

FIGURE 14.6. The common assumed relationship between motivation and action.

Action ⟶ Motivation

FIGURE 14.7. The actual relationship between motivation and action.

This psychoeducation regarding the relationship between action and motivation is a useful bridge you can use to introduce the simple behavioral technique of breaking up large tasks into small manageable chunks that will lead to the larger goal, with the explanation that once the client has achieved even one step toward completing a task, motivation will increase and the individual will be on the way to achieving the task.

Consider the case of Tyler, who used this strategy (see Figure 14.8) to deal with his procrastination over assignments (see also Handout 14.6 in Appendix 2).

Problem-Solving Techniques

Problem-solving techniques can often be useful for clients in helping to overcome perfectionism. You can introduce problem solving to clients as a tool they can take away from sessions for any situation. Emphasize that the process of writing out the steps to solve a problem is useful, as it often helps the person to gain objectivity about the problem and to think of ways of addressing the problem that might not have been considered otherwise. Figure 14.9 is an example of a completed problem-solving worksheet for the case of Sandrine, whose perfectionism regarding the cleanliness of her house interfered with her social life.

Sandrine was a 45-year-old married woman who enjoyed socializing with friends. However she held very high standards for keeping her house neat and clean, and needed to have her home looking like what she described as a "show home" before she could have friends over to visit. She said this was exhausting, as she would spend the entire day cleaning before she could have a friend over, and as a result she usually did not invite people over. Sandrine's friends teased her about never having them over and about always having her home looking perfect. They said they were afraid to go to her house, as they would not want to mess it up. Sandrine said she was embarrassed by these jokes from her friends, but that she still found it difficult to invite people over when the house was less than perfect.

1. **Define the task/goal.**
   Start assignment the week before it is due; hand it in 1 day early

2. **Break the task down into manageable chunks and rate chunks from easiest to hardest (0–100).**

   100—Hand assignment in

   90—Read over assignment for flow, check spelling errors, and make sure it sounds good

   80—Write introduction and conclusion for assignment

   70—Write main arguments for each area by expanding bullet points

   60—Summarize main points from research in bullet points under each subheading

   50—Read articles and research on each of the areas in the assignment

   40—Do research on computer to find information on each of the subheading areas

   30—Write bullet points for areas that might be included under each subheading

   20—Write subheadings that will be used throughout the assignment

   10—Save a new file name on computer for the assignment

   0—Think about assignment

FIGURE 14.8. Breaking down tasks into manageable chunks to overcome procrastination.

Time Management and Pleasant Event Scheduling

In addressing time management and scheduling of pleasant events, you can help the client understand the importance of balancing "achievement" with time for rest and relaxation. One of the most common problems in perfectionism is that clients do not allow time for relaxation or fun activities, as they always feel that they must be doing something productive and working toward achieving their goals. In addition, clients often have difficulty managing their time (e.g., they may often be extremely rushed and running late as they try to fit in too many activities). Often clients have dichotomous patterns of behavior in which they swing between times of overworking and rushing on the one hand and periods of procrastination on the other hand, in which they describe being unable to get anything useful done, wasting time, and engaging in very few tasks. Nevertheless, this time when they are engaged in procrastination and avoidance is not used for doing pleasant or fun activities. So the goal of the therapist is once again to introduce the notion of balance for the client, to use time management schedules to help clients plan their time in a more balanced way, so that they include

1. **Identify the problem.**
   Describe the problem in an objective and specific way.

   Have invited a friend for coffee but feel that I need to spend all day cleaning the house before she comes. Therefore, I feel like I want to cancel the visit.

2. **Generate potential solutions.**
   Brainstorm all of the possible solutions to the problem.

   Keep listing all the ideas you can think of without judging them as good or bad.

   Underline two or three solutions that most likely to be helpful and most possible to achieve.

   Cancel the visit, reschedule the visit, clean house entirely, clean only the room we will be in, leave house as it is

3. **Decide on a solution.**
   Consider the pros and cons of the top two or three solutions in terms of how possible it is and how likely it is to solve the problem

   Choose the solution that seems best.

   If I reschedule the visit, I will just keep my perfectionism going (which I am trying to change), and my friend will disappointed, so just cleaning the dining room where we will be sitting is the best option.

4. **Plan a solution.**
   Plan a list of action steps that need to be taken to achieve the solution.

   Shut the doors to other rooms, set a time limit for cleaning the dining room, don't do usual "spring clean" that I would do before someone comes over (e.g., no shampooing of carpet, cleaning windows and blinds).

5. **Carry out the solution.**

   Cleaned the dining room and shut the doors to other rooms, did not do a big "spring clean."

6. **Evaluate the result.**
   What was the effect of carrying out the solution?

   I felt happy with myself that I was able to break the pattern of not having friends over for coffee due to my having to clean the house perfectly. I enjoyed the visit, and even though I felt a bit uncomfortable that it was not cleaned to my usual standard it is good for me to sit with those feelings and see that being with people is more important than how clean my house is.

FIGURE 14.9. Problem solving.

time for rest, relaxation, and pleasant activities, and so that not all time is devoted to striving and achievement. This is likely to have a positive impact on clients' mood, and taking breaks to engage in pleasant events will help them to feel more refreshed, rested, and able to tackle tasks they have been putting off. It is often useful for therapists to use Socratic questions along the lines of "Which person do you think would be more likely to be productive, the one who works 12-hour days and only gets 4 hours of sleep a night, or the one who works 8-hour days and gets 8 hours of sleep?" This type of question can be informative, as clients with perfectionism often respond that people who work longer hours are more productive, as they have more time available. It can be useful to follow up with questions asking about the impact of tiredness on one's ability to work and to introduce the idea that even though they may be working longer hours, they might not be as productive as individuals who work fewer hours but are more rested, so they are more efficient and productive during the times that they do work.

Troubleshooting Difficulties with Time for Rest and Pleasant Events

If the client is reluctant to introduce rest and pleasant events into his or her schedule, it can be useful to introduce a time management schedule that includes rest and pleasant events as a behavioral experiment. Ask the client to spend half the week engaging in a normal schedule (i.e., rushing, overworking, and leaving no time for pleasant events) and half a week engaging in the new schedule that includes rest, relaxation, and pleasant events. The client's belief and prediction about what will happen to his or her productivity can be identified, and then you can ask the client to compare outcomes for each of the two schedules, including productivity, mood, and efficiency. Usually the results of such experiments are positive, and the client realizes that introducing breaks, rest, and pleasant events leads to greater efficiency, better concentration, and improved mood.

Examples of a time management schedule (Handout 14.8) and a pleasant event schedule (Handout 14.9) can be found in Appendix 2. One issue that may need to be discussed with clients is the tendency to choose pleasant events that have an achievement component and then striving to complete the task perfectly. For example, a client may choose to start a new hobby, such as learning to play the guitar, and make every effort to perfect it, seeing their new hobby as something to be "achieved" (e.g., trying to be the best at running in preparation for a fun run, or taking a cake-decorating class and spending many hours trying to perfect the new skill). After the client has selected pleasant events to introduce, you should ask if he or she is likely to be tempted to strive and apply perfectionism to the pleasant event, and if so, what might be done instead. For example, the person might choose to learn a new instrument or learn a new language and use this experience as a behavioral experiment (e.g., putting far less time than usual into practicing, practicing little, enjoying the new activity, tolerating making mistakes). It can also be useful to help clients think of doing things they would not normally do, and that they might usually deem a waste of time (e.g., watching reality TV or a soap opera, or reading a gossip magazine). Surprisingly, these types of activities can indeed be challenging for individuals with perfectionism, as they go against the grain of their beliefs about always using time well and being productive, and about how terrible it is to waste time on activities that do not matter or help to achieve goals. This is exactly why including short periods of such activities can be useful in therapy: to help clients realize that they may feel better and more rested from not striving 100% of the time, and that having downtime doing something like reading a trashy magazine is the sort of activity that people who do not have issues with perfectionism engage in all the time as a pleasant event.

Finally, you should encourage clients to engage in pleasant events that are socially focused and involve interacting with friends, family, and other supports. This is because when individuals are so driven toward achievement, their social and interpersonal life often becomes narrowed, as they have often put meeting their goals ahead of healthy social and interpersonal functioning. Hence, it is quite common for clients with perfectionism to have small social networks, and hence less social support. Often clients with perfectionism have difficulty with their intimate relationships, and it is not uncommon for them to be engaged in no intimate relationship, as they are so busy striving to achieve goals that they do not have time to socialize, or may even see socializing as a waste of time because it gets in the way of productivity. In the documentary *What it Takes*, Peter Reid, a successful world champion in Ironman distance triathlons, stated, "Sometimes the isolation really gets to me; it's the days where I have light training and you are just sitting around and it hits me—I don't have a girlfriend; I don't have anything; I am just training, every day" (Han, 2006). Although Reid was achieving at the top in the domain of sport, his life was unbalanced. His intense focus on training and achievement had come at the cost of not having an intimate relationship. A goal of therapy is to help our clients gain more balance in all areas of their lives, so that they do not miss out on important life events, developmental milestones, fun, and relaxation due to being so narrowly focused on achievement in their domains of perfectionism.

CHAPTER 15

Relapse Prevention

B efore concluding therapy for a client with perfectionism, focus some time on relapse prevention. This discussion should include standard relapse prevention techniques, as well as a brief review of the origins of perfectionism in the client's life and a reminder of how it was that the client's self-worth became dependent on achievement. Relapse prevention should also emphasize strategies for continuing to reject ideas that may have been relevant to the client early on but are less useful now.

Revisiting the Historical Review of the Origins of Perfectionism

In Chapter 13 we discussed conducting a historical review of the origins of perfectionism as a way to expand self-evaluation. When discussing relapse prevention and termination, it can be helpful to briefly revisit this historical review. This can help clients summarize how it was that their self-evaluation became dependent on performance. It can also be useful by helping them remember to separate factors that were relevant in the past from those that are relevant now (e.g., the fact that a parent criticized their performance is not necessarily relevant now as an adult). It can help to remind the client that although the perfectionism may have been helpful and functional in a previous context, perfectionism became unhelpful when the context changed, or the domains in which the perfectionism was expressed expanded.

It can be useful at this point to remind the client of strategies that can help for past-origin issues and provide a written summary of techniques that will be useful in the future. For example, clients can be encouraged to remember to use imagery when distressing images occur (e.g., using rescripting and positive imagery to cope with a memory of being teased and criticized by a teacher who had called the client "stupid"). Here it is useful for the client to remember that certain achievement-related values within their family of origin were relevant in childhood but may not continue to serve them well now. For example, family expectations of success (e.g., when child presents a report card with 80%, the parents ask, "But where is the other 20%?") and a tendency to compare the client with other family members (e.g., "Yes, but your sister has achieved more in her music and ballet") may have been part of the client's learning that lead to perfectionism. It can also be useful for clients to summarize what they learned over the course of treatment regarding their past learning from other sources, for example, teachers and coaches who pressured them to reach high standards, and parents, friends, or teachers who criticized their performance. The overarching purpose of this discussion is for the client to be reminded that he or she was sensitized to striving because of this learning, or possibly from spending time in school and work environments with exceptionally high performance expectations.

It is not necessary to spend a great deal of time on these areas when discussing relapse prevention. However, some discussion can be useful to highlight the impact of perfectionism within a historical context, and to work with the client to develop a brief list of the costs and benefits of striving across the course of his or her life. This serves as a nice bridge into a general consideration of relapse prevention and how clients can prevent themselves from going back to old patterns of striving and perfectionism and, in particular, basing their whole sense of self-worth on striving and achievement.

Relapse Prevention

The emphasis of relapse prevention should be on you and the client engaging in a collaborative plan to deal with times in the future when the client's perfectionism begins to increase again. To guide this discussion, bring out the collaborative formulation diagram again, which you referred to throughout treatment (Figure 7.2). It is useful to ask the client where he or she is now within the diagram, and if the paths that were strong at the start of treatment (e.g., the vicious cycle of self-criticism maintaining the belief that self-worth is based on achievement) are as strong now. This can have a twofold effect. First, it is useful for clients to see how their perfectionism has improved—that they have worked hard in treatment, and that many of the vicious loops that had been maintaining their perfectionism have been weakened through treatment. Second, reviewing the collaborative formulation diagram can help prompt clients to think about the potential areas where they might fall back into their perfectionism in the future. Clients should be encouraged to be on alert for cues that might signal increases in perfectionism (e.g., noticing when they achieve a goal that they reset goals higher, rather than simply reflecting on their success).

Following the summary of potential areas of relapse, therapists can then ask clients to think about which strategies they have used during treatment to help combat these maintaining factors. For example, clients with perfectionism around personal appearance and the appearance of their home might find themselves again engaging in old perfectionism behaviors of not leaving the house before their hair and makeup was perfect, and not inviting friends over for coffee until they had spent many hours cleaning the house perfectly. In these cases, clients could be encouraged to repeat a previous behavioral experiment in which they have a friend over for coffee with their personal and home appearance less than perfect. Asking the client to summarize the most important points of treatment provides him or her with a "blueprint" for the future. It is helpful at this stage to remind the client to expect some setbacks, and help the client understand that setbacks are normal. Remind clients not to engage in dichotomous thinking regarding setbacks (e.g., to view them a "complete" failure or as a sign that they have "completely relapsed").

Socratic questioning can be helpful for discussing why the client's perfectionism has had a negative impact, and why it is so important for clients to remind themselves again at the end of treatment of the importance of resisting unhelpful temptations to strive in the future. It is worth discussing with clients how they may be tempted to strive (e.g., overwork, overtrain, overstudy) at some time in the future (e.g., when changing jobs, taking part in competition, completing another degree), and how this is a signal they may get into difficulty with perfectionism again and should go back to their relapse prevention plan.

The steps toward developing a relapse prevention plan can be seen in Table 15.1. It can also be helpful to give clients Handout 15.1 in Appendix 2, which summarizes useful steps in preventing relapse, and have them complete Handout 15.2, on developing an action plan.

Future Planning for the Client to Have a Balanced Life

One of the key challenges by the end of treatment is for clients to recognize just how striving and achievement have been a main focus of their life. Because clients will have spent much of their time striving and trying to achieve, it can be a challenge for them to consider how they can have a "balanced" life, in which they have some time for striving and achievement, as well as for rest, relaxation, socializing, or other activities they have ignored. Socratic questioning can be useful for encouraging clients to think about the overall impact of perfectionism on their life.

TABLE 15.1. Major Components of Relapse Prevention Planning in Perfectionism

1. Develop an action plan.
   - Ask the client to consider which strategies he or she found to be most helpful, and summarize them.
   - Ask the client to reflect on the treatment overall and to summarize the answers to the following important questions:
     a. What changes have you made that you want to see continue to develop?
     b. What areas in your life require further attention?
   - Help the client identify a place to keep his or her action plan where it will be seen often (e.g., on the fridge, in a work diary).
   - Encourage the client to keep copies of worksheets accessible in case he or she needs to use them.

2. Discuss realistic and compassionate expectations.
   - Remind the client that perfectionism may lead him or her to interpret a "slip" or lapse in a dichotomous way (e.g., as a complete relapse) and to engage in self-criticism over the lapse.
   - Point out that it is unrealistic to expect that someone will always be improving and never have any lapses.
   - Remind your client that over the course of improving in any area, there are always natural ups and downs. These should be viewed as a normal part of learning rather than a cause for anxiety or a trigger for falling back into old habits of perfectionism.
   - Normalize times when the client needs to ask others for help during a difficult return of symptoms, and highlight that it is a sign of strength to be able to ask others for help rather than trying to do it all on one's own.

3. Dealing with setbacks: lapses and slippages.
   - Remind the client that in times of stress, such as transitions in important areas of achievement like work (e.g., getting a promotion, changing jobs), clients may be tempted to go back to old strategies. This is normal, but it is important at these times to reread one's action plan and put into place strategies that will help.

It can be helpful to present Handout 15.3 in Appendix 2, for final reflections on perfectionism, including some common quotes on the topic. These quotes help get across the idea that trying to achieve perfection is a pointless task, and once we understand that, we can learn to live a balanced life. It is helpful to discuss with the client the idea of letting go of the quest for perfection, that there is imperfection in everything in life. That is, that our lives are rich and rewarding, and that given the complexity of life we must embrace imperfection. In the final stage of therapy, we often pose the idea to clients that they have a choice. They can either keep continuing to punish themselves in the pursuit of the impossible goal of perfection (and we have lots of examples of its negative consequences provided by the client), or they can choose to take a new path in life and make the wise choice of a balanced life. Following this path, they can choose to have flexibility in their goals and thinking, guidelines rather than rules, and self-compassion. We remind clients at this point how they have managed to increase their flexibility and have not achieved less as a result. In fact, often they have achieved more as they have reduced some of the time-wasting aspects of perfectionism, such as procrastination. We end the final session with clients on a positive note, emphasizing that they now have the tools to live a life whose essence is captured by the word *freedom* rather than the constraint of rules and self-criticism. It is with this freedom from striving for perfection that clients can go on to have a more fulfilling life in their connections with others, in their sense of self as being worthwhile (and not only for what they do), and, importantly, a sense of fun and enjoyment of life, rather than always being devoted to being productive and working at all costs.

CHAPTER 16

Emerging Approaches in Treatment of Perfectionism

In many ways, the development of treatments for perfectionism is in its early days. Much more evidence is required to understand what approaches work best for which clients, and under what conditions. The transdiagnostic potential of treating perfectionism is an exciting one, and further attention to this area may yield great benefits for helping our clients, regardless of their principal diagnosis. While there are many different areas that could be further developed within our treatment for perfectionism, the purpose of this chapter is simply to outline four new and emerging approaches to the treatment of perfectionism that we believe may provide fruitful arenas of inquiry. These four areas include prevention approaches for perfectionism in children and adolescents, imagery techniques for perfectionism, mindfulness and acceptance-based approaches for intervening with perfectionism, and stepped-care approaches to the treatment of perfectionism.

Prevention Approaches for Perfectionism in Children and Adolescents

It doesn't take long working in any clinical area before one starts to think about the value of preventing the problem in the first place rather than just treating the problem in its latter stages of development. When we see the damage that psychological disorders cause in our clients' lives and know this leaves a permanent mark on many of the people we see, it becomes a dazzling and enticing vision to consider how we might effectively prevent psychopathology.

If you have the fortitude to consider the vast literature on the effectiveness of our prevention approaches to psychopathology over the years, a mixed picture emerges. In Australia alone, until 2011, there had been 19 evaluations of school-based prevention programs for depression (Nehmy, 2011). Of these, no effect was shown for 9 (47%), 8 showed a "treatment effect" (a decrease in symptom levels or diagnostic status relative to controls in pre- to postintervention analyses), and 2 had shown a "prevention effect" (with the control group showing increased symptom levels or an increased incidence of diagnoses over time relative to the intervention group, who show little evidence of increased risk). We do slightly better in the prevention of anxiety in young people (Nehmy, 2011), where 2 out of 9 studies showed a prevention effect, 6 had a treatment effect, and only 1 had no effect.

Within this context, it is somewhat encouraging to find one study (Wilksch, Durbridge, & Wade, 2008) has shown that classroom-based approaches can significantly decrease "concern over mistakes" perfectionism (the unhelpful variety of perfectionism that is associated with various forms of psychopathology) compared to both passive and active control conditions. The approach used was based on Adderholdt and Goldberg's (1999) book *What's Bad about Being Too Good?* While the result would be classified as a treatment effect rather than a "true" prevention effect, it occurred at 3-month follow-up in 15-year-old girls, indicating some longer-term effect of the intervention. Given that some people view perfectionism as a disposition, or something that can't be changed, it is encouraging to see that it can indeed be changed at a relatively young age.

Unfortunately this study didn't investigate what happened to indicators of negative affect as perfectionism decreased. However, a study by Nehmy and Wade (2014) in around 1,000 young people ages 13 to 15 years, investigating the impact of an eight-session perfectionism intervention (based partly on *Overcoming Perfectionism* by Shafran et al., 2010), showed significantly lower levels of perfectionism and negative affect at 6-month follow-up. At this early stage the results look promising, suggesting a pathway ahead for the development of effective prevention approaches for negative affect.

Imagery Techniques for Perfectionism

In Chapters 10 and 13 we briefly discussed incorporating mental imagery into therapy for perfectionism. Attention has been increasingly turning to imagery, and to a better understanding of its role in maintaining psychopathology. Imagery has generally been defined as the content of mental events that have sensory qualities. It is broader than just mental "visual" images, and can include any sensory modality (Holmes, Arntz, & Smucker, 2007).

Imagery is important to consider, as it has been shown to have a powerful impact on emotion, acting as an amplifier of negative emotional states to a greater degree than verbal-based processing (for a review see Holmes & Mathews, 2010). However, there have been no systematic studies examining the use of imagery in the treatment of perfectionism. This is important to examine, as research has shown the incorporation of mental imagery to be very useful in treatment of various disorders (e.g., Holmes, Geddes, Colom, & Goodwin, 2008; Holmes, Lang, & Shah, 2009).

Understanding the nature of imagery in perfectionism is an important area for future study, as negative intrusive imagery significantly impacts on the individual's cognitive and behavioral responses (Holmes et al., 2008). Often clients will try to avoid distressing images (Hackmann & Holmes, 2004). This avoidance of distressing imagery has been seen as a transdiagnostic factor that cuts across PTSD (Hackmann, Clark, & McManus, 2000), social anxiety disorder (Ehlers et al., 2002), unipolar depression and bipolar disorder (Holmes et al., 2009), and OCD (Hackmann et al., 2011).

Only one study to date has been published on mental imagery and perfectionism (Lee et al., 2011). In this study, using a nonclinical sample, Lee and colleagues compared groups of high and low perfectionists (as defined by a median split on the FMPS; Frost et al., 1990) on their mental imagery. Using the *Images Interview* (Hackmann et al., 2000), it was found that the high perfectionism group had a significantly higher overall imagery score compared to the low perfectionism group, as well as higher scores on the subscales of images and memories. The high perfectionism group was also found to experience more distress related to images and higher negative impact from perfectionism-related images, although there was no significant difference between groups on the frequency or intensity of images. Findings from this study suggest that it would be useful to examine the phenomenology of imagery in a clinical sample with elevated perfectionism to determine the nature and impact of imagery.

We suggest that further research is required around the use of imagery rescripting in perfectionism, as it has been found to be effective in reducing distressing imagery and symptoms in clinical and experimental studies on depression, eating disorders and social anxiety (Cooper, Todd, & Turner, 2007; Nilsson et al., 2012; Ohanian, 2002; Wheatley et al., 2007; Wheatley & Hackmann, 2011; Wild, Hackmann, & Clark, 2007, 2008). Imagery rescripting where positive imagery is encouraged can help to increase clients' sense of competence, mastery, and self-compassion (Hackmann et al., 2011).

We are currently conducting a range of experimental and clinical studies to examine the phenomenology of perfectionism in clinical samples and the impact of imagery rescripting on levels of perfectionism and symptoms. However, given the positive results for imagery rescripting in a range of disorders in which images are believed to be relevant to perfection-ism and its treatment, we suggest that therapists consider using rescripting to address images that carry strong unpleasant emotion in clients being treated for perfectionism.

Mindfulness- and Acceptance-Based Approaches for Perfectionism

Throughout this book, we have suggested that mindfulness- and acceptance-based approaches might be incorporated into the treatment of perfection-ism. There are no data so far to suggest that using these approaches alone constitutes an evidence-based approach for the treatment of perfectionism. However, in their study of clients with bulimia nervosa comparing CBT focused on perfectionism versus CBT focused on bulimia nervosa, Steele and Wade (2008) found that their control condition of mindfulness resulted in a significant decrease (with a small effect size) in "concern over mistakes" perfectionism. While this was only one-fifth the size of the decrease noted for the group that received a perfectionism intervention, it suggests that adding mindfulness along with other effective strategies could be beneficial in the treatment of perfectionism. For example, clients can be encouraged to use mindfulness-based strategies to get some distance from their own thoughts (see Segal et al., 2013).

Future research is needed on the efficacy of mindfulness-based approaches in the treatment of perfectionism. Specifically, it would be use-ful to examine the relative efficacy of a pure mindfulness/acceptance-based approach versus CBT for perfectionism. It would also be useful to compare the treatment of perfectionism using the combination of CBT and mindful-ness/acceptance-based strategies versus CBT alone, to determine the effi-cacy of adding these components to treatment. If therapists want to include more mindfulness strategies, it would be useful for them to suggest to their clients a good self-help manual with accompanying CD or downloadable materials to guide them through a range of mindfulness techniques (e.g., Orsillo & Roemer, 2011; Williams et al., 2007).

Stepped-Care Approaches to Treatment of Perfectionism

Another important area for future research is the degree to which a stepped-care approach is feasible in the treatment of perfectionism. In the United Kingdom the Improving Access to Psychological Therapies (IAPT) program was developed to increase access to psychological therapies, and one way of achieving this was to provide an alternative to face-to-face therapy, namely "low-intensity" interventions, for a proportion of clients.

In the IAPT scheme, low-intensity approaches, including self-help, are used with less complex clients (after they are screened to determine which approach is appropriate), and those with more severe problems receive a "high-intensity" approach (e.g., face-to-face CBT). Several studies have examined what may be considered to be appropriate "low-intensity" interventions for perfectionism. As described in Chapter 2, in a nonclinical sample, Pleva and Wade (2007) found that both guided and pure self-help based on the book *When Perfect Isn't Good Enough* (Antony & Swinson, 1998) were effective for reducing perfectionism, anxiety, and depression, although guided self-help was superior. Steele and Wade (2008) also found that guided self-help based on this same book was effective for reducing perfectionism, eating disorder and associated psychopathology in individuals with eating disorders. Arpin-Cribbie et al. (2008) showed that CBT for perfectionism delivered via the Internet to students with elevated perfectionism resulted in significant reductions in self-oriented perfectionism (SOP), socially prescribed perfectionism (SPP), and concern over mistakes (CM). Finally, in a recent study with participants with a range of anxiety disorders, depression, and eating disorders using the book *Overcoming Perfectionism* (Shafran, Egan, & Wade, 2010), guided self-help was found to be effective in reducing perfectionism and depression (Hoiles et al., 2014). Taken together, these studies indicate efficacy for low-intensity interventions for perfectionism. It is hoped that evaluations of stepped-care approaches may be useful in the future by increasing the ability of clients to access treatment for perfectionism and ultimately improving outcome for a range of psychological disorders.

Resources

Recommended Books and Videos

Perfectionism

SELF-HELP BOOKS

Antony, M. M., & Swinson, R. P. (2009). *When perfect isn't good enough: Strategies for coping with perfectionism* (2nd ed.). Oakland, CA: New Harbinger.

Egan, S. J., Shafran, R., & Wade, T. D. (2012). *Changing perfectionism.* Oxford, UK: Oxford Cognitive Therapy Centre. (Available from *www.octc.co.uk*)

Shafran, R., Egan, S. J., & Wade, T. D. (2010). *Overcoming perfectionism: A self-help guide using cognitive-behavioural techniques.* London: Constable & Robinson.

DVD RESOURCES

Antony, M. M. (2008). *Cognitive behavioral therapy for perfectionism over time* (DVD). Washington, DC: American Psychological Association.

Anxiety and Related Disorders

Anxiety Disorders (General)

SELF-HELP BOOKS

Abramowitz, J. S. (2012). *The stress less workbook: Simple strategies to relieve pressure, manage commitments, and minimize conflicts.* New York: Guilford Press.

Antony, M. M., & Norton, P. J. (2009). *The anti-anxiety workbook: Proven strategies to overcome worry, panic, phobias, and obsessions.* New York: Guilford Press.

Bourne, E. J. (2015). *The anxiety and phobia workbook* (6th ed.). Oakland, CA: New Harbinger.

Clark, D. A., & Beck, A. T. (2012). *The anxiety and worry workbook: The cognitive-behavioral solution.* New York: Guilford Press.
Kennerley, H. (2009). *Overcoming anxiety: A self-help guide using cognitive-behavioral techniques.* London: Constable & Robinson.
Otto, M. W., & Smits, J. A. J. (2009). *Exercise for mood and anxiety disorders* (Workbook). New York: Oxford University Press.
Shafran, R., Brosan, L., & Cooper, P. J. (Eds.). (2013). *The complete CBT guide to anxiety.* London: Constable & Robinson.

PROFESSIONAL BOOKS

Abramowitz, J. S., Deacon, B. J., & Whiteside, S. P. H. (2011). *Exposure therapy for anxiety: Principles and practice.* New York: Guilford Press.
Antony, M. M., Orsillo, S. M., & Roemer, L. (Eds.). (2001). *Practitioner's guide to empirically based measures of anxiety.* New York: Springer.
Antony, M. M., & Stein, M. B. (2009). *Oxford handbook of anxiety and related disorders.* New York: Oxford University Press.
Butler, G., Fennell, M., & Hackman, A. (2008). *Cognitive-behavioral therapy for anxiety disorders: Mastering clinical challenges.* New York: Guilford Press.
Clark, D. A., & Beck, A. T. (2010). *Cognitive therapy of anxiety disorders: Science and practice.* New York: Guilford Press.
Norton, P. J. (2012). *Group cognitive-behavioral therapy for anxiety: A transdiagnostic treatment manual.* New York: Guilford Press.
Smits, J. A. J., & Otto, M. W. (2009). *Exercise for mood and anxiety disorders* (Therapist Guide). New York: Oxford University Press.
Westra, H. A. (2012). *Motivational interviewing in the treatment of anxiety.* New York: Guilford Press.

Panic Disorder and Agoraphobia

SELF-HELP BOOKS

Antony, M. M., & McCabe, R. E. (2004). *10 simple solutions to panic: How to overcome panic attacks, calm physical symptoms, and reclaim your life.* Oakland, CA: New Harbinger.
Barlow, D. H., & Craske, M. G. (2007). *Mastery of your anxiety and panic* (4th ed.) (Workbook). New York: Oxford University Press.
Craske, M., & Barlow, D. (2006). *Mastery of your anxiety and worry* (Workbook). New York: Oxford University Press.
Silove, D. (2009). *Overcoming panic and agoraphobia: A self-help guide using cognitive-behavioral techniques.* London: Constable & Robinson.
Wilson, R. (2009). *Don't panic: Taking control of anxiety attacks* (3rd ed.). New York: HarperCollins.

PROFESSIONAL BOOKS

Craske, M. G., & Barlow, D. H. (2007). *Mastery of your anxiety and panic* (4th ed.) (Therapist Guide). New York: Oxford University Press.

Taylor, S. (2000). *Understanding and treating panic disorder: Cognitive and behavioral approaches.* Chichester, UK: Wiley.

DVD RESOURCES

AnxietyBC. (2010). *Effectively managing panic disorder* (DVD). Vancouver, British Columbia, Canada: Author. (Available from *anxietybc.com*)

Clark, D. M. (1998). *Cognitive therapy for panic disorder* (DVD). Washington, DC: American Psychological Association.

Dobson, K. S. (2010). *Cognitive therapy over time* (DVD). Washington, DC: American Psychological Association.

Rapee, R. M. (2006). *Fight or flight?: Overcoming panic and agoraphobia* (DVD). New York: Guilford Press.

Social Anxiety Disorder

SELF-HELP BOOKS

Antony, M. M. (2004). *10 simple solutions to shyness: How to overcome shyness, social anxiety, and fear of public speaking.* Oakland, CA: New Harbinger. (Available for free download at *www.martinantony.com/downloads.*)

Antony, M. M., & Swinson, R. P. (2008). *The shyness and social anxiety workbook: Proven, step-by-step techniques for overcoming your fear* (2nd ed.). Oakland, CA: New Harbinger.

Butler, G. (2008). *Overcoming social anxiety and shyness: A self-help guide using cognitive behavioral techniques.* New York: Basic Books.

Hope, D. A., Heimberg, R. G., & Turk, C. L. (2010). *Managing social anxiety: A cognitive behavioral therapy approach* (2nd ed.) (Workbook). New York: Oxford University Press.

PROFESSIONAL BOOKS

Antony, M. M., & Rowa, K. (2008). *Social anxiety disorder: Psychological approaches to assessment and treatment.* Göttingen, Germany: Hogrefe.

Beidel, D. C., & Turner, S. M. (2007). *Shy children, phobic adults: Nature and treatment of social anxiety disorder* (2nd ed.). Washington, DC: American Psychological Association.

Crozier, W. R., & Alden, L. E. (Eds.). (2005). *The essential handbook of social anxiety for clinicians.* Hoboken, NJ: Wiley.

Heimberg, R. G., & Becker, R. E. (2002). *Cognitive-behavioral group therapy for social phobia: Basic mechanisms and clinical strategies.* New York: Guilford Press.

Hofmann, S., & Otto, M. W. (2008). *Cognitive-behavior therapy of social phobia: Evidence-based and disorder-specific treatment techniques.* New York: Routledge.

Hope, D. A., Heimberg, R. G., & Turk, C. L. (2010). *Managing social anxiety: A cognitive behavioral therapy approach* (2nd ed.) (Therapist Guide). New York: Oxford University Press.

DVD RESOURCES

Albano, A. M. (2006). *Shyness and social phobia* (DVD). Washington, DC: American Psychological Association.
Rapee, R. M. (2006). *I think they think . . . . Overcoming social phobia* (DVD). New York: Guilford Press.

Generalized Anxiety Disorder

SELF-HELP BOOKS

Freeston, M., & Meares, K. (2008). *Overcoming worry: A self-help guide using cognitive behavioural techniques.* London: Constable & Robinson.
Gyoerkoe, K. L., & Wiegartz, P. S. (2006). *10 simple solutions to worry: How to calm your mind, relax your body, and reclaim your life.* Oakland, CA: New Harbinger.

PROFESSIONAL BOOKS

Dugas, M. J., & Robichaud, M. (2007). *Cognitive-behavioral treatment for generalized anxiety disorder.* New York: Routledge.
Hazlett-Stevens, H. (2008). *Psychological approaches to generalized anxiety disorder: A clinician's guide to assessment and treatment.* New York: Springer.
Marker, C. D., & Aylward, A. G. (2012). *Generalized anxiety disorder.* Göttingen, Germany: Hogrefe.
Rygh, J. L., & Sanderson, W. C. (2004). *Treating generalized anxiety disorder: Evidence-based strategies, tools, and techniques.* New York: Guilford Press.

Specific Phobia

SELF-HELP BOOKS

Antony, M. M., Craske, M. G., & Barlow, D. H. (2006). *Mastering your fears and phobias* (2nd ed.) (Workbook). New York: Oxford University Press.
Antony, M. M., & McCabe, R. E. (2005). *Overcoming animal and insect phobias: How to conquer fear of dogs, snakes, rodents, bees, spiders, and more.* Oakland, CA: New Harbinger. (Available for free download at *www.martinantony.com/downloads.*)
Antony, M. M., & Rowa, K. (2007). *Overcoming fear of heights: How to conquer acrophobia and live a life without limits.* Oakland, CA: New Harbinger. (Available for free download at *www.martinantony.com/downloads.*)
Antony, M. M., & Watling, M. (2006). *Overcoming medical phobias: How to conquer fear of blood, needles, doctors, and dentists.* Oakland, CA: New Harbinger. (Available for free download at *www.martinantony.com/downloads*)
Brown, D. (2009). *Flying without fear: Effective strategies to get you where you want to go* (2nd ed.). Oakland, CA: New Harbinger.

PROFESSIONAL BOOKS

Craske, M. G., Antony, M. M., & Barlow, D. H. (2006). *Mastering your fears and phobias* (2nd ed.) (Therapist Guide). New York: Oxford University Press.

Davis, T. E., Ollendick, T. H., & Öst, L.-G. (Eds.). (2012). *Intensive one-session treatment of specific phobias.* New York: Springer.

DVD RESOURCES

Wilson, R. (2012). *Exposure therapy for phobias* (DVD). Mill Valley, CA: Psychotherapy.net.

Posttraumatic Stress Disorder

SELF-HELP BOOKS

Herbert, C., & Wetmore, A. (2008). *Overcoming traumatic stress: A self-help guide using cognitive behavioral techniques.* London: Constable & Robinson.

Hickling, E. J., & Blanchard, E. B. (2006). *Overcoming the trauma of your motor vehicle accident: A cognitive-behavioral treatment program* (Workbook). New York: Oxford University Press.

Rothbaum, B. O., Foa, E. B., & Hembree, E. A. (2007). *Reclaiming your life from a traumatic experience* (Workbook). New York: Oxford University Press.

PROFESSIONAL BOOKS

Foa, E. B., Hembree, E. A., & Rothbaum, B. O. (2007). *Prolonged exposure therapy for PTSD: Emotional processing of traumatic experiences* (Therapist Guide). New York: Oxford University Press.

Foa, E. B., & Rothbaum, B. O. (1998). *Treating the trauma of rape: Cognitive behavioral therapy for PTSD.* New York: Guilford Press.

Hickling, E. J., & Blanchard, E. B. (2006). *Overcoming the trauma of your motor vehicle accident: A cognitive-behavioral treatment program* (Therapist Guide). New York: Oxford University Press.

Monson, C. M., & Fredman, S. J. (2012). *Cognitive-behavioral conjoint therapy for PTSD: Harnessing the healing power of relationships.* New York: Guilford Press.

Rosen, G. M., & Frueh, B. C. (Eds.). (2010). *Clinician's guide to posttraumatic stress disorder.* Hoboken, NJ: Wiley.

Taylor, S. (2006). *Clinician's guide to PTSD: A cognitive-behavioral approach.* New York: Guilford Press.

Zayfert, C., & Becker, C. B. (2007). *Cognitive-behavioral therapy for PTSD: A case formulation approach.* New York: Guilford Press.

Obsessive–Compulsive Disorder and Hoarding

SELF-HELP BOOKS

Abramowitz, J. S. (2009). *Getting over OCD: A 10-step workbook for taking back your life.* New York: Guilford Press.

Baer, L. (2012). *Getting control: Overcoming your obsessions and compulsions* (3rd ed.). New York: Plume.

Challacombe, F., Oldfield, V. B., & Salkovskis, P. (2011). *Break free from OCD: Overcoming obsessive compulsive disorder with CBT.* London: Vermilion.

Hyman, B. M., & Pedrick, C. (2010). *The OCD workbook: Your guide to breaking free from obsessive compulsive disorder* (3rd ed.). Oakland, CA: New Harbinger.

Purdon, C., & Clark, D. A. (2005). *Overcoming obsessive thoughts: How to gain control of your OCD.* Oakland, CA: New Harbinger.

Steketee, G., & Frost, R. O. (2007). *Compulsive hoarding and acquiring* (Workbook). New York: Oxford University Press.

Tolin, D., Frost, R. O., & Steketee, G. (2007). *Buried in treasures: Help for compulsive acquiring, saving, and hoarding.* New York: Oxford University Press.

Tompkins, M. A., & Hartl, T. L. (2009). *Digging out: Helping your loved one manage clutter, hoarding, and compulsive acquiring.* Oakland, CA: New Harbinger.

Yadin, E., Foa, E. B., & Lichner, T. K. (2012). *Treating your OCD with exposure and response (ritual) prevention for obsessive–compulsive disorder* (2nd ed.) (Workbook). New York: Oxford University Press.

PROFESSIONAL BOOKS

Abramowitz, J. S. (2006). *Obsessive–compulsive disorder.* Cambridge, MA: Hogrefe & Huber.

Abramowitz, J. S. (2006). *Understanding and treating obsessive–compulsive disorder: A cognitive–behavioral approach.* Mahwah, NJ: Erlbaum.

Abramowitz, J. S., & Houts, A. C. (Eds.). (2005). *Obsessive–compulsive disorder: Concepts and controversies.* New York: Springer.

Abramowitz, J. S., McKay, D., & Taylor, S. (2008). *Obsessive–compulsive disorder: Subtypes and spectrum conditions.* New York: Elsevier.

Antony, M. M., Purdon, C., & Summerfeldt, L. J. (2007). *Psychological treatment of obsessive–compulsive disorder: Fundamentals and beyond.* Washington, DC: American Psychological Association.

Clark, D. A. (2004). *Cognitive-behavioral therapy for OCD.* New York: Guilford Press.

Foa, E. B., Yadin, E., & Lichner, T. K. (2012). *Exposure and response (ritual) prevention for obsessive–compulsive disorder* (2nd ed.) (Therapist Guide). New York: Oxford University Press.

Rees, C. S. (2009). *Obsessive–compulsive disorder: A practical guide to treatment.* Melbourne, Australia: IP Communications.

Steketee, G., & Frost, R. O. (2007). *Compulsive hoarding and acquiring* (Therapist Guide). New York: Oxford University Press.
Wilhelm, S., & Steketee, G. S. (2006). *Cognitive therapy for obsessive–compulsive disorder: A guide for professionals.* Oakland, CA: New Harbinger.

DVD RESOURCES

Antony, M. M. (2009). *Behavioral therapy over time* (DVD). Washington, DC: American Psychological Association.
Wilson, R. (2012). *Cognitive therapy for obsessions* (DVD). Mill Valley, CA: Psychotherapy.net.

Health Anxiety

SELF-HELP BOOKS

Asmundson, G. J. G., & Taylor, S. (2005). *It's not all in your head: How worrying about your health could be making you sick—and what you can do about it.* New York: Guilford Press.
Owens, K. M. B., & Antony, M. M. (2011). *Overcoming health anxiety: Letting go of your fear of illness.* Oakland, CA: New Harbinger.
Veale, D., & Wilson, R. (2009). *Overcoming health anxiety: A self-help guide using cognitive behavioral techniques.* London: Constable & Robinson.

PROFESSIONAL BOOKS

Abramowitz, J. S., & Braddock, A. E. (2011). *Hypochondriasis and health anxiety.* Göttingen, Germany: Hogrefe.
Furer, P., Walker, J. R., & Stein, M. B. (2007). *Treating health anxiety and fear of death: A practitioner's guide.* New York: Springer.
Taylor, S., & Asmundson, G. J. G. (2004). *Treating health anxiety: A cognitive-behavioral approach.* New York: Guilford Press.

Trichotillomania

SELF-HELP BOOKS

Keuthen, N. J., Stein, D. J., & Christenson, G. A. (2001). *Help for hair pullers: Understanding and coping with trichotillomania.* Oakland, CA: New Harbinger.

PROFESSIONAL BOOKS

Franklin, M. E., & Tolin, D. F. (2007). *Treating trichotillomania: Cognitive-behavioral therapy for hair pulling and related problems.* New York: Springer.

Body Dysmorphic Disorder

SELF-HELP BOOKS

Wilhelm, S. (2006). *Feeling good about the way you look: A program for overcoming body image problems.* New York: Guilford Press.

PROFESSIONAL BOOKS

Phillips, K. A. (2005). *The broken mirror: Understanding and treating body dysmorphic disorder.* New York: Oxford University Press.
Veale, D., & Neziroglu, F. (2010). *Body dysmorphic disorder: A treatment manual.* West Sussex, UK: Wiley.
Wilhelm, S., Phillips, K. A., & Steketee, G. (2013). *Cognitive-behavioral therapy for body dysmorphic disorder: A treatment manual.* New York: Guilford Press.

Depression and Low Self-Esteem

SELF-HELP BOOKS

Fennell, M. (1999). *Overcoming low self-esteem.* London: Constable & Robinson.
Gilbert, P. (2009). *Overcoming depression: A self-help guide using cognitive behavioural techniques* (3rd ed.). London: Constable & Robinson.
Gilson, M., Freeman, A., Yates, J., & Freeman, S. M. (2009). *Overcoming depression: A cognitive therapy approach* (Workbook). New York: Oxford University Press.
Williams, M., Teasdale, J., Segal, Z., & Kabat-Zinn, J. (2007). *The mindful way through depression: Freeing yourself from chronic unhappiness.* New York: Guilford Press.

PROFESSIONAL BOOKS

Gilson, M., Freeman, A., Yates J., & Freeman, S. M. (2009). *Overcoming depression: A cognitive therapy approach* (Clinician's Guide). New York: Oxford University Press.
Segal, Z. V., Williams, J. M. G., & Teasdale, J. D. (2012). *Mindfulness-based cognitive therapy for depression* (2nd ed.). New York: Guilford Press.

Eating Disorders

SELF-HELP BOOKS

Cooper, P. (2009). *Overcoming bulimia nervosa and binge eating.* London: Constable & Robinson.
Fairburn, C. G. (2013). *Overcoming binge eating: The proven program to learn why you binge and how you can stop* (2nd ed.). New York: Guilford Press.
Freeman, C. (2009). *Overcoming anorexia nervosa.* London: Constable & Robinson.

Treasure, J., Smith, G., & Crane, A. (2007). *Skills-based learning for caring for a loved one with an eating disorder: The New Maudsley Method.* New York: Routledge.

PROFESSIONAL BOOKS

Agras, W. S., & Apple, R. F. (2007). *Overcoming eating disorders: A cognitive-behavioral approach for bulimia nervosa and anorexia nervosa* (Therapist Guide). New York: Oxford University Press.
Fairburn, C. G. (2008). *Cognitive behaviour therapy and eating disorders.* New York: Guilford Press.
Grilo, G. M., & Mitchell, J. E. (2011). *The treatment of eating disorders: A clinical handbook.* New York: Guilford Press.
Lock, J., & LeGrange, D. (2012). *Treatment manual for anorexia nervosa: A family-based approach* (2nd ed.). New York: Guilford Press.
Treasure, J., Schmidt, U., & Macdonald, P. (Eds.). (2009). *The clinician's guide to collaborative caring in the eating disorders: The New Maudsley Method.* New York: Routledge.
Waller, G., Cordery, H., Corstorphine, E., Hinrichesen, H., Lawson, R., Mountford, V., et al. (2007). *Cognitive behavioural therapy for eating disorders: A comprehensive treatment guide.* Cambridge, UK: Cambridge University Press.

Cognitive-Behavioral Therapy Resources (General)

SELF-HELP BOOKS

Butler, G., & Hope, T. (2007). *Managing your mind: The mental fitness guide* (2nd ed.). New York: Oxford University Press.
Greenberger, D., & Padesky, C. A. (1995). *Mind over mood: Change how you feel by changing the way you think.* New York: Guilford Press.
McKay, M., Davis, M., & Fanning, P. (2007). *Thoughts and feelings: Taking control of your moods and your life* (3rd ed.). Oakland, CA: New Harbinger.

PROFESSIONAL BOOKS

Antony, M. M., & Barlow, D. H. (Eds.). (2010). *Handbook of assessment and treatment for psychological disorders* (2nd ed.). New York: Guilford Press.
Antony, M. M., & Roemer, L. (2011). *Behavior therapy.* Washington, DC: American Psychological Association.
Barlow, D. H. (Ed.). (2014). *Clinical handbook of psychological disorders: A step-by-step treatment manual* (5th ed.). New York: Guilford Press.
Beck, J. S. (2011). *Cognitive behavior therapy: Basics and beyond* (2nd ed.). New York: Guilford Press.
Bennett-Levy, J., Butler, G., Fennell, M., & Hackman, A. (Eds.). (2011). *Oxford guide to behavioural experiments in cognitive therapy* (2nd ed.). Oxford, UK: Oxford University Press.

Bieling, P. J., McCabe, R. E., & Antony, M. M. (2006). *Cognitive-behavioral therapy in groups.* New York: Guilford Press.

Craske, M. G. (2010). *Cognitive-behavioral therapy.* Washington, DC: American Psychological Association.

Dobson, K. S. (Ed.). (2010). *Handbook of cognitive-behavioral therapies* (2nd ed.). New York: Guilford Press.

Hackmann, A., Bennett-Levy, J., & Holmes, E. (2011). *Oxford guide to imagery in cognitive therapy.* New York: Oxford University Press.

Harvey, A., Watkins, E., Mansell, W., & Shafran, R. (2004). *Cognitive behavioural processes across psychological disorders: A transdiagnostic approach to research and treatment.* Oxford, UK: Oxford University Press.

Kuyken, W., Padesky, C. A., & Dudley, R. (2009). *Collaborative case conceptualization: Working effectively with clients in cognitive-behavioral therapy.* New York: Guilford Press.

Ledley, D. R., Marx, B. P., & Heimberg, R. G. (2010). *Making cognitive-behavioral therapy work: Clinical process for new practitioners* (2nd ed.). New York: Guilford Press.

Mueller, M., Kennerley, H., McManus, F., & Westbrook, D. (2010). *Oxford guide to surviving as a CBT therapist.* New York: Oxford University Press.

Newman, C. F. (2013). *Core competencies in cognitive behavioral therapy: Becoming a highly effective and competent cognitive behavioral therapist.* New York: Routledge.

O'Donohue, W. T., & Fisher, J. E. (2012). *Cognitive behavior therapy: Core principles for practice.* Hoboken, NJ: Wiley.

Stott, R., Mansell, W., Salkovskis, P., Lavender, A., & Cartwright-Hatton, S. (2010). *Oxford guide to metaphors in CBT: Building cognitive bridges.* Oxford, UK: Oxford University Press.

Westbrook, D., Kennerley, H., & Kirk, J. (2011). *An introduction to CBT: Skills and applications* (2nd ed.). New York: Sage.

DVD RESOURCES

Beck, J. S. (2006). *Cognitive therapy* (DVD). Washington, DC: American Psychological Association.

Dobson, K. S. (2011). *Cognitive-behavioral therapy strategies* (DVD). Washington, DC: American Psychological Association.

Padesky, C. (2008). *Guided discovery using Socratic dialogue* (DVD). (Available from *www.padesky.com*)

Padesky, C. (2008). *Testing automatic thoughts with thought records* (DVD). (Available from *www.padesky.com*)

Professional Associations and Web-Based Resources

Professional Associations

Academy of Cognitive Therapy (ACT)
260 South Broad Street, 18th Floor
Philadelphia, PA 19102

Phone: 1-267-350-7683
E-mail: *info@academyofct.org*
Website: *www.academyofct.org*

An association offering professional memberships. The website has referrals to certified cognitive therapists.

Asian Cognitive Behavioral Therapy Association (ACBTA)
Website: *www.asian.weebly.com*

An association representing CBT associations throughout Asia that offers professional memberships.

Association for Behavioral and Cognitive Therapies (ABCT)
305 Seventh Avenue, 16th Floor
New York, NY 10001-6008
Phone: 1-212-647-1890
Fax: 1-212-647-1865
Website: *www.abct.org*

A U.S.-based CBT association offering professional memberships and therapist referrals for clients on its website (*www.abct.org/members/Directory/Find_A_ Therapist.cfm*).

Australian Association for Cognitive and Behaviour Therapy (AACBT)
P.O. Box 4040
Nowra East, NSW, Australia 2541
Fax: +61730410415
E-mail: *info@aacbt.org*
Website: *www.aacbt.org*

An Australian CBT association offering professional memberships. The website includes a list of CBT practitioners.

British Association for Behavioural and Cognitive Psychotherapies (BABCP)
Imperial House
Hornby Street
Bury, Lancashire BL9 5BN, United Kingdom
Phone: 0161 705 4304
Fax: 0161 705 4306
E-mail: *babcp@babcp.com*
Website: *www.babcp.com*

A U.K.-based CBT organization offering professional memberships, the website includes a "find a therapist" section for clients.

Canadian Association of Cognitive and Behavioral Therapies
260 Queen Street West
P. O. Box 60055
Toronto ON M5V OC5, Canada
Website: *www.cacbt.ca*

European Association for Behavioral and Cognitive Therapies (EABCT)
Luttenbaan 57
3524 GA Utrecht, The Netherlands
Phone: +31 30 2543054
E-mail: *office@eabct.eu*
Website: *www.eabct.org*

A European CBT association that represents 51 CBT professional associations across 38 different countries in Europe, and the website has a "find a therapist" function.

International Association of Cognitive Psychotherapy (IACP)
Website: *www.the-iacp.com*

An international association offering professional memberships, with a referral section for clients on its website (*www.the-iacp.com/therapist-referrals*).

Web-Based Resources

Anxiety Disorders, Depression, OCD, and BDD

AUSTRALIA

1. The websites *www.anxietyonline.org.au* and *www.anxietyaustralia.com.au* provide information on anxiety services and resources in Australia, including anxiety self-help groups and organizations.
2. There are online web-based self-help CBT treatment programs for anxiety and depression available on the Australian website Virtual Clinic (*www.virtualclinic.org.au*).
3. An online treatment website is available at *www.thiswayup.org.au*, which also includes information for practitioners on how to deliver evidence-based interventions for anxiety and depression.
4. The Centre for Clinical Interventions has numerous online CBT resources for clients and mental health professionals for the treatment of anxiety and depression at *www.cci.health.wa.gov.au*.

CANADA AND THE UNITED STATES

1. The Anxiety and Depression Association of America (*www.adaa.org*) provides a range of information and resources for those suffering from anxiety and depression.
2. The National Alliance on Mental Illness (*www.nami.org*) has a range of resources on mental health.
3. The Therapeutic Lifestyle Change treatment for depression has an online site providing information on treatment of depression (*www.psych.ku.edu/tlc*).
4. The Anxiety Disorders Treatment Center in North Carolina has an anxiety self-help site (*www.anxieties.com*).
5. The Depression Center (*www.depressioncenter.net*) offers a self-help web-based treatment for depression.
6. The Panic Center (*www.paniccenter.net*) has a self-help, web-based treatment for panic disorder.

7. The National Center for PTSD website (*www.ptsd.va.gov*) has information on the nature and treatment of PTSD.
8. The International OCD Foundation (IOCDF; *www.ocfoundation.org*) offers client and professional memberships and has referral lists of practitioners who treat OCD.
9. The Anxiety Disorders Association Canada (*www.anxietycanada.ca*) offers client and professional memberships and provides links to referral options.
10. A U.S.-based website that has information on BDD is *www.bddcentral.com*.

UNITED KINGDOM

1. Anxiety UK—*www.anxietyuk.org.uk*. Anxiety UK offers information and provides self-help services. They also strive to advance awareness by the general public of the causes and conditions of anxiety disorders.
2. No Panic—*www.nopanic.org.uk*. No Panic is a voluntary charity that assists people with anxiety disorders, including OCD, with self-help through recovery groups and one-to-one mentoring over the telephone, using cognitive-behavioral methods.
3. OCD-UK—*www.ocduk.org*. This website has information for clients on OCD.
4. OCD Action—*www.ocdaction.org.uk*. This website contains information and resources on OCD.
5. Depression alliance—*www.depressionalliance.org*. This U.K. charity provides information and support services to people with depression.

Eating Disorders

AUSTRALIA

1. Information on resources for eating disorders in Australia can be found on the Butterfly Foundation website—*www.thebutterflyfoundationa.org.au*—which also has a telephone support line for clients: 1-800-334-673.

CANADA AND UNITED STATES

1. Information on resources for eating disorders in the United States can be found at *www.nationaleatingdisorders.org*.
2. Information on resources for eating disorders in Canada can be found at the National Eating Disorder Information Center (*www.nedic.ca*).

UNITED KINGDOM

1. Information on resources for eating disorders in the United Kingdom can be found at *www.eating-disorders.org.uk*.
2. The Oxford University Department of Psychiatry CREDO (Centre for Research on Eating Disorders at Oxford) website makes worksheets and self-report measures available for practitioners to use in the cognitive-behavioral treatment of eating disorders at *www.credo-oxford.com*.

APPENDIX 2

Handouts

Goal Setting

To help you set goals, it is useful to first brainstorm all of the steps that are involved in goal setting, including what the goal is, why you want to achieve the goal, who is involved in the goal, where the goal is, and any requirements or constraints for the goal.

Once you have considered the background to your goals, ensure that when you set your goals, they are SMARTER—*Specific, Measurable, Attainable, Relevant,* and *Time-bound*— and that once you have carried out your goal, you *Evaluate* and *Reevaluate* the outcome.

Steps to Setting Specific Goals

- *What:* What do you want to accomplish?
- *Why:* Specific reasons, purpose or benefits of accomplishing the goal.
- *Who:* Who is involved?
- *Where:* Identify a location.
- *Which:* Identify requirements and constraints.

Cognitive-Behavioral Formulation of Perfectionism

Answer the following questions to help you design a personalized formulation. Give examples of each of these areas in the spaces below.

1. **Self-worth:** Does how you feel about yourself depend on achievement?

   _____

   _____

   _____

2. **Inflexible standards:** Do you have very high standards that can be inflexible in the form of rules (e.g., anything less than 80% on a test is a failure)?

   _____

   _____

   _____

3. **Cognitive biases:** Do you judge things in an all-or-nothing manner? Do you notice negative aspects of your performance and ignore positive aspects?

   _____

   _____

   _____

4. **Performance-related behavior:** Do you avoid, procrastinate, check your work repeatedly, or check your work compared to others? Are you overly detailed or thorough?

   _____

   _____

   _____

5. **Temporarily meets standards:** Think of a recent time when you met your standard: did you think it was no big deal, that anyone could do it, and that you needed to try harder next time?

   _____

   _____

   _____

(continued)

6. **Fails to meet standards:** Can you think of a recent time you failed to meet a standard?

_____

_____

_____

7. **Counterproductive behavior and self-criticism:** If you fail to meet a standard, are you hard on yourself? Do you engage in performance-related behavior like checking or procrastination, and do you criticize yourself (e.g., think you are a failure)?

_____

_____

_____

8. **Avoidance:** Do you sometimes not even try to meet standards at all because you are concerned about not doing well?

_____

_____

_____

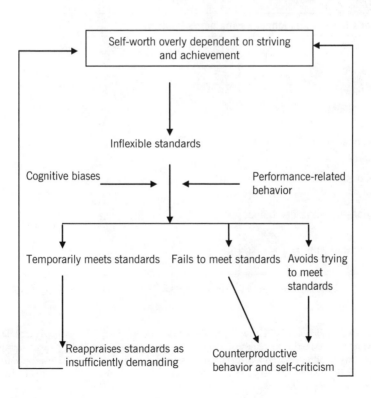

Consider the Long-Term Costs and Benefits of Perfectionism

Consider the continued impact of perfectionism on different areas of your life, and what your life would look like in these areas if you did not have perfectionism.

In 1 year's time . . . still having perfectionism	
Area of life	*What will have happened in this area?*
My social life	
My work/education	
My emotional health	
My relationship with my partner	
My relationship with close friends	
My relationship with family	

In 1 year's time . . . no longer having perfectionism	
Area of life	*What will have happened in this area?*
My social life	
My work/education	
My emotional health	
My relationship with my partner	
My relationship with close friends	
My relationship with family	

Adapted from Shafran, Egan, and Wade (2010). Copyright 2010 by Constable & Robinson. Adapted by permission.

Self-Monitoring Perfectionism

1. Record the area of perfectionism and what rules you have for your performance.
2. Record what self-critical thoughts you had regarding your performance and what feelings the thoughts resulted in.
3. Record your behaviors (what you did) as a result of the thoughts.

Perfectionism area and situation	Rules (rate 0–100% how much you believe them at the time)	Self-critical thoughts	Feelings (0–100% intensity)	What do you do? (rate 0–100%)

(continued)

Adapted from Shafran, Egan, and Wade (2010). Copyright 2010 by Constable & Robinson. Adapted by permission.

Perfectionism area and situation	Rules (rate 0–100% how much you believe them at the time)	Self-critical thoughts	Feelings (0–100% intensity)	What do you do? (rate 0–100%)

Challenging Perfectionism Beliefs through Surveys

1. The purpose of this worksheet is to help you use surveys to challenge your perfectionism beliefs. The aim of a survey is to find out information about a belief that you hold. Think of a belief that you hold that would be useful to challenge, then design a question to ask others.
2. Once you have the responses, draw conclusions about the range of responses you receive and what you can conclude as a result.

EXAMPLES

Belief: "I make more mistakes than other people at work." This survey would be given to people who are successful in your workplace.

Survey Questions:
1. How many mistakes have you made at work in the past month?
2. Can you give examples of the mistakes you have made at work?
3. Do you think others at work make similar mistakes?
4. What is your opinion of others who make mistakes at work?

Belief: "I am more prone to make serious mistakes compared to others at work." This survey would be given to people who are successful in your workplace.

Survey Questions:
1. How many mistakes have you made at work in the past year?
2. How many of these mistakes were serious?
3. What examples do you have of serious mistakes you have made at work?
4. What were the negative consequences of your serious mistakes?
5. What is the worst consequence you have ever had due to serious mistakes?

Belief: "I should be available for work calls all times of the day and night even when I'm on vacation." This survey could be given to people in your workplace and others whom you respect.

Survey Questions:
1. How often do you take your work phone with you on vacation?
2. What do you think of people who do take their work phone with them on vacation?
3. What do you think of people who do not take their work phone with them on vacation?
4. Do you answer your work phone at night and on weekends?
5. What do you think of people who do answer their work phone at night and on weekends?
6. What do you think of people who do not answer their work phone at night and on weekends?

(continued)

Belief: "I am a failure because I didn't get that job." This survey could be given your friends.

Survey Questions:
1. Have you ever not gotten a job that you interviewed for?
2. If so, what did you think of yourself for not getting the job?
3. What do you think of others who do not get jobs they have applied for?
4. Do you think someone is a failure if they do not get a job they apply for?

Belief: "The way to better myself is to constantly keep striving." This survey could be given to people at work and friends.

Survey Questions:
1. Do you think that successful people have time off and rest time away from work?
2. Do you think successful people strive all of the time and don't let themselves have time off?
3. Do you think it is important to constantly push yourself in order to keep achieving?
4. Have you had any examples in your life where constantly striving resulted in you being less successful?

Belief: "Successful people do not read trashy magazines." This survey could be given to anyone you think is successful, either at work or among friends.

Survey Questions:
1. Do you read gossip magazines?
2. What do you think of others who read gossip magazines?
3. Do you think reading magazines is a waste of time?

CONSTRUCT YOUR OWN SURVEY

Belief: _____

_____

Survey Questions:

1. _____

2. _____

3. _____

4. _____

Conclusions: _____

_____

_____

_____

_____

_____

ABC Thought Diary

1. Think of a recent time when you were upset. Record the event (A) and the beliefs (B) that were going through your mind about the event that resulted in the emotional consequences (C).
2. Identify any thinking errors that may be present (see Handouts 10.2–10.6).

A—Activating event	B—Beliefs (rate 0–100%)	C—Consequences (emotions—rate 0–100%)

(continued)

A—Activating event	B—Beliefs (rate 0–100%)	C—Consequences (emotions—rate 0–100%)

Thinking Errors in Perfectionism

The following is a list of common thinking errors that occur in perfectionism. Read through the list and see if you can recognize yourself thinking these.

Dichotomous thinking—One of the most common thinking styles in perfectionism. It involves judging things in an all-or-nothing way (e.g., "Because I stumbled over a few words at the start of my speech the entire talk was ruined and I am a complete failure"; "Because I weigh 105 pounds and that is above my goal weight of 100 pounds I am completely fat and a failure").

Selective attention—Focusing in on the negative aspects of your performance and noticing mistakes, and at the same time discounting the positive aspects of your performance and not recognizing your successes (e.g., "Because I made a bad dessert the whole meal was ruined").

Double standards—Holding a set of harsher rules for yourself than for other people (e.g., "It is okay for others to make spelling mistakes but not okay for me").

Overgeneralizing—Generalizing from one mistake or flaw in performance to conclude that you are a failure overall (e.g., "Because I made a mistake at work, I am a failure as a person").

"Should" statements—Saying "should" and "must" regarding meeting your standards (e.g., "I should always push myself"; "I should do a better job").

Catastrophizing—Associated with "what if" statements that lead to imagining the worst-case scenario, which makes you feel anxious (e.g., "What if I lose my job because I stumbled over my words in a presentation?").

Emotional reasoning—When you view a situation based on feelings rather than on facts (e.g., "I feel anxious; therefore, I know I am going to give a bad talk").

Labeling—Associated with self-critical thinking, often occurs when you feel that you have failed to meet your standards or goals, and includes negative self-labels such as "failure," "loser," "screw up," "useless," and "idiot."

Personalization—Involves taking full responsibility for events and outcomes in which responsibility is actually shared, and without taking into account all of the factors that contribute to the outcome (e.g., "If my work team does not win the bid, it is entirely my fault").

Mind reading—Occurs when you assume you can guess what others around you are thinking (e.g., "I know my colleagues thought my presentation was bad and boring, because some of them were staring out of the window").

Predictive thinking—Involves having a strong negative prediction about the future (e.g., "I know I am going to do a bad presentation"; "I know I am not going to do well in the race").

Thinking Errors in Perfectionism: Selective Attention

Selective attention involves focusing in on the negative aspects of your performance and noticing mistakes, while at the same time discounting the positive aspects of your performance and not recognizing your successes.

Identifying Selective Attention

- When you think about your performance, what do you tend to focus on?

- How much do you notice mistakes in performance? Do you notice successes?

- How do you react to positive aspects of performance?

- How do you feel when you meet a goal or standard? Do you feel satisfied? Not satisfied? How long does that last?

- Do you discount your goals when you meet them as being too easy, or feel that anyone could have done that?

- After you meet your goals, do you set the goals for next time higher, lower, or the same?

Challenging Selective Attention

- What does focusing in on your mistakes and discounting your successes do to your mood?

- How does focusing on your flaws and discounting the positive aspects of your performance impact how much you base your sense of self-worth on achievement?

- If you constantly set your goals higher even after you have done well and discount your achievements by saying "it was no big deal," how will you ever feel satisfied with your performance?

- What effect do you think it has on other people when you brush off meeting your goals as no big deal?

- If you constantly followed a friend around as a "critical judge," pointed out everything he or she did wrong, and never commented on what your friend did well, what do you think would start to happen to your friend's mood and self-esteem? What would the judge actually need to do instead in order for your friend to feel like a success?

Thinking Errors in Perfectionism: Double Standards

Double standards involve holding a set of harsher rules for yourself than for other people.

Identifying Double Standards

- Do you have one set of rules for yourself, and another set of rules for other people?
- Are the rules for yourself harder than your rules for others?

Challenging Double Standards

- Is it fair to have harsher rules for yourself that are different from your rules for everyone else?
- What is the impact when people hold standards for themselves that are different from the standards they hold for other people?
- What does it do to you always giving yourself these hard standards to meet but thinking it is okay for others not to meet them?
- What would you say to a friend who had a harder set of rules for him- or herself than for other people?
- How does it follow that rules need to be harder for you than for other people?
- What does holding double standards do to your self-esteem and mood?

Thinking Errors in Perfectionism: Overgeneralizing

Overgeneralizing involves concluding from one mistake or flaw in performance that you are a failure overall.

Identifying Overgeneralizing

- What do you think of yourself as a person overall when you make even just a small mistake?

- What happens to your self-esteem when your performance has not met your standards?

Challenging Overgeneralizing

- How does it follow that someone's worth as a person can be judged on one instance of not meeting a goal or making a mistake?

- What is the universal definition that people in society would hold of a "failure"? How do you compare to that definition? In what ways are you similar or different?

- What do most people judge as important in making up a person's worth?

- How is it that making a small mistake or error (e.g., a spelling mistake in an e-mail) can reflect on a person's worth overall?

- What does overgeneralizing from one small mistake to say you are a failure as a person do to your self-esteem and mood?

Thinking Errors in Perfectionism: Should Statements

Should statements involve saying "should" and "must" regarding meeting your standards (e.g., "I should always push myself"; "I should do a better job").

Identifying "Should" Statements

- What do you say to yourself to really get yourself going when you think you have to get something done?

- What runs through your mind when you think of the to-do list that you have to get through?

- How often do you say "should" and "must" to yourself when you are thinking of everything you have to do?

Challenging "Should" Statements

- How does saying "should" to yourself constantly make you feel? In what way does it impact on your sense of self?

- If a friend wanted to engage in exercise more, how would he feel if he said to himself, "I should exercise 7 days a week"? What would it do to his sense of pressure on himself? Now consider if he said to himself, "I would like to engage in exercise more regularly if I can." Which one do you think would make him feel more stressed? Which statement would make him more likely to engage in exercise?

Complete Thought Diary

1. Think about a recent time when you were upset. Record the event (A) and the beliefs (B) that were going through your mind about the event that resulted in the emotional consequences (C).
2. Identify any thinking errors that may be present (see thinking errors handouts).
3. Challenge the unhelpful beliefs (D) and evaluate the outcome (E).

A—Activating event	B—Beliefs (rate 0–100%)	C— Consequences (rate 0–100%)	D—Disputation	E—Evaluate outcome
What was the event, situation, thought, image, or memory?	What went through my mind? What does it say about me as a person? Am I using unhelpful thinking styles?	What was I feeling?	What would a friend say? Is there another way of viewing this thought?	How do I feel now?

(continued)

A—Activating event	B—Beliefs (rate 0–100%)	C—Consequences (rate 0–100%)	D—Disputation	E—Evaluate outcome
What was the event, situation, thought, image, or memory?	What went through my mind? What does it say about me as a person? Am I using unhelpful thinking styles?	What was I feeling?	What would a friend say? Is there another way of viewing this thought?	How do I feel now?

Challenging Core Beliefs 1

1. Record the core belief (choose a belief from a thought record) and ask yourself, "What was the worst thing about that?" "If that were true, what would that mean about me and what does it say about me as a person?").
2. Record evidence that shows the belief is not true (think of what a friend would say about you).
3. Write a new more helpful core belief.

Core belief:

Evidence that shows this belief is not true:

Helpful new core belief:

Challenging Core Beliefs 2

1. Specify core belief and think of an experiment to test your predictions based on the core belief.
2. Record the outcome of the experiment and a revised core belief.

Core belief:
Experiment:
Prediction:
Outcome:
Helpful new core belief:

Challenging Selective Attention

1. Record negative thoughts and rate them from 0% belief to 100% belief in the thought, then identify ways to broaden your attention to include *all* of the information by asking yourself (a) "What positive aspects of my performance am I missing?" and (b) "How can I focus my attention on things other than negative flaws?"
2. Record the outcome.

Situation	Noticing the negative thoughts (rate 0–100%)	Ways to broaden my attention in the situation	Outcome

Adapted from Shafran, Egan, and Wade (2010). Copyright 2010 by Constable & Robinson. Adapted by permission.

HANDOUT 11.5

Diary of Positive Comments and Lack of Negative Comments

Think of recent situations where people have commented on your performance. For example, this might be at work, at home, or with friends. Then record this evidence as follows:

1. Record positive comments and evidence regarding performance.
2. Record lack of negative evidence regarding performance.

Area	Positive evidence	Lack of negative evidence

Challenging Dichotomous Thinking through Continua

The purpose of this worksheet is to identify your all-or-nothing thinking and consider an example when a thought or behavior was not completely all-or-nothing.

1. Identify the all-or-nothing thought.
2. Specify the categories on the continuum.
3. Think of examples of evidence that fall at various points along the continuum and make an X mark along the horizontal line reflecting, for example, being low to high on the continuum.
4. Reflect.

1. What is my all-or-nothing thought?

2. Specify the all-or-nothing categories on the continuum.

$\vdash$————————————————————$\dashv$

3. Examples of evidence that fall at various points along the continuum in the thought/ behavior:

$\vdash$————————————————————$\dashv$

$\vdash$————————————————————$\dashv$

$\vdash$————————————————————$\dashv$

4 . What I learned from the continua:

Adapted from Shafran, Egan, and Wade (2010). Copyright 2010 by Constable & Robinson. Adapted by permission.

Behavioral Experiment Record Sheet

The purpose of a behavioral experiment is to gather evidence to test a specific prediction that you have based on a belief. For example, if someone believed that she must always appear perfectly well groomed, a specific prediction may be that if she did not go out without perfect hair and makeup, her friends would say she was not looking good. An experiment to test this prediction would be to go out with friends will little makeup and not having perfect hair.

Belief to be tested (rate degree of belief 0–100%):

Is there an alternative belief? (rate degree of belief 0–100% if applicable):

Experiment that will test the belief (specify what you will do in detail, including when, where, and how):

Specify the prediction precisely (specify behaviors and rate intensity of beliefs and emotions):

What problems might occur, and how will you overcome them?

(continued)

Experiment—what did you actually do?

Results—what happened?

Rerate the predictions made: What can you conclude?

Rerate the belief you were testing and the alternative belief (if you had one):

Reflection (including plans for any follow-up experiments):

Revised belief/behavior:

Broadening Self-Evaluation 1: Pie Charts

1. **Consider what areas of life constitute how you view yourself as a person (self-worth).** Divide the pie into sections based on your view of yourself (e.g., 75% of your self-worth may be derived from work and the remainder from other areas such as family or friends).

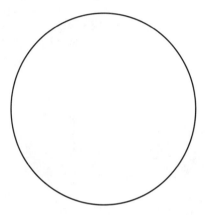

2. **Consider a more balanced view of what areas of life constitute how you view yourself as a person—a view that relies not only on one main area of performance but also on other domains, including those that do not involve achievement.** Divide the pie again, but consider more "slices" of the pie and any new areas.

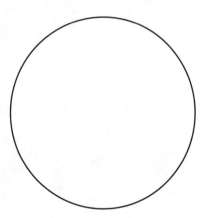

Broadening Self-Evaluation 2

Record what areas you used to evaluate yourself. Focus on the new domains identified in your more balanced pie chart (#2 in Handout 13.1) or areas in your life that do not involve performance—for example, listening to music or being with friends.

Day	What area did you use to evaluate yourself?	Record the thoughts that you had about evaluating yourself.	Describe how you felt and rate the intensity of the feelings from 0 (low) to 100 (high).

Challenging Self-Criticism 1: Identifying Self-Critical Thoughts Using the Downward-Arrow Technique

Record your thoughts that are leading to negative feelings in three different situations. Then, for each one, ask yourself what the worst thing is that could happen and what it says about you as a person to uncover your "if . . . then . . ." self-critical rules.

Situation 1:	Situation 2:	Situation 3:
Feeling:	Feeling:	Feeling:
Thought:	Thought:	Thought:
First question: What does it mean if this happens? Answer:	First question: What does it mean if this happens? Answer:	First question: What does it mean if this happens? Answer:

(continued)

Second question:	**Second question:**	**Second question:**
If that was true, what would that mean about you?	If that was true, what would that mean about you?	If that was true, what would that mean about you?
Answer:	**Answer:**	**Answer:**
Third question:	**Third question:**	**Third question:**
What is the "if . . . then . . ." statement?	What is the "if . . . then . . ." statement?	What is the "if . . . then . . ." statement?
Answer:	**Answer:**	**Answer:**

Challenging Self-Criticism 2: Determining Your Values
That Guide How Others Should Be Treated

Here are some examples of values used to treat other people.

Acceptance: To accept my friends no matter what they do	**Caring:** To be caring toward others	**Compassion:** To feel concern for others
Courtesy: To be polite and considerate to others	**Forgiveness:** To be forgiving of others	**Generosity:** To give people the benefit of the doubt
Helpfulness: To be helpful to others	**Hope:** To keep believing in my friends	**Fun:** To have fun with friends and share a sense of humor with them
Justice: To treat my friends fairly	**Service:** To be of service to others	**Respect:** To treat my friends with respect and not put them down

Consider what values guide the way you treat other people. Fill in the blank cells with values and specific examples.

Adapted from Shafran, Egan, and Wade (2010). Copyright 2010 by Constable & Robinson. Adapted by permission.

Challenging Self-Criticism 3:
Generating Self-Compassionate Responses

Record self-critical thoughts as well as helpful, self-compassionate responses. For each self-critical thought:

1. Record your self-critical thought.
2. Write challenges to the thought based on self-kindness, common humanity, and mindfulness.

Self-critical thought	Exercising self-kindness	Exercising common humanity	Exercising mindfulness

Procrastination 1: Understanding Areas of Procrastination

The purpose of this handout is to consider in which areas of your life you procrastinate and to identify examples of your procrastination.

1. Circle your area(s) of perfectionism.
2. Identify examples of your procrastination.

IN WHICH AREAS OF MY LIFE DO I PROCRASTINATE?

Perfectionism area/ behavior	Example	My procrastination behavior
Eating/shape/weight	Delay trying on clothes	_____
Social performance	Put off phoning a friend	_____
Organization	Delay writing to-do lists	_____
House cleanliness, neatness	Delay starting cleaning	_____
Appearance	Delay ironing clothes	_____
Artistic performance	Postpone new painting	_____
Musical performance	Postpone violin practice	_____
Athletic performance	Put off training	_____
Academic performance	Ask for extension	_____
Work performance	Delay starting report	_____
Intimate relationships	Put off asking for a date	_____
Parenting	Delaying choice of school	_____
Health, fitness	Put off going for a walk	_____
Entertaining	Delay cooking for party	_____
Other perfectionism areas:		_____
_____	_____	_____
_____	_____	_____
_____	_____	_____
_____	_____	_____

Adapted from Shafran, Egan, and Wade (2010). Copyright 2010 by Constable & Robinson. Adapted by permission.

Procrastination 2: Self-Monitoring Procrastination

The purpose of this handout is to identify what procrastination behaviors you do as a result of your predictions about what will happen. For example, if someone had a prediction "I will not be able to write a report to an excellent standard," their procrastination behavior might be to read e-mails all day instead of starting the report, and leave writing it until the night before it was due.

Follow these steps:

1. Record the situation.
2. Record your perfectionistic predictions. Ask yourself: "What was going through my mind when I decided to delay the task?" Rate how strongly you believe the thought (0% = do not believe; 100% = completely believe).
3. Record your behavior.
4. Record your feelings. Examples include: anxious, sad, angry, ashamed, depressed, scared, embarrassed, irritated, happy, disappointed, excited. Rate the intensity of your feelings (0% = no feeling; 100% = strongest feeling).

Perfectionism area and situation	Perfectionist prediction	Procrastination behavior	Feelings (rate 0–100%)

(continued)

Adapted from Shafran, Egan, and Wade (2010). Copyright 2010 by Constable & Robinson. Adapted by permission.

Perfectionism area and situation	Perfectionist prediction	Procrastination behavior	Feelings (rate 0–100%)

Procrastination 3: Understanding How Procrastination Is Maintained by Increasing Belief in Perfectionistic Predictions

The purpose of this worksheet is to help you understand how procrastination keeps going by increasing your belief in your perfectionistic predictions. Record the area of perfectionism, your perfectionistic prediction, your procrastination behaviors, and how procrastination is maintained by increasing your belief in the predictions. For example, if someone had the prediction "I will not be able to write reports to an excellent standard," they might procrastinate by delaying writing the reports and writing detailed lists instead of doing the reports. Their procrastination would be maintained by increasing belief in the prediction, as the more the person procrastinated the less time he would have to do the report, and thus he would not do as good a job, confirming the prediction of not doing reports well and making it more likely he will procrastinate again.

Example	Perfectionism area	Perfectionistic prediction	Procrastination behaviors	How procrastination keeps going by increasing belief in predictions

(continued)

Adapted from Shafran, Egan, and Wade (2010). Copyright 2010 by Constable & Robinson. Adapted by permission.

Example	Perfectionism area	Perfectionistic prediction	Procrastination behaviors	How procrastination keeps going by increasing belief in predictions

Procrastination 4:
Behavioral Experiment to Overcome Procrastination

The purpose of a behavioral experiment is to gather evidence to test a specific prediction that you have based on a belief. For example, if someone believed "I work best under pressure; leaving an assignment to the last minute helps me do better," his prediction may be "If I start an assignment early, I will do a poorer job." An experiment could be (1) start an assignment 1 week before it is due and hand it in early and (2) start and assignment 1 day before it is due and hand it 5 minutes before the deadline, and compare which one leads to a better performance.

Belief to be tested (rate degree of belief 0–100%):

Alternative belief to be tested (rate degree of belief 0–100%):

Experiment that will test the belief (specify what you will do in detail, including when, where, and how):

Specify the prediction (specify behaviors and rate intensity of beliefs and emotions):

(continued)

From *Cognitive-Behavioral Treatment of Perfectionism* by Sarah J. Egan, Tracey D. Wade, Roz Shafran, and Martin M. Antony. Copyright 2014 by The Guilford Press. Permission to photocopy this handout is granted to purchasers of this book for personal use only (see copyright page for details). Purchasers can download and print a larger version of this handout from *www.guilford.com/egan-forms*.

What problems might occur and how will you overcome them?

Experiment—what did you actually do?

Results—what happened?

Rerate the predictions made: What can you conclude? Rerate the belief you tested, as well as the alternative, if you had one:

Alternative belief to be tested (rate degree of belief 0–100%):

Reflection, including plans for any follow-up experiments:

Revised belief:

Procrastination 5: Helpful Reminders for Procrastination

1. Consider the list of reminders to help decrease procrastination.
2. Write your own list of reminders to help you reduce procrastination and post this list prominently in a place where you work.

"I feel better once I start something."

"I feel less anxious once I get going with a task I am putting off."

"If I put it off I will feel worse."

"Getting started with a task gives me more confidence to keep going."

"I am not a failure because of procrastinating; if I make a small start I will feel better."

"Procrastination makes me feel anxious, so it's best to not put things off."

My own helpful reminders for procrastination:

_____

_____

_____

_____

_____

_____

_____

_____

_____

_____

_____

_____

_____

Procrastination 6: Breaking Down Tasks into Manageable Chunks to Overcome Procrastination

1. Define the task/goal:

2. **Break the task down in to manageable chunks.** Then list the chunks in the order in which they need to be accomplished. Then give each step a rating (0 = easiest to 100 = hardest) according to how difficult you expect it to be.

Problem Solving

The purpose of this handout is to generate solutions to a problem. Follow the steps below to think about how you might solve any problem you are experiencing.

1. **Identify the problem.**

   Describe the problem in an objective and specific way.

2. **Generate potential solutions.**

   Brainstorm all of the possible solutions to the problem.

   Keep listing all of the ideas you can think of without judging them as good or bad.

   Underline two or three solutions that seem most likely to be helpful and most possible to achieve.

3. **Decide on a solution.**

   Consider the pros and cons of the top two or three solutions in terms of how possible they are and how likely they are to solve the problem.

   Choose the solution that seems best.

(continued)

4. **Plan a solution.**

   Plan a list of action steps that need to be taken to achieve the solution.

5. **Carry out the solution.**

6. **Evaluate the result.**

   What was the effect of carrying out the solution?

Time Management Schedule

The purpose of this schedule is to balance things you need to do and achievement with time for relaxation, fun, and rest. Try to schedule some things in your week that are not about achievement and striving to meet your goals.

	Monday	Tuesday	Wednesday	Thursday	Friday	Saturday	Sunday
7–8							
8–9							
9–10							
10–11							
11–12							
12–1							

(continued)

Time Management Schedule *(page 2 of 2)*

	Monday	Tuesday	Wednesday	Thursday	Friday	Saturday	Sunday
1–2							
2–3							
3–4							
4–5							
5–6							
6–7							
7–8							
8–9							
9–10							

List of Pleasant Events

The following list contains some typical events that might be fun, enjoyable, or relaxing. Try one of these events or think of events of your own that you find pleasant and notice how you feel after you do the event.

1. Download some music
2. Cook a nice meal
3. Go bike riding
4. Go to a football game
5. Learn a language
6. Watch TV
7. Listen to music
8. Go swimming
9. Join a new club
10. Watch a downloaded movie
11. Buy a bunch of flowers and arrange them
12. Play golf
13. Go for a walk
14. Have a bath
15. Plan a vacation
16. Buy a gift for someone
17. Play cards
18. Do meditation
19. Go on a vacation
20. Join a book club
21. Read a magazine
22. Play tennis
23. Do a crossword puzzle

24. Light a candle
25. Have a coffee at your favorite café
26. Read a book
27. Play with a pet
28. Meet a friend for a meal
29. Play a board game
30. Start a new hobby
31. Listen to the radio
32. Play squash
33. Go for a drive
34. Go to a museum or art gallery
35. Do woodwork
36. Go dancing
37. Play cricket
38. Go on a picnic
39. Exercise
40. Get a manicure
41. Play football
42. Draw or paint
43. Play a musical instrument
44. Go to a movie
45. Surf the web
46. Go window shopping
47. Go for a jog

(continued)

48. Have friends over for dinner
49. Go to the park
50. Sing
51. Buy something new for house
52. Boil cinnamon
53. Play computer games
54. Bake a cake
55. Have a quiet evening at home
56. Go hiking in the outdoors
57. Buy some new clothes
58. Join a community group to help others
59. Arrange old photos
60. Phone a friend
61. Do something nice for someone else
62. Listen to a relaxation track

63. Take time to read the newspaper
64. Burn scented oils
65. E-mail a friend
66. Do yoga
67. _____
68. _____
69. _____
70. _____
71. _____
72. _____
73. _____
74. _____
75. _____
76. _____
77. _____

Relapse Prevention

- Develop an action plan for future problems—anticipate future stressors and situations that might cause perfectionism to appear again.

- Catch the problem quickly. The earlier you start to work on a problem that reoccurs, the easier it will be to deal with the problem before it has a chance to "set in" again. Don't panic. Instead, remember that lapses will happen, and just see them as an opportunity for further practice of the skills you learned in therapy.

- If you have experienced a lapse, think about what help you need, and from whom you need support (e.g., a friend? a therapist?).

- If you experience a lapse, put your action plan into place.

- Once the stress has settled a little, try to identify the exact trigger that set off the lapse to see if it is something that can be dealt with to prevent problems in the future.

- Remember to practice self-compassion—congratulate yourself on having noticed the lapse and putting techniques back into action to combat it.

Relapse Prevention: My Action Plan for the Future

The purpose of this handout is to consider what the main messages are that you learned in treatment, what areas you need to look out for in the future regarding perfectionism becoming a problem again and what you need to do in response, and ways to maintain balance in your life by including fun, rest, and relaxation.

In a couple of sentences, what might I say to summarize the main message that I have taken away from treatment? _____

_____

_____

_____

_____

In what situations is perfectionism likely to arise in the future? What do I need to look out for? _____

_____

_____

_____

_____

What are the most effective strategies that I learned in treatment? (Remember to use these strategies when I get an "attack" of perfectionism in the future!) _____

_____

_____

_____

_____

What do I need to do so that I have a balanced life (i.e., maintain a balance between striving to achieve and other areas of my life, such as socializing, fun, relaxation, and rest)?

_____

_____

_____

_____

_____

Final Reflections on Perfectionism

Consider these quotes about perfectionism:

Striving for excellence motivates you; striving for perfection is demoralizing.—*Harriet Braiker*

A man would do nothing if he waited until he could do it so well that no one could find fault.—*John Henry Newman*

When you aim for perfection, you discover it's a moving target.—*George Fisher*

Perfection has one grave defect: it is apt to be dull.—*W. Somerset Maugham*

The pursuit of perfection often impedes improvement.—*George Will*

No one is perfect . . . that's why pencils have erasers.—*Author Unknown*

A life spent making mistakes is not only more honorable, but more useful than a life spent doing nothing.—*George Bernard Shaw*

Be thankful for your mistakes. They will teach you valuable lessons.—*Author Unknown*

Record any final reflections regarding perfectionism that can help you in the future. For example, what would be the main messages you can use to remind yourself why striving for perfection is problematic? _____

_____

_____

_____

_____

_____

_____

_____

_____

_____

_____

Self-Report Measures

Scoring instructions for each measure are included in Chapter 5.

Adaptive/Maladaptive Perfectionism Scale

Please read each statement. **Circle** the answer that best describes you.
If you think that the statement is really **unlike** you, circle 1.
If you think that the statement is somewhat **unlike** you, circle 2.
If you think that the statement is somewhat **like** you, circle 3.
If you think that the statement is really **like** you, circle 4.

1 = really unlike me
2 = somewhat unlike me
3 = somewhat like me
4 = really like me

1. I feel super when I do well at something.	1	2	3	4
2. I am fearful of making mistakes.	1	2	3	4
3. I like for things to always be in order.	1	2	3	4
4. I like to be praised for my work because then others will want to be like me.	1	2	3	4
5. I do not get mad if I make a mistake.	1	2	3	4
6. I take a long time to do something because I check it many times.	1	2	3	4
7. Once I do well at something, I am pleased.	1	2	3	4
8. When I make a mistake, I feel so bad that I want to hide.	1	2	3	4
9. I always make a list of things and check them off after I do them.	1	2	3	4
10. I do not get excited when I do a good job.	1	2	3	4
11. I do good work so that others think I am great.	1	2	3	4
12. I get mad when I see a mistake in my work.	1	2	3	4
13. I have certain places where I always put my things.	1	2	3	4
14. I never feel good about my work.	1	2	3	4
15. Mistakes are OK to make.	1	2	3	4
16. I want to be known as the best at what I do.	1	2	3	4

(continued)

17. I become sad when I see a mistake on my paper.   1 2 3 4

18. I like to help others after I do something well.   1 2 3 4

19. I want to be perfect so that others will like me.   1 2 3 4

20. I notice more what I do right than what I do wrong.   1 2 3 4

21. After doing an activity, I feel happy.   1 2 3 4

22. I cannot relax until I have done all my work.   1 2 3 4

23. When one thing goes wrong, I wonder if I can do anything right.   1 2 3 4

24. My work is never done well enough to be praised.   1 2 3 4

25. I only like to do one task at a time.   1 2 3 4

26. Making one mistake is as bad as making ten mistakes.   1 2 3 4

27. I like to share my ideas with others.   1 2 3 4

Almost Perfect Scale—Revised

Instructions: The following items are designed to measure attitudes people have toward themselves, their performance, and toward others. There are no right or wrong answers. Please respond to all of the items. Use your first impression and do not spend too much time on individual items in responding.

Respond to each of the items using the scale below to describe your degree of agreement with each item. Record your response on the line to the left of each item.

1	2	3	4	5	6	7
Strongly Disagree	Disagree	Slightly Disagree	Neutral	Slightly Agree	Agree	Strongly Agree

_____ 1. I have high standards for my performance at work or at school.

_____ 2. I am an orderly person.

_____ 3. I often feel frustrated because I can't meet my goals.

_____ 4. Neatness is important to me.

_____ 5. If you don't expect much out of yourself, you will never succeed.

_____ 6. My best just never seems to be good enough for me.

_____ 7. I think things should be put away in their place.

_____ 8. I have high expectations for myself.

_____ 9. I rarely live up to my high standards.

_____ 10. I like to always be organized and disciplined.

_____ 11. Doing my best never seems to be enough.

_____ 12. I set very high standards for myself.

_____ 13. I am never satisfied with my accomplishments.

_____ 14. I expect the best from myself.

(continued)

_____ 15. I often worry about not measuring up to my own expectations.

_____ 16. My performance rarely measures up to my standards.

_____ 17. I am not satisfied even when I know I have done my best.

_____ 18. I try to do my best at everything I do.

_____ 19. I am seldom able to meet my own high standards of performance.

_____ 20. I am hardly ever satisfied with my performance.

_____ 21. I hardly ever feel that what I've done is good enough.

_____ 22. I have a strong need to strive for excellence.

_____ 23. I often feel disappointment after completing a task because I know I could have done better.

Behavioral Domains Questionnaire

The purpose of this questionnaire is to obtain information on your behavior and how it relates to perfectionist behavior. Please indicate the number that best corresponds to your behavior with each question below using the rating system provided. Please read each question carefully.

Guide for the rating scale: **Rarely** (twice or less in the last four weeks)

Sometimes (3-4 times in the last four weeks)

Often (5 or more times in the last four weeks)

Please consider the following questions in relation to your behavior **over the past four weeks . . .**	Never	Rarely	Sometimes	Often	Always
1. How often have you spent more than 5 minutes making your bed (not changing the sheets)?	1	2	3	4	5
2. How often have you spent more than 30 minutes cleaning the kitchen in one go?	1	2	3	4	5
3. How often have you cleaned inside the fridge?	1	2	3	4	5
4. How often have you cleaned your windows?	1	2	3	4	5
5. How often have you ironed your underwear?	1	2	3	4	5
6. How often have you found it difficult to stop cleaning the house because you have been striving to complete it to your personal standards?	1	2	3	4	5
7. How often have you checked the cleanliness of your house over and over again?	1	2	3	4	5
8. How often have you not trusted someone other than yourself to clean the house because of your cleaning standards?	1	2	3	4	5
9. How often have you overpacked when going away/on a day-to-day basis to allow for every eventuality?	1	2	3	4	5
10. How often have you compared you achievements at work with other people?	1	2	3	4	5

(continued)

Please consider the following questions in relation to your behavior **over the past four weeks . . .**	Never	Rarely	Sometimes	Often	Always
11. How often have your personal standards interfered with the completion of a task?	1	2	3	4	5
12. How often have you checked your work over and over for mistakes?	1	2	3	4	5
13. How often have you put off doing work because you know that you're overly thorough and it will take a long time?	1	2	3	4	5
14. How often have you worked overtime to complete a task to your standards?	1	2	3	4	5
15. How often have you found it difficult to stop work because you are striving to complete it to your personal standards?	1	2	3	4	5
16. How often have you found it difficult starting tasks because you're afraid of failing?	1	2	3	4	5
17. How often have you spent more than 15 minutes making written plans for your day/week?	1	2	3	4	5
18. How often have you thought about past social interactions and checked to see if your behavior met your personal standards?	1	2	3	4	5
19. How often have you avoided social interactions?	1	2	3	4	5
20. How often have you arrived early for social meetings to make sure you are not late?	1	2	3	4	5
21. How often have you continually checked for reassurance from your friends that you are a likeable person?	1	2	3	4	5
22. How often have you thought about/planned conversations in advance?	1	2	3	4	5
23. How often have you made yourself busy to avoid social interactions?	1	2	3	4	5
24. How often have you written lists to make sure you haven't forgotten anything?	1	2	3	4	5
25. How often have you chosen not to say anything in social interactions for fear of saying something wrong?	1	2	3	4	5
26. How often have you spent more than 1 hour preparing for your hobbies/interests?	1	2	3	4	5

(continued)

Please consider the following questions in relation to your behavior **over the past four weeks . . .**	Never	Rarely	Sometimes	Often	Always
27. How often have you avoided group activities because you wanted to achieve the best and were afraid of being compared?	1	2	3	4	5
28. How often have you compared your achievements in a hobby/interest to other people's achievements?	1	2	3	4	5
29. How often have you found it difficult stopping activities because you are striving to be perfect at them?	1	2	3	4	5
30. How often have you checked your performance in hobbies/interests for mistakes?	1	2	3	4	5
31. How often have you overprepared for your hobbies/interests to allow for every eventuality?	1	2	3	4	5
32. How often have you spent more than 1 hour washing yourself?	1	2	3	4	5
33. How often have you brushed your teeth for longer than 5 minutes?	1	2	3	4	5
34. How often have you found it difficult leaving for work/school in the morning because of the way you look?	1	2	3	4	5
35. How often have you spent more time staying in than going out because of your appearance?	1	2	3	4	5
36. How often have you checked your appearance in a mirror more than 5 times in a day?	1	2	3	4	5
37. How often have you spent so much time getting ready that you decided not to go out?	1	2	3	4	5

Please answer these questions in full sentences, using as many words as necessary.

Are there any particular day-to-day activities that take you a really long time? _____

_____

_____

_____

_____

_____

(continued)

What sort of checks do you make on a day-to-day basis? _____

_____

_____

_____

_____

_____

Are there any specific perfectionist behaviors that you carry out? _____

_____

_____

_____

_____

_____

Thank you for completing this questionnaire. If you have any additional comments please use overleaf.

Clinical Perfectionism Questionnaire

INSTRUCTIONS: This questionnaire is concerned with "perfectionism." **By perfectionism, we mean trying to meet really high standards whether or not you actually succeed in reaching them. In this questionnaire we are only concerned with perfectionism that affects areas of life other than your eating, weight, or appearance.**

Have you been trying to achieve high standards over the past month *whether or not you have succeeded* (excluding standards for your eating, weight, or appearance)? Please circle YES or NO.

YES / NO

If so, in what areas of your life (other than eating, weight, or appearance) has this applied?

For example, it might have been in your performance at work, at sport, at music, at home, etc. Please note these below:

_____

_____

_____

Now, please place an "X" in the column below that best describes you over the past month. Remember, do not count standards for your eating, weight, or appearance.

Over the past month . . .	Not at all	Some of the time	Most of the time	All of the time
1. Over the past month, have you pushed yourself really hard to meet your goals?				
2. Over the past month, have you tended to focus on what you <u>have</u> achieved, rather than on what you have not achieved?				
3. Over the past month, have you been told that your standards are too high?				
4. Over the past month, have you felt a failure as a person because you have not succeeded in meeting your goals?				

(continued)

Over the past month . . .	Not at all	Some of the time	Most of the time	All of the time
5. Over the past month, have you been afraid that you might not reach your standards?				
6. Over the past month, have you raised your standards because you thought they were too easy?				
7. Over the past month, have you judged yourself on the basis of your ability to achieve high standards?				
8. Over the past month, have you done just enough to get by?				
9. Over the past month, have you <u>repeatedly</u> checked how well you are doing at meeting your standards (for example, by comparing your performance with that of others)?				
10. Over the past month, do you think that other people would have thought of you as a "perfectionist"?				
11. Over the past month, have you kept trying to meet your standards, even if this has meant that you have missed out on things?				
12. Over the past month, have you avoided any tests of your performance (at meeting your goals) in case you failed?				

Consequences of Perfectionism Scale

1 = **Extremely Untrue of Me**
2 = **Somewhat Untrue of Me**
3 = **Neither True nor Untrue of Me**
4 = **Somewhat True of Me**
5 = **Extremely True of Me**

	Untrue				**True**
1. Being perfectionistic gets me to stay on track in my performance.	1	2	3	4	5
2. Being perfectionistic gets me to concentrate worse.	1	2	3	4	5
3. Being perfectionistic hinders me from staying on track in my performance.	1	2	3	4	5
4. Being perfectionistic drives me to be motivated.	1	2	3	4	5
5. Being perfectionistic gets me to be less on top of things.	1	2	3	4	5
6. Being perfectionistic pushes me to achieve more.	1	2	3	4	5
7. Being perfectionistic gets me to be on top of things.	1	2	3	4	5
8. Being perfectionistic pushes me to pursue my goals.	1	2	3	4	5
9. Being perfectionistic gets me to decrease my productivity.	1	2	3	4	5
10. Being perfectionistic encourages me to be successful.	1	2	3	4	5

Dyadic Almost Perfect Scale

The following items are designed to measure attitudes people have about romantic/intimate relationships. There are no right or wrong answers. Please respond to all of the items. Use your first impression and do not spend too much time on individual items. The terms "significant other" and "partner" are used interchangeably. If you do not have a current significant other or partner, please use someone who has filled that role for you in the past.

Instructions: Respond on the answer line to the left of each item by using the scale below to describe your degree of agreement or disagreement with each statement.

1	2	3	4	5	6	7
Strongly Disagree	Disagree	Slightly Disagree	Neutral	Slightly Agree	Agree	Strongly Agree

_____ 1. I often feel disappointment after my partner completes a task because I know that she/he could have done better.

_____ 2. I expect my significant other to be an orderly person.

_____ 3. My significant other can generally meet the standards that I have set for him/her.

_____ 4. My significant other rarely lives up to my standards.

_____ 5. I have very high standards for my significant other.

_____ 6. My partner's best rarely seems to be enough for me.

_____ 7. Neatness should be important to my significant other.

_____ 8. I expect the best from my significant other.

_____ 9. I am rarely satisfied with my partner's accomplishments.

_____ 10. I often feel frustrated because my significant other does not meet the goals I have for him/her.

_____ 11. I expect my partner to try to do her/his best at everything she/he does.

_____ 12. I have trouble with my partner leaving things incomplete.

_____ 13. My partner's best never seems to be good enough for me.

_____ 14. I have high standards for my significant other's performance at work or at school.

(continued)

_____ 15. My significant other often does not measure up to my expectations.

_____ 16. I usually feel like what my partner has done is good enough.

_____ 17. I think my partner should be organized.

_____ 18. I am hardly ever satisfied with my partner's performance.

_____ 19. I have a strong need for my partner to strive for excellence.

_____ 20. My significant other is seldom able to meet my standards for performance.

_____ 21. I usually feel pretty satisfied with what my significant other does.

_____ 22. I expect my partner to think things should be put away in their place.

_____ 23. My partner's performance rarely measures up to my standards.

_____ 24. I am not satisfied, even when I know my significant other has done his/her best.

_____ 25. I have high expectations of my significant other.

_____ 26. I can get pretty upset when my partner doesn't do as well as I think she/he should.

Family Almost Perfect Scale

Instructions: The following items are designed to measure your perceptions of the attitudes, beliefs, and values your family has and conveyed to you. There are no right or wrong answers. Please respond to all of the items. Use your first impression and do not spend too much time on individual items in responding.

Respond to each of the items using the scale below to describe your degree of agreement with each item.

1	2	3	4	5	6	7
Strongly Disagree	Disagree	Slightly Disagree	Neutral	Slightly Agree	Agree	Strongly Agree

_____ 1. My family has high standards for my performance at work or at school.

_____ 2. My family expects me to be an orderly person.

_____ 3. Neatness is important to my family.

_____ 4. My best just never seems to be good enough for my family.

_____ 5. My family thinks things should be put away in their place.

_____ 6. My family has high expectations for me.

_____ 7. I rarely live up to my family's high standards.

_____ 8. My family expects me to always be organized and disciplined.

_____ 9. Doing my best never seems to be enough for my family.

_____ 10. My family sets very high standards for me.

_____ 11. Nothing short of perfect is acceptable in my family.

_____ 12. My family expects the best from me.

_____ 13. My performance rarely measures up to my family's standards.

_____ 14. My family expects me to try to do my best at everything I do.

_____ 15. I am seldom able to meet my family's high standards of performance.

_____ 16. I am aware that my family sets standards that are unrealistically high.

_____ 17. My family expects me to have a strong need to strive for excellence.

Frost et al. Multidimensional Perfectionism Scale

Please circle the number that best corresponds to your agreement with each statement below. Use this rating system:

Strongly Disagree   1   2   3   4   5   Strongly Agree

	Strongly Agree				Strongly Disagree
1. My parents set very high standards for me.	1	2	3	4	5
2. Organization is very important to me.	1	2	3	4	5
3. As a child, I was punished for doing things less than perfectly.	1	2	3	4	5
4. If I do not set the highest standards for myself, I am likely to end up a second-rate person.	1	2	3	4	5
5. My parents never tried to understand my mistakes.	1	2	3	4	5
6. It is important to me that I be thoroughly competent in everything that I do.	1	2	3	4	5
7. I am a neat person.	1	2	3	4	5
8. I try to be an organized person.	1	2	3	4	5
9. If I fail at work/school, I am a failure as a person.	1	2	3	4	5
10. I should be upset if I make a mistake.	1	2	3	4	5
11. My parents wanted me to be the best at everything.	1	2	3	4	5
12. I set higher goals than most people.	1	2	3	4	5
13. If someone does a task at work/school better than I, then I feel like I failed the whole task.	1	2	3	4	5
14. If I fail partly, it is as bad as being a complete failure.	1	2	3	4	5
15. Only outstanding performance is good enough in my family.	1	2	3	4	5
16. I am very good at focusing my efforts on attaining a goal.	1	2	3	4	5

(continued)

	Strongly Agree				Strongly Disagree
17. Even when I do something very carefully, I often feel that it is not quite right.	1	2	3	4	5
18. I hate being less than best at things.	1	2	3	4	5
19. I have extremely high goals.	1	2	3	4	5
20. My parents have expected excellence from me.	1	2	3	4	5
21. People will probably think less of me if I make a mistake.	1	2	3	4	5
22. I never felt like I could meet my parents' expectations.	1	2	3	4	5
23. If I do not do as well as other people, it means I am an inferior human being.	1	2	3	4	5
24. Other people seem to accept lower standards from themselves than I do.	1	2	3	4	5
25. If I do not do well all the time, people will not respect me.	1	2	3	4	5
26. My parents have always had higher expectations for my future than I have.	1	2	3	4	5
27. I try to be a neat person.	1	2	3	4	5
28. I usually have doubts about the simple everyday things I do.	1	2	3	4	5
29. Neatness is very important to me.	1	2	3	4	5
30. I expect higher performance in my daily tasks than most people.	1	2	3	4	5
31. I am an organized person.	1	2	3	4	5
32. I tend to get behind in my work because I repeat things over and over.	1	2	3	4	5
33. It takes me a long time to do something "right."	1	2	3	4	5
34. The fewer mistakes I make, the more people will like me.	1	2	3	4	5
35. I never felt like I could meet my parents' standards.	1	2	3	4	5

Multidimensional Parenting Perfectionism Questionnaire—Part A

INSTRUCTIONS: Listed below are several statements that concern the topic of parenting. Please read each item carefully and decide to what extent it is characteristic of you. Whenever possible, answer the questions with your current children in mind. If you have never had children, answer in terms of what you think your responses would most likely be if you were to ever have children. Then, for each statement indicate your response on the line to the left of each item using this scale:

0 = <u>Not at all</u> characteristic of me.
1 = Slightly characteristic of me.
2 = Somewhat characteristic of me.
3 = Moderately characteristic of me.
4 = Very characteristic of me.

I plan to respond to the following statements based on (check one):

_____ Currently being a parent.

_____ Imagining what I would be like as a future parent.

_____ 1. I set very high standards for myself as a parent.

_____ 2. Only if I am "perfect" as a parent will society consider me to be a good parent.

_____ 3. My partner sets very high standards of excellence for herself/himself as a parent.

_____ 4. My partner expects me to be a perfect parent.

_____ 5. I expect my partner to always be a top-notch and competent parent.

_____ 6. I must always be successful as a parent.

_____ 7. Most people in society expect me to always be a perfect parent.

_____ 8. My partner is perfectionistic in that she/he expects to be a perfect parent all the time.

_____ 9. My partner demands nothing less than perfection of me as a parent.

_____ 10. My partner should never let me down when it comes to being a parent.

_____ 11. One of my goals is to be a "perfect" parent.

_____ 12. Most people expect me to always be an excellent parent.

(continued)

_____ 13. It makes my partner uneasy for him/her to be less than a perfect parent.

_____ 14. My partner always wants me to be a perfect parent.

_____ 15. I cannot stand for my partner to be less than a competent parent.

_____ 16. I always feel the need to be a "perfect" parent.

_____ 17. I have to be a perfect parent in order for most people to regard me as okay.

_____ 18. My partner sets very high, perfectionistic goals for herself (himself) as a parent.

_____ 19. My partner pressures me to be a perfect parent.

_____ 20. I expect nothing less than "parental perfectionism" from my partner.

_____ 21. I always pressure myself to be the best parent in the world.

_____ 22. In order for people to accept me, I have to be the greatest parent in the world.

_____ 23. My partner is always trying to be totally perfect as a parent.

_____ 24. My partner has very high perfectionistic goals for me as a parent.

_____ 25. I will appreciate my partner, but only if she/he is a perfect parent.

_____ 26. I have very high perfectionistic goals for myself as a parent.

_____ 27. Most people expect me to be perfectionistic when it comes to being a parent.

_____ 28. My partner always feels that she/he has to be the best possible parent.

_____ 29. In order for my partner to appreciate me, I have to be a perfect parent.

_____ 30. I expect my partner to try to be perfectionistic when it comes to parenting behavior.

Multidimensional Parenting Perfectionism Questionnaire—Part B

INSTRUCTIONS: Listed below are several statements that concern the topic of parenting. Please read each item carefully and decide to what extent it is characteristic of you. Whenever possible, answer the questions with your current children in mind. If you have never had children, answer in terms of what you think your responses would most likely be if you were to ever have children. Then, for each statement indicate your response on the line to the left of each item using this scale:

> 0 = <u>Not at all</u> characteristic of me.
> 1 = <u>Slightly</u> characteristic of me.
> 2 = <u>Somewhat</u> characteristic of me.
> 3 = <u>Moderately</u> characteristic of me.
> 4 = <u>Very</u> characteristic of me.

I plan to respond to the following statements based on (check one):

_____ Currently being a parent.

_____ Imagining what I would be like as a future parent.

_____ 1. My spouse/partner sets very high parenting standards for me.

_____ 2. Being organized as a parent is very important to me.

_____ 3. My spouse/partner has criticized me for being less than a perfect parent.

_____ 4. If I do not set the highest standards for myself, I am likely to end up a second rate parent.

_____ 5. My spouse/partner never tries to understand my mistakes/shortcomings as a parent.

_____ 6. It is important to me that I am thoroughly competent in everything I do as a parent.

_____ 7. I am rather neat (i.e., not messy) as a parent.

_____ 8. I try to take an organized approach to being a parent.

_____ 9. If I fail to rear my children well, I would be a total failure as a person.

_____ 10. I should be upset if I make a mistake in rearing my children.

_____ 11. My spouse/partner wants me to be the best possible parent in the entire world.

_____ 12. I set higher goals for myself as a parent than do most people.

(continued)

_____ 13. If someone were a better parent than I, then I would feel like a complete failure as a parent.

_____ 14. If I fail in even a small way to be a totally good parent, it is as bad as being completely inadequate.

_____ 15. Only when I am an "outstanding" parent is it good enough for my spouse/partner.

_____ 16. I am very good at focusing my efforts and time at being a good parent.

_____ 17. Even when I am very careful as a parent, I often feel that I failed to do something quite right.

_____ 18. I hate being less than the best possible parent.

_____ 19. I have extremely high goals for myself as a parent.

_____ 20. My spouse/partner expects "parenting excellence" from me.

_____ 21. My spouse/partner would probably think less of me if I made a mistake in parenting.

_____ 22. I never feel like I can meet my spouse/partner's expectations for me as a parent.

_____ 23. If I am not as good a parent as other people, it means I am an inferior parent.

_____ 24. Other people seem to accept less from themselves as a parent than I do for myself.

_____ 25. If I do not constantly attend to our children, my spouse/partner will not respect me as a parent.

_____ 26. My spouse/partner has always had higher expectations for me as a parent than I have.

_____ 27. I try to be an organized and neat parent.

_____ 28. I usually have doubts about even the simple things I do and say as a parent.

_____ 29. As a parent, orderliness (and neatness) is very important to me.

_____ 30. I expect more of myself as a parent than most people.

_____ 31. I take an organized approach to being a parent.

_____ 32. I tend to have problems as a parent, because I keep doing things the same old way.

_____ 33. It takes me a long time to do something "right" as a parent.

_____ 34. The fewer mistakes I make as a parent, the more my spouse/partner will like me.

_____ 35. I never feel like I can meet my spouse/partner's standards for good parenting behavior.

Multidimensional Perfectionism Cognitions Inventory

Listed below are a variety of thoughts about perfectionism that sometimes pop into people's heads. Please read each thought and indicate how frequently, if at all, the thought occurred to you over the last week. Read each item carefully and choose the appropriate number, using the scale shown below.

	Never	Sometimes	Frequently	Always
1. I can't be satisfied unless I make it perfect.	1	2	3	4
2. I must be perfect at any cost.	1	2	3	4
3. The higher my goal, the better.	1	2	3	4
4. It's a shame to make a mistake.	1	2	3	4
5. It's to my own benefit to set high standards for myself.	1	2	3	4
6. I feel miserable if I make a mistake.	1	2	3	4
7. I can't feel satisfied unless things are done perfectly.	1	2	3	4
8. I'm going to aim for the highest standards.	1	2	3	4
9. I'll blame myself if I make a mistake.	1	2	3	4
10. The higher the goal is, the more challenging.	1	2	3	4
11. There is meaning in "doing something perfectly."	1	2	3	4
12. If I can't do this well, it means I'm below average.	1	2	3	4
13. Things shouldn't be imperfect.	1	2	3	4
14. It's important to set high standards for myself.	1	2	3	4
15. I would feel worthless if I fail.	1	2	3	4

Perfectionism Inventory

Please use the following options to rate how much you generally agree with each statement.

1	2	3	4	5
Strongly Disagree	Disagree Somewhat	Neither Agree nor Disagree	Agree Somewhat	Strongly Agree

_____ 1. My work needs to be perfect, in order for me to be satisfied. (se1)

_____ 2. I am oversensitive to the comments of others. (na1)

_____ 3. I usually let people know when their work isn't up to my standards. (hso1)

_____ 4. I am well organized. (o1)

_____ 5. I think through my options carefully before making a decision. (p1)

_____ 6. If I make mistakes, people might think less of me. (cm1)

_____ 7. I've always felt pressure from my parent(s) to be the best. (pp1)

_____ 8. If I do something less than perfectly, I have a hard time getting over it. (r1)

_____ 9. All my energy is put into achieving a flawless result. (se2)

_____ 10. I compare my work to others and often feel inadequate. (na2)

_____ 11. I get upset when other people don't maintain the same standards I do. (hso2)

_____ 12. I think things should be put away in their place. (o2)

_____ 13. I find myself planning many of my decisions. (p2)

_____ 14. I am particularly embarrassed by failure. (cm2)

_____ 15. My parents hold me to high standards. (pp2)

_____ 16. I spend a lot of time worrying about things I've done, or things I need to do. (r2)

_____ 17. I can't stand to do something halfway. (se3)

_____ 18. I am sensitive to how others respond to my work. (na3)

_____ 19. I'm not very patient with people's excuses for poor work. (hso3)

_____ 20. I would characterize myself as an orderly person. (o3)

_____ 21. Most of my decisions are made after I have had time to think about them. (p3)

_____ 22. I overreact to making mistakes. (cm3)

_____ 23. My parent(s) are difficult to please. (pp3)

(continued)

_____ 24. If I make a mistake, my whole day is ruined. (r3)

_____ 25. I have to be the best in every assignment I do. (se4)

_____ 26. I'm concerned with whether or not other people approve of my actions. (na4)

_____ 27. I'm often critical of others. (hso4)

_____ 28. I like to always be organized and disciplined. (o4)

_____ 29. I usually need to think things through before I know what I want. (p4)

_____ 30. If someone points out a mistake I've made, I feel like I've lost that person's respect in some way. (cm4)

_____ 31. My parent(s) have high expectations for achievement. (pp4)

_____ 32. If I say or do something dumb I tend to think about it for the rest of the day. (r4)

_____ 33. I drive myself rigorously to achieve high standards. (se5)

_____ 34. I often don't say anything, because I'm scared I might say the wrong thing. (na5)

_____ 35. I am frequently aggravated by the lazy or sloppy work of others. (hso5)

_____ 36. I clean my home often. (o5)

_____ 37. I need time to think up a plan before I take action. (p5)

_____ 38. If I mess up on one thing, people might start questioning everything I do. (cm5)

_____ 39. Growing up, I felt a lot of pressure to do everything right. (pp5)

_____ 40. When I make an error, I generally can't stop thinking about it. (r5)

_____ 41. I must achieve excellence in everything I do. (se6)

_____ 42. I am self-conscious about what others think of me. (na6)

_____ 43. I have little tolerance for other people's careless mistakes. (hso6)

_____ 44. I make sure to put things away as soon as I'm done using them. (o6)

_____ 45. I tend to deliberate before making up my mind. (p6)

_____ 46. To me, a mistake equals failure. (cm6)

_____ 47. My parent(s) put a lot of pressure on me to succeed. (pp6)

_____ 48. I often obsess over some of the things I have done. (r6)

_____ 49. I am often concerned that people will take what I say the wrong way. (na7)

_____ 50. I often get frustrated over other people's mistakes. (hso7)

_____ 51. My closet is neat and organized. (o7)

_____ 52. I usually don't make decisions on the spot. (p7)

(continued)

_____ 53. Making mistakes is a sign of stupidity. (cm7)

_____ 54. I always felt that my parent(s) wanted me to be perfect. (pp7)

_____ 55. After I turn a project in, I can't stop thinking of how it could have been better. (r7)

_____ 56. My workspace is generally organized. (o8)

_____ 57. If I make a serious mistake, I feel like I'm less of a person. (cm8)

_____ 58. My parent(s) have expected nothing but my best. (pp8)

_____ 59. I spend a great deal of time worrying about other people's opinion of me. (na8)

Physical Appearance Perfectionism Scale

Please read each statement and decide how much you agree or disagree. If you strongly agree, circle 5. If you strongly disagree, circle 1. If you feel somewhere in between, circle one of the numbers from 2 to 4. If you feel neutral or are not sure, circle the middle number, which is 3. Thank you.

Strongly Disagree   1   2   3   4   5   Strongly Agree

1. I am not satisfied with my appearance.	1	2	3	4	5
2. I hope my body shape is perfect.	1	2	3	4	5
3. I am never happy with my appearance no matter how I dress.	1	2	3	4	5
4. I hope that I look attractive.	1	2	3	4	5
5. I worry that my appearance is not good enough.	1	2	3	4	5
6. I hope others admire my appearance.	1	2	3	4	5
7. I hope others find me attractive.	1	2	3	4	5
8. I wish I could completely change my appearance.	1	2	3	4	5
9. My appearance is far from my expectations.	1	2	3	4	5
10. I worry about others' being critical of my appearance.	1	2	3	4	5
11. I often think about shortcomings of my appearance.	1	2	3	4	5
12. I hope I am handsome/beautiful.	1	2	3	4	5

Positive and Negative Perfectionism Scale

Please circle the appropriate number under the column that applies best to each of the following statements.

1 = Strongly Disagree
2 = Disagree
3 = Don't Know
4 = Agree
5 = Strongly Agree

1. When I start something I feel anxious that I might fail.	1	2	3	4	5
2. My family and friends are proud of me when I do really well.	1	2	3	4	5
3. I take pride in being meticulous when doing things.	1	2	3	4	5
4. I set impossibly high standards for myself.	1	2	3	4	5
5. I try to avoid the disapproval of others at all costs.	1	2	3	4	5
6. I like the acclaim I get for an outstanding performance.	1	2	3	4	5
7. When I am doing something I cannot relax until it's perfect.	1	2	3	4	5
8. It feels as though my best is never good enough for other people.	1	2	3	4	5
9. Producing a perfect performance is a reward in its own right.	1	2	3	4	5
10. The problem of success is that I must work even harder to please others.	1	2	3	4	5
11. If I make a mistake I feel that the whole thing is ruined.	1	2	3	4	5
12. I feel dissatisfied with myself unless I am working towards a higher standard all the time.	1	2	3	4	5
13. I know the kind of person I ought or want to be, but feel I always fall short of this.	1	2	3	4	5
14. Other people respect me for my achievements.	1	2	3	4	5
15. As a child however well I did, it never seemed good enough to please my parents.	1	2	3	4	5
16. I think everyone loves a winner.	1	2	3	4	5

(continued)

17. Other people expect nothing less than perfection of me.　　　1　2　3　4　5

18. When I'm competing against others, I'm motivated by wanting to be the best.　　　1　2　3　4　5

19. I feel good when pushing out the limits.　　　1　2　3　4　5

20. When I achieve my goals I feel dissatisfied or disillusioned.　　　1　2　3　4　5

21. My high standards are admired by others.　　　1　2　3　4　5

22. If I fail people, I fear they will cease to respect or care for me.　　　1　2　3　4　5

23. I like to please other people by being successful.　　　1　2　3　4　5

24. I gain great approval from others by the quality of my accomplishments.　　　1　2　3　4　5

25. My successes spur me on to greater achievements.　　　1　2　3　4　5

26. I feel guilty or ashamed if I do less than perfectly.　　　1　2　3　4　5

27. No matter how well I do I never feel satisfied with my performance,　　　1　2　3　4　5

28. I believe that rigorous practice makes for perfection.　　　1　2　3　4　5

29. I enjoy the glory gained by my successes.　　　1　2　3　4　5

30. I gain deep satisfaction when I have perfected something.　　　1　2　3　4　5

31. I feel I have to be perfect to gain people's approval.　　　1　2　3　4　5

32. My parents encouraged me to excel.　　　1　2　3　4　5

33. I worry what others think if I make mistakes.　　　1　2　3　4　5

34. I get fulfilment from totally dedicating myself to a task.　　　1　2　3　4　5

35. I like it when others recognize that what I do requires great skill and effort to perfect.　　　1　2　3　4　5

36. The better I do, the better I am expected to do by others.　　　1　2　3　4　5

37. I enjoy working towards greater levels of precision and accuracy.　　　1　2　3　4　5

38. I would rather not start something than risk doing it less than perfectly.　　　1　2　3　4　5

39. When I do things I feel others will judge critically the standard of my work.　　　1　2　3　4　5

40. I like the challenge of setting very high standards for myself.　　　1　2　3　4　5

Sport Multidimensional Perfectionism Scale–2

INSTRUCTIONS: The purpose of this questionnaire is to identify how players view certain aspects of their competitive experiences in sport. Please help us to more fully understand how players view a variety of their competitive experiences by indicating the extent to which you **agree or disagree** with the following statements. (Circle one response option to the right of each statement.) Some of the questions relate to your sport experiences in general, while others relate specifically to experiences on the team that you have most recently played with. **There are no right or wrong answers** so please don't spend too much time on any one statement; simply choose the answer that best describes how you view each statement.

To what extent do you agree or disagree with the following statements?	Strongly Disagree	Disagree	Neither Agree nor Disagree	Agree	Strongly Agree
1. If I do not set the highest standards for myself in my sport, I am likely to end up a second-rate player.	1	2	3	4	5
2. Even if I fail slightly in competition, for me, it is as bad as being a complete failure.	1	2	3	4	5
3. I usually feel uncertain as to whether or not my training effectively prepares me for competition.	1	2	3	4	5
4. My parents set very high standards for me in my sport.	1	2	3	4	5
5. On the day of competition I have a routine that I try to follow.	1	2	3	4	5
6. I feel like my coach criticizes me for doing things less than perfectly in competition.	1	2	3	4	5
7. In competition, I never feel like I can quite meet my parents' expectations.	1	2	3	4	5
8. I hate being less than the best at things in my sport.	1	2	3	4	5
9. I have and follow a pre-competitive routine.	1	2	3	4	5
10. If I fail in competition, I feel like a failure as a person.	1	2	3	4	5
11. Only outstanding performance during competition is good enough in my family.	1	2	3	4	5

Please complete the remaining items in this questionnaire on the next page.

(continued)

Sport Multidimensional Perfectionism Scale–2 *(page 2 of 3)*

To what extent do you agree or disagree with the following statements?	Strongly Disagree	Disagree	Neither Agree nor Disagree	Agree	Strongly Agree
12. I usually feel unsure about the adequacy of my pre-competition practices.	1	2	3	4	5
13. Only outstanding performance in competition is good enough for my coach.	1	2	3	4	5
14. I rarely feel that my training fully prepares me for competition.	1	2	3	4	5
15. My parents have always had higher expectations for my future in sport than I have.	1	2	3	4	5
16. The fewer mistakes I make in competition, the more people will like me.	1	2	3	4	5
17. It is important to me that I be thoroughly competent in everything I do in my sport.	1	2	3	4	5
18. I follow preplanned steps to prepare myself for competition.	1	2	3	4	5
19. I feel like I am criticized by my parents for doing things less than perfectly in competition.	1	2	3	4	5
20. Prior to competition, I rarely feel satisfied with my training.	1	2	3	4	5
21. I think I expect higher performance and greater results in my daily sport-training than most players.	1	2	3	4	5
22. I feel like I can never quite live up to my coach's standards.	1	2	3	4	5
23. I feel that other players generally accept lower standards for themselves in sport than I do.	1	2	3	4	5
24. I should be upset if I make a mistake in competition.	1	2	3	4	5
25. In competition, I never feel like I can quite live up to my parents' standards.	1	2	3	4	5
26. My coach sets very high standards for me in competition.	1	2	3	4	5
27. I follow a routine to get myself into a good mindset going into competition.	1	2	3	4	5
28. If a teammate or opponent (who plays a similar position to me) plays better than me during competition, then I feel like I failed to some degree.	1	2	3	4	5

Please complete the remaining items in this questionnaire on the next page.

(continued)

Sport Multidimensional Perfectionism Scale–2 *(page 3 of 3)*

To what extent do you agree or disagree with the following statements?	Strongly Disagree	Disagree	Neither Agree nor Disagree	Agree	Strongly Agree
29. My parents expect excellence from me in my sport.	1	2	3	4	5
30. My coach expects excellence from me at all times: both in training and competition.	1	2	3	4	5
31. I rarely feel that I have trained enough in preparation for a competition.	1	2	3	4	5
32. If I do not do well all the time in competition, I feel that people will not respect me as an athlete.	1	2	3	4	5
33. I have extremely high goals for myself in my sport.	1	2	3	4	5
34. I develop plans that dictate how I want to perform during competition.	1	2	3	4	5
35. I feel like my coach never tries to fully understand the mistakes I sometimes make.	1	2	3	4	5
36. I set higher achievement goals than most athletes who play my sport.	1	2	3	4	5
37. I usually have trouble deciding when I have practiced enough heading into a competition.	1	2	3	4	5
38. I feel like my parents never try to fully understand the mistakes I make in competition.	1	2	3	4	5
39. People will probably think less of me if I make mistakes in competition.	1	2	3	4	5
40. My parents want me to be better than all other players who play my sport.	1	2	3	4	5
41. I set plans that highlight the strategies I want to use when I compete.	1	2	3	4	5
42. If I play well but only make one obvious mistake in the entire game, I still feel disappointed with my performance.	1	2	3	4	5

Sport Perfectionism Scale

Please respond to each question using five responses and indicate the extent to which you agree or disagree with each statement.

| —— 1 —————— 2 —————— 3 —————— 4 —————— 5 —— |
| Strongly   Disagree   Neither Disagree   Agree   Strongly |
| Disagree   nor Agree   Agree |

_____ 1. As a child, I was punished for doing things less than perfect.

_____ 2. If I do not set the highest standards for myself, I am likely to end up a second-rate person.

_____ 3. If I perform poorly as an athlete, I feel I have failed as a person.

_____ 4. I feel I should be upset after making an error.

_____ 5. I set higher goals for myself than most people set for themselves.

_____ 6. It is as bad as being a complete failure if I partly fail.

_____ 7. I feel that I had a bad game or match if I made an error during the contest.

_____ 8. Even after I perform well I think about something I could have done better during the competition.

_____ 9. I tend to hate being less than the best at things.

_____ 10. I have extremely high goals.

_____ 11. My parents always expected excellence from me as an athlete.

_____ 12. People such as coaches, teammates, and spectators will think less of me if I make an error.

_____ 13. If someone has better skills at a particular sport than I do, then I feel like I am inferior in all skills or sports.

_____ 14. Other people seem to accept lower standards from themselves than I do.

_____ 15. If I do not perform well all the time, people will not respect me.

_____ 16. My parents always had very high expectations of my future performance in sport.

(continued)

_____ 17. I usually have doubts about the simple everyday things I do.

_____ 18. I tend to get behind in my activities because I repeat things over and over.

_____ 19. The fewer mistakes I make, the more people will like me.

_____ 20. I become frustrated or angry if I make a mistake during competition.

_____ 21. After the contest, I usually have regrets about what I should have done differently.

_____ 22. My coach would become angry with me or punish me if I performed below his expectations.

_____ 23. Even after I perform successfully, my coach tends to point out my mistakes during the competition.

_____ 24. I concentrate on making up for my mistakes during the contest.

_____ 25. Usually I am not very happy with my performance, no matter what others say.

_____ 26. No matter how well I perform, my coach asks me to perform better.

_____ 27. Making a mistake, even a "small" one, bothers me.

_____ 28. When I am working on something, I cannot relax until it is perfect.

_____ 29. My coach usually expects me to perform perfectly.

_____ 30. If I win the competition or generally perform well, I tend to criticize myself if I have made an error.

_____ 31. My goals guide my every move during competition.

_____ 32. When I evaluate myself as an athlete, I tend to think about my weaknesses rather than my strengths.

_____ 33. My parents want me to reach the top or be the best I could be in my sport.

_____ 34. My coach's standards tend to be too high for me.

_____ 35. My coach rarely compliments me on my performance.

References

Abramowitz, J. S., Deacon, B. J., & Whiteside, S. P. H. (2011). *Exposure therapy for anxiety: Principles and practice.* New York: Guilford Press.

Adderholdt, M., & Goldberg, J. (1999). *Perfectionism: What's bad about being too good?* Minneapolis, MN: Free Spirit Publishing.

Aldea, M., Rice, K., Gormley, B., & Rojas, A. (2010). Telling perfectionists about their perfectionism: Effects of providing feedback on emotional reactivity and psychological symptoms. *Behaviour Research and Therapy, 48,* 1194–1203.

Alloy, L. B., Abramson, L. Y., Walshaw, P. D., Gerstein, R. K., Keyser, J. D., Whitehouse, W. G., et al. (2009). Behavioral approach system (BAS)—Relevant cognitive styles and bipolar spectrum disorders: Concurrent and prospective associations. *Journal of Abnormal Psychology, 118,* 459–471.

American Psychiatric Association. (2013). *Diagnostic and statistical manual of mental disorders* (5th ed.). Arlington, VA: Author.

Anderluh, M. B., Tchanturia, K., Rabe-Hesketh, S., & Treasure, J. (2003). Childhood obsessive–compulsive personality traits in adult women with eating disorders: Defining a broader eating disorder phenotype. *American Journal of Psychiatry, 160,* 242–247.

Anshel, M. H., & Eom, H. J. (2002). Exploring the dimensions of perfectionism in sport. *International Journal of Sport Psychology, 34,* 255–271.

Anshel, M. H., Kim, J. K., & Henry, R. (2009). Reconceptualizing indicants of sport perfectionism as a function of gender. *Journal of Sport Behavior, 32,* 395–418.

Anshel, M. H., Weatherby, N. L., Kang, M., & Watson, T. (2009). Rasch calibration of a unidimensional perfectionism inventory for sport. *Psychology of Sport and Exercise, 10,* 210–216.

Antony, M. M., & Barlow, D. H. (Eds.). (2010). *Handbook of assessment and treatment planning for psychological disorders* (2nd ed.). New York: Guilford Press.

Antony, M. M., Purdon, C. L., Huta, V., & Swinson, R. P. (1998). Dimensions of perfectionism across the anxiety disorders. *Behaviour Research and Therapy, 36,* 1143–1154.

Antony, M. M., & Swinson, R. P. (1998). *When perfect isn't good enough: Strategies for coping with perfectionism.* Oakland, CA: New Harbinger.

Antony, M. M., & Swinson, R. P. (2009). *When perfect isn't good enough: Strategies for coping with perfectionism* (2nd ed.). Oakland, CA: New Harbinger.

Arntz A., & Weertman, A. (1999). Treatment of childhood memories: Theory and practice. *Behaviour Research and Therapy, 37,* 715–740.

Arpin-Cribbie, C. A, Irvine, J., Ritvo, P., Cribbie, R. A., Flett, G. L., & Hewitt, P. L. (2008). Perfectionism and psychological distress: A modeling approach to understanding their therapeutic relationship. *Journal of Rational-Emotive and Cognitive Behavior Therapy, 26,* 151–167.

Ashbaugh, A., Antony, M. M., Liss, A., Summerfeldt, L. J., McCabe, R. E., & Swinson, R. P. (2007). Changes in perfectionism following cognitive-behavioral treatment for social phobia. *Depression and Anxiety, 24,* 169–177.

Atkinson, M. J., & Wade, T. D. (2012). Impact of metacognitive acceptance on body dissatisfaction and negative affect: Engagement and efficacy. *Journal of Consulting and Clinical Psychology, 80,* 416–425.

Azrin, N. H., & Nunn, R. G. (1973). Habit-reversal: A method of eliminating nervous habits and tics. *Behaviour Research and Therapy, 11,* 619–628.

Baer, R. A. (2003). Mindfulness training as a clinical intervention: A conceptual and empirical review. *Clinical Psychology: Science and Practice, 10,* 125–143.

Bardone-Cone, A. M., Abramson, L. Y., Vohs, K. D., Heatherton, T. F., & Joiner, T. E. (2006). Predicting bulimic symptoms: An interactive model of self-efficacy, perfectionism, and perceived weight status. *Behaviour Research and Therapy, 44,* 27–42.

Bardone-Cone, A. M., Sturm, K., Lawson, M. A., Robinson, D. P., & Smith, R. (2010). Perfectionism across stages of recovery from eating disorders. *International Journal of Eating Disorders, 43,* 139–148.

Bardone-Cone, A. M., Wonderlich, S. A., Frost, R. O., Bulik, C. M., Mitchell, J. E., Uppala, S., et al. (2007). Perfectionism and eating disorders: Current status and future directions. *Clinical Psychology Review, 27,* 384–405.

Barlow, D. H., Farchione, T. J., Fairholme, C. P., Ellard, K. K., Boisseau, C. L., Allen, L. B., et al. (2011). *Unified protocol for transdiagnostic treatment of emotional disorders.* New York: Oxford University Press.

Barrow, J. C., & Moore, C. A. (1983). Group interventions with perfectionistic thinking. *Personnel and Guidance Journal, 61,* 612–615.

Bartsch, D. (2007). Prevalence of body dysmorphic disorder symptoms and associated clinical features among Australian university students. *Clinical Psychologist, 11,* 16–23.

Bastiani, A. M., Rao, R., Weltzin, T., & Kaye, W. H. (1995). Perfectionism in anorexia nervosa. *International Journal of Eating Disorders, 17,* 147–152.

Beck, A. T., Epstein, N., Brown, G., & Steer, R. A. (1988). An inventory for measuring clinical anxiety: Psychometric properties. *Journal of Consulting and Clinical Psychology, 56,* 893–897.

Beck, A. T., Rush, A. J., Shaw, B. F., & Emery, G. (1979). *Cognitive therapy of depression.* New York: Guilford Press.

Beck, A. T., Steer, R. A., & Brown, G. K. (1996). *Manual for the Beck Depression Inventory* (2nd ed.). San Antonio, TX: Pearson Assessment.

Beck, J. S. (2011). *Cognitive behavior therapy: Basics and beyond* (2nd ed.). New York: Guilford Press.

Beevers, C. G., & Miller, I. W. (2004). Perfectionism, cognitive bias and hopelessness as prospective predictors of suicidal ideation. *Suicide and Life-Threatening Behavior, 34*, 126–137.

Bennett-Levy, J., Butler, G., Fennell, M., Hackmann, A., Mueller, M., & Westbrook, D. (Eds.). (2004). *Oxford guide to behavioural experiments in cognitive therapy.* Oxford, UK: Oxford University Press.

Bieling, P. J., Israeli, A., & Antony, M. M. (2004). Is perfectionism good, bad, or both?: Examining models of the perfectionism construct. *Personality and Individual Differences, 36*, 1373–1385.

Bieling, P. J., McCabe, R. E., & Antony, M. M. (2006). *Cognitive-behavioral therapy in groups.* New York: Guilford Press.

Bieling, P. J., Summerfeldt, L. J., Israeli, A. L., & Antony, M. M. (2004). Perfectionism as an explanatory construct in comorbidity of axis I disorders. *Journal of Psychopathology and Behavioral Assessment, 26*, 193–201.

Bizuel, C., Sadowsky, N., & Riguad, D. (2001). The prognostic value of EDI scores in anorexia nervosa patients: A prospective follow-up study of 5–10 years. *European Psychiatry, 16*, 232–238.

Blackburn, I. M., James, I. A., Milne, D. L., Baker, C., Standart, S., Garland, A., et al. (2001). The revised Cognitive Therapy Scale (CTS-R): Psychometric properties. *Behavioral and Cognitive Psychotherapy, 29*, 431–446.

Blatt, S. J. (1995). The destructiveness of perfectionism. Implications for the treatment of depression. *American Psychologist, 50*, 1003–1020.

Blatt, S. J., D'Afflitti, J. P., & Quinlan, D. M. (1976). Experiences of depression in normal young adults. *Journal of Abnormal Psychology, 85*, 383–389.

Blatt, S. J., Quinlan, D. M., Pilkonis, P. A., & Shea, M. T. (1995). Impact of perfectionism and need for approval on the brief treatment of depression: The National Institute of Mental Health Treatment of Depression Collaborative Research program revisited. *Journal of Consulting and Clinical Psychology, 63*, 125–132.

Blatt, S. J., & Zuroff, D. (2005). Empirical evaluation of the assumptions in identifying evidence based treatments in mental health. *Clinical Psychology Review, 25*, 459–486.

Blatt, S. J., Zuroff, D. C., Bondi, C. M., Sanislow, C. A., & Pilkonis, P. A. (1998). When and how perfectionism impedes the brief treatment of depression: Further analyses of the National Institute of Mental Health Treatment of Depression Collaborative Research Program. *Journal of Consulting and Clinical Psychology, 66*, 423–428.

Bordin, E. S. (1979). The generalizability of the psychoanalytic concept of the working alliance. *Psychotherapy: Theory, Research and Practice, 16*, 252–260.

Borkovec, T. D., Alcaine, O. M., & Behar, E. (2004). Avoidance theory of worry and generalized anxiety disorder. In R. G. Heimberg, C. I. Turk, & D. S. Mennin (Eds.), *Generalized anxiety disorder: Advances in research and practice* (pp. 77–108). New York: Guilford Press.

Bossieau, C. L., Farchione, T., Fairholme, C. P., Ellard, K. E., & Barlow, D. (2010). The development of the unified protocol for the transdiagnostic treatment of emotional disorders: A case study. *Cognitive and Behavioral Practice, 17*, 102–113.

Broman-Fulks, J. J., Hill, R. W., & Green, B. A. (2008). Is perfectionism categorical or dimensional?: A taxometric analysis. *Journal of Personality Assessment, 90*, 481–490.

Bruch, H. (1978). *The golden cage: The enigma of anorexia nervosa*. Cambridge, MA: Harvard University Press.

Buhlmann, U., Etcoff, N. L., & Wilhelm, S. (2008). Facial attractiveness ratings and perfectionism in body dysmorphic disorder and obsessive–compulsive disorder. *Journal of Anxiety Disorders, 22*, 540–547.

Burns, D. D. (1980, November). The perfectionist's script for self-defeat. *Psychology Today, 14*(6), 34–52.

Burns, L. R., & Fedewa, B. A. (2005). Cognitive styles: Links with perfectionistic thinking. *Personality and Individual Differences, 38*, 103–113.

Butcher, J. N., Dahlstrom, W. G., Graham, J. R., Tellegen, A., & Kaemmer, B. (2001). *MMPI-2: Minnesota Multiphasic Personality Inventory-2: Manual for administration, scoring, and interpretation* (Rev. ed.). Minneapolis: University of Minnesota Press.

Byrne, S. M., Fursland, A., Allen, K. L., & Watson, H. (2011). The effectiveness of Enhanced Cognitive Behavioural Therapy for eating disorders: An open trial. *Behaviour Research and Therapy, 49*, 219–226.

Castonguay, L. G., Constantino, M. J., & Holtforth, M. G. (2006). The working alliance: Where are we and where should we go? *Psychotherapy: Theory, Research, Practice, Training, 43*, 271–279.

Chadwick, P. D. J., Birchwood, M. J., & Trower, P. (1996). *Cognitive therapy for delusions, voices and paranoia*. Chichester, UK: Wiley.

Chan, D. W. (2010). Perfectionism among Chinese gifted and non-gifted students in Hong Kong: The use of the Revised Almost Perfect Scale. *Journal for the Education of the Gifted, 34*, 68–98.

Chang, E. C., Ivezaj, V., Downey, C. A., Kashima, Y., & Morady, A. R. (2008). Complexities of measuring perfectionism: Three popular perfectionism measures and their relations with eating disturbances and health behaviors in a female college student sample. *Eating Behaviors, 9*, 102–110.

Chang, E. C., & Sanna, L. J. (2012). Evidence for the validity of the Clinical Perfectionism Questionnaire in a nonclinical population: More than just negative affectivity. *Journal of Personality Assessment, 94*, 102–108.

Chelminski, R. (2005). *The perfectionist: Life and death in haute cuisine*. New York: Penguin.

Chik, H. M., Whittal, M. L., & O'Neill, M. P. (2008). Perfectionism and treatment outcome in obsessive–compulsive disorder. *Cognitive Therapy and Research, 32*, 376–388.

Clara, I. P., Cox, B. J., & Enns, M. W. (2007). Assessing self-critical perfectionism in clinical depression. *Journal of Personality Assessment, 88*, 309–316.

Clark, S., & Coker, S. (2009). Perfectionism, self-criticism and maternal criticism: A study of mothers and their children. *Personality and Individual Differences, 47*, 321–325.

Cockell, S. J., Hewitt, P. L., Seal, B., Sherry, S., Goldner, E. M., Flett, G. L., et al. (2002). Trait and self-presentational dimensions of perfectionism among women with anorexia nervosa. *Cognitive Therapy and Research, 26,* 745–758.

Cohen, J. (1988). *Statistical power for the behavioural sciences* (2nd ed.). Hillsdale, NJ: Erlbaum.

Cohen, S., Kamarck, T., & Mermelstein, R. (1983). A global measure of perceived stress. *Journal of Health and Social Behavior, 24,* 385–396.

Coles, M. E., Frost, R. O., Heimberg, R. G., & Rheaume, J. (2003). "Not just right experiences": Perfectionism, obsessive–compulsive features and general psychopathology. *Behaviour Research and Therapy, 41,* 681–700.

Coles, M. E., Pinto, A., Mancebo, M. C., Rasmussen, M. A., & Eisen, J. L. (2008). OCD with comorbid OCPD: A subtype of OCD? *Journal of Psychiatric Research, 42,* 289–296.

Cook, L. C., & Kearney, C. A. (2009). Parent and youth perfectionism and internalizing psychopathology. *Personality and Individual Differences, 46,* 325–330.

Cooper, M. J., Todd, G., & Turner, H. (2007). The effects of using imagery to modify core emotional beliefs in bulimia nervosa: An experimental pilot study. *Journal of Cognitive Psychotherapy, 21,* 117–122.

Coull, G., & Morris, P. G. (2011). The clinical effectiveness of CBT-based guided self-help interventions for anxiety and depressive disorders: A systematic review. *Psychological Medicine, 41,* 2239–2252.

Cox, B. J., & Enns, M. W. (2003). Relative stability of dimensions of perfectionism in depression. *Canadian Journal of Behavioural Sciences, 35,* 124–132.

Cox, B. J., Enns, M. W., & Clara, I. P. (2002). The multidimensional structure of perfectionism in clinically distressed and college student samples. *Psychological Assessment, 14,* 365–373.

Craske, M., Farchione, T. J., Allen, L. B., Barrios, V., Stoyanova, M., & Rose, R. (2007). Cognitive behavioral therapy for panic disorder and comorbidity: More of the same or less of more? *Behaviour Research and Therapy, 45,* 1095–1109.

Craske, M. G., Hermans, D., & Vansteenwegen, D. (2006). *Fear and learning: From basic processes to clinical implications.* Washington, DC: American Psychological Association.

Deary, V., & Chalder, T. (2010). Personality and perfectionism in chronic fatigue syndrome: A closer look. *Psychology and Health, 25,* 465–475.

Deci, E. L., & Ryan, R. M. (2000). The "what" and "why" of goal pursuits: Human needs and the self-determination of behavior. *Psychological Inquiry, 11,* 227–268.

Derogatis, L. R., & Melisaratos, N. (1983). The Brief Symptom Inventory: An introductory report. *Psychological Medicine, 13,* 595–605.

DiBartolo, P. M., Dixon, A., Almodovar, S., & Frost, R. O. (2001). Can cognitive restructuring reduce the disruption associated with perfectionistic concerns? *Behavior Therapy, 32,* 167–184.

DiBartolo, P. M., Li, C. Y., & Frost, R. O. (2008). How do the dimensions of perfectionism relate to mental health? *Cognitive Therapy and Research, 32,* 401–417.

Dickie, L., Surgenor, L. J., Wilson, M., & McDowall, J. (2012). The structure and reliability of the Clinical Perfectionism Questionnaire. *Personality and Individual Differences, 52,* 865–869.

Dimidjian S., & Dobson, K. S. (2004). Process of change in cognitive therapy. In M. A. Reinecke & D. A. Clark (Eds.), *Cognitive therapy across the lifespan* (pp. 477–506). Cambridge, UK: Cambridge University Press.

DiPrima, A. J., Ashby, J. S., Gnilka, P. B., & Noble, C. L. (2011). Family relationships and perfectionism in middle-school students. *Psychology in the Schools, 48,* 815–827.

Dray J., & Wade, T. D. (2012). Is the transtheoretical model and motivational interviewing approach applicable to the treatment of eating disorders?: A review. *Clinical Psychology Review, 32,* 558–565.

D'Souza, F., Egan, S. J., & Rees, C. S. (2011). The relationship between perfectionism, stress and burnout in clinical psychologists. *Behaviour Change, 28,* 17–27.

Dunkley, D. M., Blankstein, K. R., Masheb, R. M., & Grilo, C. M. (2006). Personal standards and evaluative concerns dimensions of "clinical" perfectionism: A reply to Shafran et al. (2002, 2003) and Hewitt et al. (2003). *Behaviour Research and Therapy, 44,* 63–84.

Dunkley, D. M., Sanislow, C. A., Grilo, C. M., & McGlashan, T. H. (2006). Perfectionism and depressive symptoms three years later: Negative social interactions, avoidant coping, and perceived social support as mediators. *Comprehensive Psychiatry, 47,* 106–115.

Dunkley, D. M., Sanislow, C. A., Grilo, C. M., & McGlashan, T. H. (2009). Self-criticism vs. neuroticism in predicting depression and psychosocial impairment for 4 years in a clinical sample. *Comprehensive Psychiatry, 50,* 335–346.

Dunn, J. G. H., Causgrove Dunn, J. L., & Syrotuik, D. G. (2002). Relationship between multidimensional perfectionism and goal orientations in sport. *Journal of Sport and Exercise Psychology, 24,* 376–395.

Egan, S. J., Hattaway, M., & Kane, R. T. (2014). The relationship between perfectionism and rumination in posttraumatic stress disorder. *Behavioural and Cognitive Psychotherapy, 42,* 211–213.

Egan, S. J., & Hine, P. (2008). Cognitive behavioural treatment of perfectionism: A single case experimental design series. *Behaviour Change, 25,* 245–258.

Egan, S. J., Piek, J. P., Dyck, M. J., & Kane, R. T. (2011). Reliability and validity of the Positive and Negative Perfectionism Scale. *Clinical Psychologist, 15,* 121–132.

Egan, S. J., Piek, J. P., Dyck, M. J., & Rees, C. S. (2007). The role of dichotomous thinking and rigidity in perfectionism. *Behaviour Research and Therapy, 45,* 1813–1822.

Egan, S. J., Piek, J. P., Dyck, M. J., Rees, C. S., & Hagger, M. S. (2013). A qualitative investigation of motivation to change standards and cognitions about failure in clinical perfectionism. *Behavioural and Cognitive Psychotherapy, 41*(5), 565–578.

Egan, S. J., Shafran, R., Lee, M., Fairburn, C. G., Cooper, Z., Doll, H. A., Palmer, R., & Watson, H. J. (2014). The reliability and validity of the Clinical Perfectionism Questionnaire in eating disorder and community samples. *Behavioural and Cognitive Psychotherapy.* Manuscript under review.

Egan, S., & Stout, S. (2007, November). *Group cognitive behavioural therapy for clinical perfectionism: A preliminary investigation.* Poster presented at the meeting of the Association for Behavioral and Cognitive Therapies, Philadelphia, PA.

Egan, S. J., van Noort, E., Chee, A., Hoiles, K. J., Kane, R. T., Willan, V., et al. (2014). *A randomized controlled trial of individual face to face versus online pure self-help treatment for clinical perfectionism.* Manuscript under review.

Egan, S. J., Wade, T. D., & Shafran, R. (2011). Perfectionism as a transdiagnostic process. *Clinical Psychology Review, 31,* 203–212.

Egan, S. J., Wade, T. D., & Shafran, R. (2012). The transdiagnostic process of perfectionism. *Revista de Psicopatologia y Psicologia Clinicia, 17,* 279–294.

Ehlers, A., Clark, D. M., Hackmann, A., McManus, F., Fennell, M., Herbert, C., et al. (2003). A randomized controlled trial of cognitive therapy, a self-help booklet, and repeated assessments as early interventions for posttraumatic stress disorder. *Archives of General Psychiatry, 60,* 1024–1032.

Ehlers, A., Hackmann, A., Steil, R., Clohessy, S., Wenninger, K., & Winter, H. (2002). The nature of intrusive memories after trauma: The warning signal hypothesis. *Behaviour Research and Therapy, 40,* 995–1002.

Elkin, I. (1994). The NIMH Treatment of Depression Collaborative Research Program: Where we began and where we are now. In A. E. Bergin & S. L. Garfield (Eds.), *Handbook of psychotherapy and behavior change* (4th ed., pp. 114–135). New York: Wiley.

Elkin, I., Shea, M. T., Watkins, J. T., Imber, S. D., Sotsky, S. M., Collins, J. F., et al. (1989). NIMH Treatment of Depression Collaborative Research Program: General effectiveness of treatments. *Archives of General Psychiatry, 46,* 971–983.

Ellard, K. K., Fairholme, C. P., Bossieau, C. L., Farchione, T., & Barlow, D. (2010). Unified protocol for the transdiagnostic treatment of emotional disorders: Protocol development and initial outcome data. *Cognitive and Behavioral Practice, 17,* 88–101.

Ellis, A. (1997). Must masturbation and demandingness lead to emotional disorders? *Psychotherapy: Theory, Research, Practice, Training, 34,* 95–98.

Ellis, A., & Harper, R. (1961). *A guide to rational living.* New York: Riverhead Books.

Emery, S., McLean, S., & Wade, T. D. (2009). Associations among therapist beliefs, personal resources and burnout in clinical psychologists. *Behaviour Change, 26,* 83–96.

English, H. B., & English, A. C. (1958). *A comprehensive dictionary of psychological and psychoanalytical terms.* New York: Longmans, Green.

Enns, M. W., Cox, B. J., & Borger, S. C. (2001). Correlates of analogue and clinical depression: A further test of the phenomenological continuity hypothesis. *Journal of Affective Disorders, 66,* 175–183.

Enns, M. W., Cox, B. J., & Clara, I. (2002). Adaptive and maladaptive perfectionism: Developmental origins and association with depression proneness. *Personality and Individual Differences, 33,* 921–935.

Fairburn, C. G. (2008). *Cognitive behavior therapy and eating disorders.* New York: Guilford Press.

Fairburn, C. G. (2013). *Overcoming binge eating* (2nd ed.). New York: Guilford Press.

Fairburn, C. G., Cooper, Z., Doll, H. A., O'Connor, M. E., Bohn, K., Hawker, D. M., et al. (2009). Transdiagnostic cognitive-behavioral therapy for patients with eating disorders: A two-site trial with 60-week follow-up. *American Journal of Psychiatry, 166,* 311–319.

Fairburn, C. G., Cooper, Z., & Shafran, R. (2003a). Cognitive behaviour therapy for eating disorders: A "transdiagnostic" theory and treatment. *Behaviour Research and Therapy, 41,* 509–528.

Fairburn, C. G., Cooper, Z., & Shafran, R. (2003b). *Clinical Perfectionism Questionnaire*. Unpublished scale, University of Oxford, Oxford, UK.

Farchione, T. J., Fairholme, C. P., Ellard, K. K., Boisseau, C. L., Thompson-Hollands, J., Carl, J. R., et al. (2012). Unified protocol for transdiagnostic treatment of emotional disorders: A randomized controlled trial. *Behavior Therapy, 3,* 666–678.

Fennell, M. (1999). *Overcoming low self-esteem: A self-help guide using cognitive behavioral techniques*. London: Robinson.

Ferguson, K. L., & Rodway, G. R. (1994). Cognitive-behavioral treatment of perfectionism: Initial evaluation studies. *Research on Social Work Practice, 4,* 283–308.

Ferrari, J. R., & Mautz, W. T. (1997). Predicting perfectionism: Applying tests of rigidity. *Journal of Clinical Psychology, 53,* 1–6.

Field, A., Javaras, K. M., Aneja, P., Kitos, N., Camargo, C. A., Taylor, C. B., et al. (2008). Family, media, and peer predictors of becoming eating disordered. *Archives of Pediatric and Adolescent Medicine, 162,* 574–579.

Finn, S., & Tonsager, E. (1992). Therapeutic effects of providing MMPI-2 test feedback to college students awaiting therapy. *Psychological Assessment, 4,* 278–287.

First, M. B., Williams, J. B. W., Karg, R. S., & Spitzer, R. L. (2014). *Structured clinical interview for DSM-5 disorders—Patient edition (SCID-5)*. New York: Biometrics Research Department, New York State Psychiatric Institute.

Flett, G. L., Hewitt, P. L., Blankstein, K. R., & Gray, L. (1998). Psychological distress and the frequency of perfectionistic thinking. *Journal of Personality and Social Psychology, 75,* 1363–1381.

Flett, G. L., Hewitt, P. L., Boucher, D. J., Davidson, L. A., & Munro, Y. (2000). *The Child–Adolescent Perfectionism Scale: Development, validation, and association with adjustment*. Unpublished scale, York University, Toronto, ON.

Flett, G. L., Hewitt, P. L., Whelan, T., & Martin, T. R. (2007). The Perfectionism Cognitions Inventory: Psychometric properties and associations with distress and deficits in cognitive self-management. *Journal of Rational Emotive and Cognitive Behaviour Therapy, 25,* 255–277.

Fredtoft, T., Poulsen, S., Bauer, M., & Malm, M. (1996). Dependency and perfectionism: Short term dynamic group psychotherapy for university students. *Psychodynamic Counselling, 24,* 476–497.

Freeman, A., & Dolan, M. (2001). Revisiting Prochaska and DiClemente's Stages of Change theory: An expansion and specification to aid in treatment planning and outcome evaluation. *Cognitive and Behavioral Practice, 8,* 224–234.

Frost, R. O., Heimberg, R. G., Holt, C. S., Mattia, J. I., & Newbauer, A. L. (1993).

A comparison of two measures of perfectionism. *Personality and Individual Differences, 14,* 119–126.

Frost, R. O., Lahart, C., & Rosenblate, R. (1991). The development of perfectionism: A study of daughters and their parents. *Cognitive Therapy and Research, 15,* 469–489.

Frost, R. O., Marten, P., Lahart, C., & Rosenblate, R. (1990). The dimensions of perfectionism. *Cognitive Therapy and Research, 14,* 449–468.

Frost, R. O., Novara, C., & Rheaume, J. (2002). Perfectionism in obsessive–compulsive disorder. In R. O. Frost & G. Steketee (Eds.), *Cognitive approaches to obsessions and compulsions* (pp. 91–105). New York: Pergamon.

Frost, R. O., & Steketee, G. (1997). Perfectionism in obsessive–compulsive disorder patients. *Behaviour Research and Therapy, 35,* 291–296.

Frost, R. O., Steketee, G., Cohn, L., & Greiss, K. (1994). Personality traits in subclinical and non-obsessive–compulsive volunteers and their parents. *Behaviour Research and Therapy, 32,* 47–56.

Garner, D. M. (1991). *Eating Disorder Inventory-2 Professional Manual.* Odessa, FL: Psychological Assessment Resources.

Garner, D. M., Olmsted, M. P., & Polivy, J. (1983). Development and validation of a multidimensional eating disorder inventory for anorexia nervosa and bulimia. *International Journal of Eating Disorders, 2,* 15–34.

Geller, J. (2002). Estimating readiness for change in anorexia nervosa: Comparing clients, clinicians and research assessors. *International Journal of Eating Disorders, 31,* 251–260.

Gilbert, P. (2010). *The compassionate mind.* London: Constable & Robinson.

Gilbert, P., & Irons, C. (2005). Focused therapies for shame and self-attacking, using cognitive, behavioral, emotional, imagery and compassionate mind training. In P. Gilbert (Ed.), *Compassion: Conceptualisations, research and use in psychotherapy* (pp. 263–325). London, UK: Brunner-Routledge.

Glover, D. S., Brown, G. P., Fairburn, C. G., & Shafran, R. (2007). A preliminary evaluation of cognitive-behaviour therapy for clinical perfectionism: A case series. *British Journal of Clinical Psychology, 46,* 85–94.

Gotwals, J. K., & Dunn, J. G. H. (2009). A multi-method multi-analytic approach to establishing internal construct validity evidence: The Sport Multidimensional Perfectionism Scale 2. *Measurement in Physical Education and Exercise Science, 13,* 71–92.

Gotwals, J. K., Dunn, J. G. H., Causgrove Dunn, J. L., & Gamache, V. (2010). Establishing the validity evidence for the Sport Multidimensional Perfectionism Scale-2 in intercollegiate sport. *Psychology of Sport and Exercise, 11,* 423–432.

Greenspon, T. S. (2008). Making sense of error: A view of the origins and treatment of perfectionism. *American Journal of Psychotherapy, 62,* 263–283.

Haase, A. M., & Prapavessis, H. (2004). Assessing the factor structure and composition of the Positive and Negative Perfectionism Scale in sport. *Personality and Individual Differences, 36,* 1725–1740.

Hackmann, A., Bennett-Levy, J., & Holmes, E. A. (2011). *Oxford guide to imagery in cognitive therapy.* Oxford, UK: Oxford University Press.

Hackmann, A., Clark, D. M., & McManus, F. (2000). Recurrent images and early memories in social phobia. *Behaviour Research and Therapy, 38,* 601–610.

Hackmann, A., & Holmes, E. A. (2004). Reflecting on imagery: A clinical perspective and overview of the special issue of memory on mental imagery and memory in psychopathology. *Memory, 12,* 389–402.

Halmi, K. A., Sunday, S. R., Strober, M., Kaplan, A., Woodside, D. B., Fichter M., et al. (2000). Perfectionism in anorexia nervosa: Variation by clinical subtype, obsessionality, and pathological eating behavior. *American Journal of Psychiatry, 157,* 1799–1805.

Halmi, K. A., Tozzi, F., Thornton, L. M., Crow, S., Fichter, M. M., Kaplan, A. S., et al. (2005). The relation among perfectionism, obsessive–compulsive personality disorder and obsessive–compulsive disorder in individuals with eating disorders. *International Journal of Eating Disorders, 38,* 371–374.

Hamachek, D. E. (1978). Psychodynamics of normal and neurotic perfectionism. *Psychology: A Journal of Human Behavior, 15,* 27–33.

Han, P. (Director). (2006). *What it takes: A documentary about four world-class triathletes' quest for greatness.* United States: Wit Media.

Handley, A. K., Egan, S. J., Kane, R. T., & Rees, C. S. (2014). The relationship between perfectionism, pathological worry and generalised anxiety disorder. *BMC Psychiatry, 14*(98).

Handley, A., Egan, S. J., Kane, R. T., & Rees, C. S. (2014). *A randomized controlled trial of group cognitive behavioural therapy for clinical perfectionism.* Manuscript under review.

Hannan, C., Lambert, M. J., Harmon, C., Nielsen, S. L., Smart, D. W., Shimokawa, K., et al. (2005). A lab test and algorithms for identifying clients at risk for treatment failure. *Journal of Clinical Psychology, 61*(2), 155–163.

Harvey, A., Watkins, E., Mansell, W., & Shafran, R. (2004). *Cognitive behavioural processes across psychological disorders: A transdiagnostic approach to research and treatment.* Oxford, UK: Oxford University Press.

Hawkins, C. C., Watt, H. H., & Sinclair, K. E. (2006). Psychometric properties of the Frost Multidimensional Perfectionism Scale with Australian adolescent girls: Clarification of multidimensionality and perfectionist typology. *Educational and Psychological Measurement, 66,* 1001–1022.

Hawkins, P., & Shohet, R. (2000). *Supervision in the helping professions: An individual, group, and organisational approach.* Buckingham: Open University Press.

Hawley, L. L., Ho, M.-H. R., Zuroff, D. C., & Blatt, S. J. (2006). The relationship of perfectionism, depression, and therapeutic alliance during treatment for depression: Latent difference score analysis. *Journal of Consulting and Clinical Psychology, 74,* 930–942.

Heimberg, R. G., Juster, H. R., Hope, D. A., & Mattia, J. I. (1995). Cognitive behavioral group treatment: Description, case presentation, and empirical support. In M. B. Stein (Ed.), *Social phobia: Clinical and research perspectives* (pp. 293–321). Washington, DC: American Psychiatric Press.

Hewitt, P. L., Blasberg, J. S., Flett, G. L., Besser, A., Sherry, S. B., Caelian, C., et al. (2011). Perfectionistic self-presentation in children and adolescents: Development and validation of the Perfectionistic Self-Presentation Scale—Junior Form. *Psychological Assessment, 23,* 125–142.

Hewitt, P. L., & Flett, G. L. (1991a). Dimensions of perfectionism in unipolar depression. *Journal of Abnormal Psychology, 100,* 98–101.

Hewitt, P. L., & Flett, G. L. (1991b). Perfectionism in the self and social contexts: Conceptualization, assessment, and association with psychopathology. *Journal of Personality and Social Psychology, 60,* 456–470.

Hewitt, P. L., Flett, G. L., Besser, A., Sherry, S. B., & McGee, B. (2003). Perfectionism is multidimensional: A reply to Shafran, Cooper and Fairburn (2002). *Behaviour Research and Therapy, 41,* 1221–1236.

Hewitt, P. L., Flett, G. L., & Ediger, E. (1996). Perfectionism and depression: Longitudinal assessment of a specific vulnerability hypothesis. *Journal of Abnormal Psychology, 105,* 276–280.

Hewitt, P. L., Flett, G. L., Sherry, S. B., & Caelian, C. (2006). Trait perfectionism dimensions and suicidal behavior. In T. Ellis (Ed.), *Cognition and suicide: Theory, research and therapy* (pp. 215–230). Washington, DC: American Psychological Association.

Hewitt, P. L., Flett, G. L., Sherry, S. B., Habke, M., Parkin, M., Lam, R. W., et al. (2003). The interpersonal expression of perfection: Perfectionistic self-presentation and psychological distress. *Journal of Personality and Social Psychology, 84,* 1303–1325.

Hewitt, P. L., Flett, G. L., Turnbull-Donovan, W., & Mikhail, S. F. (1991). The Multidimensional Perfectionism Scale: Reliability, validity, and psychometric properties in psychiatric samples. *Psychological Assessment, 3,* 464–468.

Hewitt, P. L., Flett, G. L., & Weber, C. (1994). Dimensions of perfectionism and suicide ideation. *Cognitive Therapy and Research, 18,* 439–460.

Hewitt, P. L., Norton, R., Flett, G. L., Callander, L., & Cowan, T. (1998). Dimensions of perfectionism, hopelessness, and attempted suicide in a sample of alcoholics. *Suicide and Life-Threatening Behavior, 28,* 395–406.

Hill, R. W., Huelsman, T. J., Furr, R. M., Kibler, J., Vicente, B. B., & Kennedy, C. (2004). A new measure of perfectionism: The Perfectionism Inventory. *Journal of Personality Assessment, 82,* 80–91.

Himle, J. A., Van Etten, M., & Fischer, D. J. (2003). Group cognitive behavioral therapy for obsessive–compulsive disorder (OCD): A controlled study. *International Journal of Psychiatry in Clinical Practice, 9,* 257–263.

Hirsch, C. R., & Hayward, P. (1998). The perfect patient: Cognitive behavioural therapy for perfectionism. *Behavioural and Cognitive Psychotherapy, 26,* 359–364.

Hoffman, S. G., & Otto, M. W. (2008). *Cognitive behavioral therapy for social anxiety disorder: Evidence-based and disorder-specific treatment techniques.* New York: Routledge.

Hoiles, K., Egan, S. J., & Kane, R. T. (2012). The validity of the transdiagnostic cognitive behavioural model of eating disorders in predicting dietary restraint. *Eating Behaviors, 13,* 123–126.

Hoiles, K., Egan, S. J., Kane, R. T., & Rees, C. S. (2014). *A randomized controlled trial of guided self-help treatment for clinical perfectionism.* Manuscript in preparation.

Hollender, M. H. (1965). Perfectionism. *Comprehensive Psychiatry, 6,* 94–103.

Holliday, J., Tchanturia, K., Landau, S., Collier, D., & Treasure, J. (2005). Is impaired set-shifting an endophenotype of anorexia nervosa? *American Journal of Psychiatry, 162,* 2269–2275.

Holmes, E. A., Arntz, A., & Smucker, M. R. (2007). Imagery rescripting in cognitive behaviour therapy: Images, treatment techniques and outcomes. *Journal of Behavior Therapy and Experimental Psychiatry, 38*, 297–305.

Holmes, E. A., Geddes, J. R., Colom, F., & Goodwin, G. M. (2008). Mental imagery as an emotional amplifier: Application to bipolar disorder. *Behaviour Research and Therapy, 46*, 1251–1258.

Holmes, E. A., Lang, T. J., & Shah, D. M. (2009). Developing interpretation bias modification as a "cognitive vaccine" for depressed mood: Imagining positive events makes you feel better than thinking about them verbally. *Journal of Abnormal Psychology 118*, 76–88.

Holmes, E. A., & Mathews, A. (2010). Mental imagery in emotion and emotional disorders. *Clinical Psychology Review, 30*, 349–362.

Holmes, E. A., Mathews, A., Dalgleish, T., & Mackintosh, B. (2006). Positive interpretation training: Effects of mental imagery versus verbal training on positive mood. *Behavior Therapy, 37*, 237–247.

Holtforth, M. G., & Castonguay, L. G. (2005). Relationship and techniques in cognitive-behavioral therapy: A motivational approach. *Psychotherapy: Theory, Research, Practice, Training, 42*(4), 443–455.

Horney, K. (1950). *Neurosis and human growth: The struggle toward self-realization.* New York: Norton.

Huprich, S. K., Porcerelli, J., Keaschuk, R., Binienda, J., & Engle, B. (2008). Depressive personality disorder, dysthymia, and their relationship to perfectionism. *Depression and Anxiety, 25*, 207–217.

Iketani, T., Kiriike, N., Stein, M. B., Nagao, K., Nagata, T., Minamikawa, N., et al. (2002). Relationship between perfectionism and agoraphobia in patients with panic disorder. *Cognitive Behaviour Therapy, 31*, 119–128.

Jacobi, C., Hayward, C., de Zwaan, M., Kraemer, H. C., & Agras, W. S. (2004). Coming to terms with risk factors for eating disorders: Application of risk terminology and suggestions for general taxonomy. *Psychological Bulletin, 130*, 19–65.

Jacobs, M. J., Roesch, S., Wonderlich, S. A., Crosby, R., Thornton, L., Wilfley, D. E., et al. (2009). Anorexia nervosa trios: Behavioral profiles of individuals with anorexia nervosa and their parents. *Psychological Medicine, 39*, 451–461.

Jacobs, R. H., Silva, S. G., Reinecke, M. A., Curry, J. F., Ginsburg, G. S., Kratochvil, C. J., et al. (2009). Dysfunctional Attitudes Scale perfectionism: A predictor and partial mediator of acute treatment outcome among clinically depressed adolescents. *Journal of Clinical Child and Adolescent Psychology, 38*(6), 803–813.

Johnson, J. G., Cohen, P., Kasen, S., & Brook, J. S. (2002). Eating disorders during adolescence and the risk for physical and mental disorders during early adulthood. *Archives of General Psychiatry, 59*, 545–552.

Jones, L. (2011, May 16). My shoulders are so bony I look ill. But I'd still rather be dead than fat. *Daily Mail.* Retrieved from *www.dailymail.co.uk/femail/article-1387364/Anorexia-nervosa-My-shoulders-bony-I-look-ill-Id-dead-fat.html.*

Jones, L., Scott, J., Haque, S., Gordon-Smith, K., Heron, J., Caesar, S., et al. (2005). Cognitive styles in bipolar disorder. *British Journal of Psychiatry, 187*, 431–437.

Juster, H. R., Heimberg, R. G., Frost, R. O., Holt, C. S., Mattia, J. I., & Faccenda,

K. (1996). Social phobia and perfectionism. *Personality and Individual Differences, 21,* 403–410.

Kawamura, K. Y., Frost, R. O., & Harmatz, M. G. (2002). The relationship between perceived parenting styles to perfectionism. *Personality and Individual Differences, 32,* 317–327.

Kawamura, K. Y., Hunt, S. L., Frost, R. O., & DiBartolo, P. M. (2001). Perfectionism, anxiety and depression: Are the relationships independent? *Cognitive Therapy and Research, 25,* 291–301.

Kempke, S., Van Houdenhove, B., Luyten, P., Goosens, L., Bekaert, P., & Van Wambeke, P. (2011). Unraveling the role of perfectionism in chronic fatigue syndrome: Is there a distinction between adaptive and maladaptive perfectionism? *Psychiatry Research, 186,* 373–377.

Kennerley, H. (2007). *Socratic method.* Oxford, UK: Oxford Cognitive Therapy Centre.

Kessler, R. C., Chiu, W. T., Demler, O., Merikangas, K. R., & Walters, E. E. (2005). Prevalence, severity, and comorbidity of 12-month DSM-IV disorders in the national comorbidity survey replication. *Archives of General Psychiatry, 62,* 617–627.

Khawaja, N. G., & Armstrong, K. A. (2005). Factor structure and psychometric properties of the Frost Multidimensional Perfectionism Scale: Developing shorter versions using an Australian sample. *Australian Journal of Psychology, 57,* 129–138.

Kim, J. M. (2010). *The conceptualization and assessment of the perceived consequences of perfectionism.* Unpublished honors thesis, University of Michigan, Ann Arbor. Retrieved from *http://hdl.handle.net/2027.42/77633.*

Kim, J. M., & Chang, E. C. (2010). *Consequences of perfectionism scale.* Unpublished scale. Ann Arbor, MI: University of Michigan.

Klibert, J. J., Langhinrichsen-Rohling, J., & Saito, M. (2005). Adaptive and maladaptive aspects of self-oriented versus socially prescribed perfectionism. *Journal of College Student Development, 46,* 141–156.

Kobori, O. (2006). *A cognitive model of perfectionism: The relationship of perfectionism personality to psychological adaptation and maladaptation.* Unpublished doctoral dissertation, University of Tokyo, Tokyo, Japan. Retrieved January 2, 2013, from *https://sites.google.com/site/cbtiapt/english/publication.*

Kobori, O., Hayakawa, M., & Tanno, Y. (2009). Do perfectionists raise their standards after success?: An experimental examination of the revaluation of standard-setting in perfectionism. *Journal of Behavior Therapy and Experimental Psychiatry, 40,* 515–521.

Kolb, D. A. (1984). *Experiential learning: Experience as the source of learning and development.* Englewood Cliffs, NJ: Prentice-Hall.

Kraemer, H. C., Morgan, G. A., Leech, N. L., Gliner, J. A., Vaske, J. J., & Harmon, R. J. (2003). Measures of clinical significance. *Journal of the American Academy of Child and Adolescent Psychiatry, 42,* 1524–1529.

Kutlesa, N., & Arthur, N. (2008). Overcoming negative aspects of perfectionism through group treatment. *Journal of Rational-Emotive and Cognitive Behavior Therapy, 26,* 134–150.

Kuyken, W., Watkins, E., Holden, E., White, K., Taylor, R. S., Byford, S., et al.

(2010). How does mindfulness-based cognitive therapy work? *Behaviour Research and Therapy, 48,* 1105–1112.

Kyrios, M., Hordern, C., Nedeljokovic, M., Bhar, S., Moulding, R., & Doron, G. (2007, November). *Prediction of outcome following individual manualised cognitive-behaviour therapy for obsessive–compulsive disorder.* Paper presented at the World Psychiatric Association Conference, Melbourne, Australia.

Lambert, M. J., Whipple, J. L., Vermeersch, D. A., Smart, D. W., Hawkins, E. J., Nielsen, S. L., et al. (2002). Enhancing psychotherapy outcomes via providing feedback on client progress: A replication. *Clinical Psychology and Psychotherapy, 9,* 91–103.

Lampard, A. M., Byrne, S. M., McLean, N., & Fursland, A. (2012). The Eating Disorder Inventory-2 Perfectionism Scale: Factor structure and associations with dietary restraint and weight and shape concern in eating disorders. *Eating Behaviors, 13,* 49–53.

Leary, M. R., Tate, E. B., Adams, C. E., Allen, A. B., & Hancock, J. (2007). Self-compassion and reactions to unpleasant self-relevant events: The implications of treating oneself kindly. *Journal of Personality and Social Psychology, 92,* 887.

Lee, M., Roberts-Collins, C., Coughtrey, A., Phillips, L., & Shafran, R. (2011). Behavioral expressions, imagery and perfectionism. *Behavioural and Cognitive Psychotherapy, 39,* 413–425.

Lilenfeld, L. R., Stein, D., Bulik, C. M., Strober, M., Plotnicov, K., Pollice, C., et al. (2000). Personality traits among currently eating disordered, recovered and never ill first-degree female relatives of bulimic and control women. *Psychological Medicine, 30,* 1399–1410.

Lilenfeld, L. R., Wonderlich, S., Riso, L. P., Crosby, R., & Mitchell, J. (2006). Eating disorders and personality: A methodological and empirical review. *Clinical Psychology Review, 26,* 299–320.

Linehan, M. M. (1993). *Cognitive-behavioral treatment of borderline personality disorder.* New York: Guilford Press.

Lopez, C., Tchanturia, K., Stahl, D., & Treasure, J. (2008). Central coherence in women with bulimia nervosa. *International Journal of Eating Disorders, 41*(4), 340–347.

Lovibond, P. F., & Lovibond, S. H. (1995). The structure of negative emotional states: Comparison of the depression and anxiety inventories. *Behaviour Research and Therapy, 33,* 335–343.

Lundh, L. G., & Öst, L. G. (2001). Attentional bias, self-consciousness and perfectionism in social phobia before and after cognitive-behaviour therapy. *Scandinavian Journal of Behaviour Therapy, 30,* 4–16.

McLean, S., Wade, T. D., & Encel, J. (2003). The contribution of therapist beliefs to psychological distress in therapists: An investigation of vicarious traumatisation, burnout and symptoms of avoidance and intrusion. *Behavioural and Cognitive Psychotherapy, 31,* 417–428.

McManus, F., van Doorn, K., & Yiend, J. (2012). Examining the effects of thought records and behavioral experiments in instigating belief change. *Journal of Behavior Therapy and Experimental Psychiatry, 43,* 540–547.

Miller, J. L., & Vaillancourt, T. (2007). Relation between childhood victimization and adult perfectionism: Are victims of indirect aggression more perfectionistic? *Aggressive Behavior, 33,* 230–241.

Miller, S. D., Duncan, B. L., Brown, J., Sparks, J., & Claud, D. (2003). The Outcome Rating Scale: A preliminary study of the reliability, validity, and feasibility of a brief visual analog measure. *Journal of Brief Therapy, 2,* 91–100.

Miller, W. R., & Rollnick, S. (2013). *Motivational interviewing: Helping people change* (3rd ed.). New York: Guilford Press.

Millon, T. (2004). *Millon Index of Personality Styles—Revised* (manual). San Antonio, TX: Pearson Assessment.

Milne, D. (2009). *Evidence-based clinical supervision: Principles and practice.* London: British Psychological Society and Blackwell Publishing.

Mitzman, S. F., Slade, P., & Dewey, M. E. (1994). Preliminary development of a questionnaire designed to measure neurotic perfectionism in the eating disorders. *Journal of Clinical Psychology, 50,* 516–522.

Mobley, M., Slaney, R. B., & Rice, K. G. (2005). Cultural validity of the Almost Perfect Scale—Revised for African American college students. *Journal of Counseling Psychology, 52,* 629–639.

Moretz, M. W., & McKay, D. (2009). The role of perfectionism in obsessive–compulsive symptoms: "Not just right" experiencing and checking compulsions. *Journal of Anxiety Disorders, 23,* 640–644.

Moser, J. S., Slane, J. D., Alexandra Burt, S., & Klump, K. L. (2012). Etiologic relationships between anxiety and dimensions of maladaptive perfectionism and young adult female twins. *Depression and Anxiety, 29,* 47–53.

Mussell, M. P., Mitchell, J. E., Crosby, R. D., Fulkerson, J. A., Hoberman, H. M., & Romano, J. L. (2000). Commitment to treatment goals in prediction of group cognitive-behavioral therapy treatment outcome for women with bulimia nervosa. *Journal of Consulting and Clinical Psychology, 68,* 432–437.

Neff, K. D. (2003). The development and validation of a scale to measure self-compassion. *Self and Identity, 2,* 223–250.

Neff, K. D., Hsieh, Y-P., & Dejitterat, K. (2005). Self-compassion, achievement goals, and coping with academic failure. *Self and Identity, 43,* 263–287.

Nehmy, T. J. (2011). School-based prevention of depression and anxiety in Australia: Current state and future directions. *Clinical Psychologist, 14,* 74–83.

Nehmy, T., & Wade, T. D. (2014). *Transdiagnostic universal prevention of adolescent depression, anxiety and disordered eating.* Manuscript in preparation.

Newman, M., & Greenway, P. (1997). Therapeutic effects of providing MMPI-2 test feedback to clients at a university counseling service: A collaborative approach. *Psychological Assessment, 9,* 122–131.

Nilsson, J. E., Lundh, L. G., & Viborg, G. (2012). Imagery rescripting of early memories in social anxiety disorder: An experimental study. *Behaviour Research and Therapy, 50*(6), 387–392.

Nilsson, K., Sundbom, E., & Hagglof, B. (2008). A longitudinal study of perfectionism in adolescent onset anorexia nervosa–restricting type. *European Eating Disorders Review, 16,* 386–394.

Norman, R. M. G., Davies, F., Nicholson, I. R., Cortese, L., & Malla, A. K. (1998). The relationship of two aspects of perfectionism with symptoms in a psychiatric outpatient population. *Journal of Social and Clinical Psychology, 17,* 50–68.

378

References

Norton P. J., & Philipp, L. M. (2008). Transdiagnostic approaches to the treatment of anxiety disorders: A quantitative review. *Psychotherapy: Theory, Research, Practice and Training, 45*, 214–226.

Obsessive Compulsive Cognitions Working Group. (1997). Cognitive assessment of obsessive–compulsive disorder. *Behaviour Research and Therapy, 35*, 667–681.

Obsessive Compulsive Cognitions Working Group. (2001). Development and initial validation of the obsessive beliefs questionnaire and the interpretation of intrusions inventory. *Behaviour Research and Therapy, 39*, 987–1006.

O'Connor, K. P., Brault, M., Robillard, S., Loiselle, J., Borgeat, F., & Stip, E. (2001). Evaluation of a cognitive-behavioural program for the management of chronic tic and habit disorders. *Behaviour Research and Therapy, 39*, 667–681.

O'Connor, R. C., Dixon, D., & Rasmussen, S. (2009). The structure and temporal stability of the Child and Adolescent Perfectionism Scale. *Psychological Assessment, 21*, 437–443.

O'Connor, R. C., Rasmussen, S., & Hawton, K. (2010). Predicting depression, anxiety and self-harm in adolescents: The role of perfectionism and acute life stress, *Behaviour Research and Therapy, 48*, 52–59.

Ohanian, V. (2002). Imagery rescripting within cognitive behavior therapy for bulimia nervosa: An illustrative case report. *International Journal of Eating Disorders, 31*, 352–357.

Orsillo, S. M., & Roemer, L. (2011). *A mindful way through anxiety: Break free from chronic worry and reclaim your life*. New York: Guilford Press.

Owens, R. G., & Slade, P. D. (2008). So perfect it's positively harmful?: Reflections on the adaptiveness and maladaptive miss of positive and negative perfectionism. *Behavior Modification, 32*, 928–937.

Oxford Dictionaries (2013). *Perfectionism*. Retrieved from *http://oxforddictionaries.com/definition/american_english/perfectionism*.

Padesky, C. (1990). Schema as self prejudice. *International Cognitive Therapy Newsletter, 6*, 6–7.

Padesky, C. A. (1994). Schema change processes in cognitive therapy. *Clinical Psychology and Psychotherapy, 1*, 267–278.

Padesky, C. A. (1996). *Developing cognitive therapist competency: Teaching and supervision models*. In P. M. Salkovskis (Ed.), *Frontiers of cognitive therapy* (pp. 266–292). New York: Guilford Press.

Padesky, C. A., & Greenberger, D. (1995). *Mind over mood: Change how you feel by changing the way you think*. New York: Guilford Press.

Parker, G., & Crawford, J. (2009). Personality and self-reported treatment effectiveness in depression. *Australian and New Zealand Journal of Psychiatry, 43*, 518–525.

Pinto, A., Liebowitz, M. R., Foa, E. B., & Simpson, H. B. (2011). Obsessive compulsive personality disorder as a predictor of exposure and ritual prevention outcome for obsessive compulsive disorder. *Behaviour Research and Therapy, 49*, 453–458.

Pinto, A., Mancebo, M. C., Eisen, J. L., Pagano, M. E., & Rasmussen, S. A. (2006). The Brown Longitudinal Obsessive Compulsive Study: Clinical features and symptoms of the sample at intake. *Journal of Clinical Psychiatry, 67,* 703–711.

Pla, C., & Toro, J. (1999). Anorexia nervosa in a Spanish adolescent sample: An 8-year longitudinal study. *Acta Psychiatrica Scandinavica, 100,* 441–446.

Pleva, J., & Wade, T. D. (2007). Guided self-help versus pure self-help for perfectionism: A randomised controlled trial. *Behaviour Research and Therapy, 45,* 849–861.

Piacentini J. C., & Chang, S. W. (2006). Behavioral treatments for tic suppression: Habit reversal training. *Advances in Neurology, 99,* 227–233.

Powers, T., Koestner, R., Lacaille, N., Kwan, L., & Zuroff, D. (2009). Self-criticism, motivation, and goal progress of athletes and musicians: A prospective study. *Personality and Individual Differences, 47,* 279–283.

Powers, T. A., Koestner, R., & Zuroff, D. C. (2007). Self-criticism, goal motivation, and goal progress. *Journal of Social and Clinical Psychology, 26,* 826–840.

Rachman, S., & de Silva, P. (1978). Abnormal and normal obsessions. *Behaviour Research and Therapy, 16,* 233–248.

Rachman, S., Radomsky, A. S., & Shafran, R. (2008). Safety behaviour: A reconsideration. *Behaviour Research and Therapy, 46,* 163–73.

Radhu, N., Zafiris, J. D., Arpin-Cribbie, C. A., Irvine, J., & Ritvo, P. (2012). Evaluating a web-based cognitive-behavioral therapy for maladaptive perfectionism in university students. *Journal of American College Health, 60,* 357–366.

Radomsky, A. S., Shafran, R., Coughtrey, A. E., & Rachman, S. (2010). Cognitive-behavior therapy for compulsive checking in OCD. *Cognitive and Behavioural Practice, 17,* 119–131.

Raes, F., Pommier, E., Neff, K. D., & Van Gucht, D. (2011). Construction and factorial validation of a short form of the Self-Compassion Scale. *Clinical Psychology and Psychotherapy, 18,* 250–255.

Rasmussen, S. A., O'Connor, R. C., & Brodie, D. (2008). The role of perfectionism and autobiographical memory in a sample of parasuicide patients: An exploratory study. *Crisis, 29,* 64–72.

Resick, P. A., & Schnicke, M. K. (1996). *Cognitive processing therapy for rape victims.* London, UK: Sage.

Rhéaume, J., Freeston, M. H., Ladouceur, R., Bouchard, C., Gallant, L., Talbot, F., et al. (2000). Functional and dysfunctional perfectionists: Are they different on compulsive-like behaviors? *Behaviour Research and Therapy, 38,* 119–128.

Rice, K. G., & Ashby, J. S. (2007). An efficient method for classifying perfectionists. *Journal of Counseling Psychology, 54,* 72–85.

Rice, K. G., Kubal, A. E., & Preusser, K. J. (2004). Perfectionism in children's self-concept: Further validation of the Adaptive/Maladaptive Perfectionism Scale. *Psychology in the Schools, 41,* 279–290.

Rice, K. G., & Preusser, K. J. (2002). The Adaptive/Maladaptive Perfectionism Scale. *Measurement and Evaluation in Counseling and Development, 34,* 210–222.

Rice, K. G., Richardson, C. M. E., & Tueller, S. (in press). The short form of the Revised Almost Perfect Scale. *Journal of Personality Assessment.*

Rice, K. G., & Stuart, J. (2010). Differentiating adaptive and maladaptive perfectionism on the MMPI-2 and MIPS Revised. *Journal of Personality Assessment, 92,* 158–167.

Riley, C., Lee, M., Cooper, Z., Fairburn, C., & Shafran, R. (2007). A randomised controlled trial of cognitive-behaviour therapy for clinical perfectionism: A preliminary study. *Behaviour Research and Therapy, 45,* 2221–2231.

Riley, C., & Shafran, R. (2005). Clinical perfectionism: A preliminary qualitative analysis. *Behavioural and Cognitive Psychotherapy, 33,* 369–374.

Robins, C. J., Ladd, J. S., Welkowitz, J., Blaney, P. H., Diaz, R., & Kutcher, G. (1994). The Personal Style Inventory: Preliminary validation studies of a new measure of sociotropy and autonomy. *Journal of Psychopathology and Behavioral Assessment, 16,* 277–300.

Saboonchi, F., Lundh, L., & Öst, L. (1999). Perfectionism and self-consciousness in social phobia and panic disorder with agoraphobia. *Behaviour Research and Therapy, 37,* 799–808.

Safran, J. D., & Muran, J. C. (2000). *Negotiating the therapeutic alliance.* New York: Guilford Press.

Safran, J. D., Muran, J. C., Samstag, L. W., & Stevens, C. (2001). Repairing alliance ruptures. *Psychotherapy: Theory, Research, Practice, Training, 38,* 406–412.

Salkovskis, P. M. (1996). The cognitive approach to anxiety: Threat beliefs, safety-seeking behaviour, and the special case of health anxiety and obsessions. In P. M. Salkovskis (Ed.), *Frontiers of cognitive therapy* (pp. 48–74). New York: Guilford Press.

Salkovskis, P. M. (1999). Understanding and treating obsessive–compulsive disorder. *Behaviour Research and Therapy, 37,* S29–S52.

Salkovskis, P. M. (2002). Empirically grounded clinical interventions: Cognitive-behavioral therapy progresses through a multi-dimensional approach to clinical science. *Behavioural and Cognitive Psychotherapy, 30,* 1–10.

Samuels, J., Nestadt, G., Bienvenu, O. J., Costa, P. T., Jr., Riddle, M. A., Liang, K. Y., et al. (2000). Personality disorders and normal personality dimensions in obsessive-compulsive disorder. *British Journal of Psychiatry, 177,* 457–462.

Santanello, A. W., & Gardner, F. L. (2007). The role of experiential avoidance in the relationship between maladaptive perfectionism and worry. *Cognitive Therapy and Research, 30,* 319–332.

Sassaroli, S., Lauro, L. J. R., Ruggiero, G. M., Mauri, M. C., Vinai, P., & Frost, R. (2008). Perfectionism in depression, obsessive–compulsive disorder and eating disorders. *Behaviour Research and Therapy, 46,* 757–765.

Schmidt, U., Bone, G., Hems, S., Lessem, J., & Treasure, J. (2002). Structured therapeutic writing tasks as an adjunct to treatment in eating disorders. *European Eating Disorders Review, 10,* 299–315.

Schmidt, U., & Treasure, J. (2006). Anorexia nervosa: valued and visible. A cognitive-interpersonal maintenance model and its implications for research and practice. *British Journal of Clinical Psychology, 45,* 343–366.

Segal, Z. V., Williams, J. M. G., & Teasdale, J. D. (2013). *Mindfulness-based cognitive therapy for depression* (2nd ed.). New York: Guilford Press.

Sexton, J. D., & Pennebaker, J. W. (2009). The healing powers of expressive writing. In S. B. Kaufman & J. C. Kaufman (Eds.), *The psychology of creative writing* (pp. 264–273). New York: Cambridge University Press.

Shafran, R., Cooper, Z., & Fairburn, C. G. (2002). Clinical perfectionism: A cognitive behavioural analysis. *Behaviour Research and Therapy, 40,* 773–791.

Shafran, R., Cooper, Z., & Fairburn, C. G. (2003). "Clinical perfectionism" is not "multidimensional perfectionism": A reply to Hewitt, Flett, Besser, Sherry, & McGee. *Behaviour Research and Therapy, 41,* 1217–1220.

Shafran, R., Egan, S. J., & Wade, T. D. (2010). *Overcoming perfectionism: A self-help guide using cognitive-behavioural techniques.* London: Constable & Robinson.

Shafran, R., Lee, M., & Fairburn, C. G. (2004). Clinical perfectionism: A case report. *Behavioural and Cognitive Psychotherapy, 32,* 353–357.

Shafran, R., Lee, M., Payne, E., & Fairburn, C. G. (2006). The impact of manipulating personal standards on eating attitudes and behaviour. *Behaviour Research and Therapy, 44,* 897–906.

Shafran, R., & Mansell, W. (2001). Perfectionism and psychopathology: A review of research and treatment. *Clinical Psychology Review, 21,* 879–906.

Shahar, G. (2006). An investigation of the perfectionism/self-criticism domain of the Personal Style Inventory. *Cognitive Therapy and Research, 30,* 185–200.

Shahar, G., Blatt, S. J., Zuroff, D. C., Krupnick, J. L., & Sotsky, S. M. (2004). Perfectionism impedes social relations and response to brief treatment for depression. *Journal of Social and Clinical Psychology, 23,* 140–154.

Shahar, G., Kalnitzki, E., Shulman, S., & Blatt, S. J. (2006). Personality, motivation, and the construction of goals during the transition to adulthood. *Personality and Individual Differences, 40,* 53–63.

Shawyer, F., Meadows, G. N., Judd, F., Martin, P. R., Segal, Z., & Piterman, L. (2012). The DARE study of relapse prevention in depression: Design for a phase 1/2 translational randomised controlled trial involving mindfulness-based cognitive therapy and supported self monitoring. *BMC Psychiatry, 12*(3). Retrieved from *www.biomedcentral.com/1471-244X/12/3.*

Shea, A. J., & Slaney, R. B. (1999). The *Dyadic Almost Perfect Scale.* Unpublished scale. Pennsylvania State University, University Park, PA.

Shea, A. J., Slaney, R. B., & Rice, K. G. (2006). Perfectionism in intimate relationships: The Dyadic Almost Perfect Scale. *Measurement and Evaluation in Counseling and Development, 39,* 107–125.

Sheehan, D. V., Lecrubier, Y., Sheehan, K. H., Amorim, P., Janavs, J., Weiller, E., et al. (1998). The Mini-International Neuropsychiatric Interview (M.I.N.I.): The development and validation of a structured diagnostic psychiatric interview for DSM-IV and ICD–10. *Journal of Clinical Psychiatry, 59*(Suppl. 20), 22–33.

Singer, A. R., & Dobson, K. S. (2007). An experimental investigation of the cognitive vulnerability to depression. *Behaviour Research and Therapy, 45,* 563–575.

Singer, A. R., & Dobson, K. S. (2009). The effect of the cognitive style of acceptance on negative mood in a recovered depressed sample. *Depression and Anxiety, 26,* 471–479.

Slade, P. (1982). Towards a functional analysis of anorexia nervosa and bulimia nervosa. *British Journal of Clinical Psychology, 21,* 167–179.

Slade, P. D., & Owens, R. G. (1998). A dual process model of perfectionism based on reinforcement theory. *Behavior Modification, 22,* 372–390.

Slaney, R. B., & Johnson, D. G. (1992). *The Almost Perfect Scale.* Unpublished scale, Pennsylvania State University, University Park, PA.

Slaney, R. B., Rice, K. G., & Ashby, J. (2002). A programmatic approach to measuring perfectionism. In G. L. Flett & P. L. Hewitt (Eds.), *Perfectionism: Theory, research, and treatment* (pp. 63–88). Washington, DC: American Psychological Association.

Slaney, R. B., Rice, K. G., Mobley, M., Trippi, J., & Ashby, J. S. (2001). The Revised Almost Perfect Scale. *Measurement and Evaluation in Counseling and Development, 34,* 130–145.

Snell, W. E., Overbey, G. A., & Brewer, A. L. (2005). Parenting perfectionism and the parenting role. *Personality and Individual Differences, 39,* 613–624.

Somov, P. (2010). *Present perfect: A mindfulness approach to letting go of perfectionism and the need for control.* Oakland, CA: New Harbinger.

Sorotzkin, B. (1998). Understanding and treating perfectionism in religious adolescents. *Psychotherapy, 35,* 87–95.

Southgate, L., Tchanturia, K., Collier, D., & Treasure, J. (2008). The development of the Childhood Retrospective Perfectionism Questionnaire (CHIRP) in an eating disorder sample. *European Eating Disorders Review, 16,* 451–462.

Srinivasagam, N. M., Kaye, W. H., Plotnicov, K. H., Greeno, C., Welzin, T. E., & Rao, R. (1995). Persistent perfectionism, symmetry, and exactness after long-term recovery from anorexia nervosa. *American Journal of Psychiatry, 152,* 1630–1634.

Steele, A. L., Bergin, J. L., & Wade, T. D. (2011). Self-efficacy as a robust predictor of outcome in guided self-help treatment for broadly defined bulimia nervosa. *International Journal of Eating Disorders, 44,* 389–396.

Steele, A. L., O'Shea, A., Murdock, A., & Wade, T. D. (2011). Perfectionism and its relation to overvaluation of weight and shape and depression in an eating disorder sample. *International Journal of Eating Disorders, 4,* 459–464.

Steele, A. L., & Wade, T. D. (2008). A randomised trial investigating guided self-help to reduce perfectionism and its impact on bulimia nervosa: A pilot study. *Behaviour Research and Therapy, 46,* 1316–1323.

Steele, A. L., Waite, S., Egan, S. J., Finnigan, J., Handley, A., & Wade, T. D. (2013). Psychoeducation and group cognitive-behavioural therapy for clinical perfectionism: A case-series evaluation. *Behavioural and Cognitive Psychotherapy, 41,* 129–143.

Stice, E. (2002). Risk and maintenance factors for eating pathology: A meta-analytic review. *Psychological Bulletin, 128,* 825–848.

Stoeber, J. (2011). Perfectionism, efficiency, and response bias in proof-reading performance: Extension and replication. *Personality and Individual Differences, 50,* 426–429.

Stoeber, J., & Damian, L. E. (2014). The Clinical Perfectionism Questionnaire: Further evidence for two factors capturing perfectionistic strivings and concerns. *Personality and Individual Differences, 61–62,* 38–42.

Stoeber, J., Harris, R. A., & Moon, P. S. (2007). Perfectionism and the experience of pride, shame, and guilt: Comparing healthy perfectionists, unhealthy perfectionists, and non-perfectionists. *Personality and Individual Differences, 43,* 131–141.

Stoeber, J., Hoyle, A., & Last, F. (2013). The Consequences of Perfectionism Scale: Factorial structure and relationships with perfectionism, performance perfectionism, affect, and depressive symptoms. *Measurement and Evaluation in Counseling and Development, 46,* 178–191.

Stoeber, J., & Joorman, J. (2001). Worry, procrastination and perfectionism: Differentiating amount of worry, pathological worry, anxiety and depression. *Cognitive Therapy and Research, 25,* 49–60.

Stoeber, J., Kempe, T., & Keogh, E. J. (2008). Facets of self-oriented and socially prescribed perfectionism and feelings of pride, shame and guilt following success and failure. *Personality and Individual Differences, 44,* 1506–1516.

Stoeber, J., Kobori, O., & Tanno, Y. (2010). The Multidimensional Perfectionism Cognitions Inventory—English (MPCI-E): Reliability, validity, and relationships with positive and negative affect. *Journal of Personality Assessment, 92,* 16–25.

Stott, R., Mansell, W., Salkovskis, P. M., Lavender, A., & Cartwright-Hatton, S. (2010). *Oxford guide to metaphors in CBT: Building cognitive bridges.* Oxford, UK: Oxford University Press.

Summerfeldt, L. J., Kloosterman, P. H., & Antony, M. M. (2010). Structured and semi-structured interviews. In M. M. Antony & D. H. Barlow (Eds.), *Handbook of assessment and treatment planning for psychological disorders* (2nd ed., pp. 95–137). New York: Guilford Press.

Sutandar-Pinnock, K., Woodside, D. B., Carter, J. C., Olmsted, M. P., & Kaplan, A. S. (2003). Perfectionism in anorexia nervosa: A 6–24-month follow-up study. *International Journal of Eating Disorders, 33,* 225–229.

Terry-Short, L. A., Owens, R. G., Slade, P. D., & Dewey, M. E. (1995). Positive and negative perfectionism. *Personality and Individual Differences, 18,* 663–668.

Tozzi, F., Aggen, S. H., Neale, B. M., Anderson, C. B., Mazzeo, S. E., Neale, M. C., et al. (2004). The structure of perfectionism: A twin study. *Behavior Genetics, 34,* 483–494.

Van Dam, N. T., Sheppard, S. C., Forsyth, J. P., & Earleywine, M. (2011). Self-compassion is a better predictor than mindfulness of symptom severity and QOL in mixed anxiety and depression. *Journal of Anxiety Disorders, 25,* 123–130.

Vandiver, B. J., & Worrell, F. C. (2002). The reliability and validity of scores on the Almost Perfect Scale—Revised with academically talented middle school students. *Journal of Secondary Gifted Education, 13,* 108–119.

Wade, T. D., Frayne, A., Edwards, S. A., Robertson, T., & Gilchrist, P. (2009). Motivational change in an inpatient anorexia nervosa population and implications for treatment. *Australian and New Zealand Journal of Psychiatry, 43,* 235–243.

Wade, T. D., & Schmidt, U. (2009). Writing therapies for eating disorders. In S. Paxton & P. Hay (Eds.), *Treatment approaches for body dissatisfaction and eating disorders: Evidence and practice* (pp. 251–267). Melbourne, Australia: IP Communications.

Wade, T. D., Treasure, J., & Schmidt, U. (2011). A case series evaluation of the Maudsley model for treatment of adults with anorexia nervosa. *European Eating Disorder Review, 19,* 382–389.

Wade, T. D., Treloar, S. A., & Martin, N. G. (2008). Shared and unique risk factors between lifetime purging and objective binge eating: A twin study. *Psychological Medicine, 38*, 1455–1464.

Waller, G. (2012). The myths of motivation: Time for a fresh look at some received wisdom in the eating disorders? *International Journal of Eating Disorders, 45*, 1–16.

Waller G., Cordery, E., Corstorphine, H., Hinrichsen, R., Lawson, R., Mountford, V., et al. (2007). *Cognitive behavioral therapy for eating disorders: A comprehensive treatment guide.* Cambridge, UK: Cambridge University Press.

Waller, G., Mountford, V., Lawson, R., Gray, E., Cordery, H., & Hinrichsen, H. (2010). *Beating your eating disorder: A cognitive-behavioural self-help guide for adult sufferers and their carers.* Cambridge, UK: Cambridge University Press.

Wang, K. T. (2010). The Family Almost Perfect Scale: Development, psychometric properties, and comparing Asian and European Americans. *Asian American Journal of Psychology, 1*, 186–199.

Wang, K. T., Methikalam, B., & Slaney, R. B. (2010). *Family Almost Perfect Scale.* Unpublished scale. Pennsylvania State University, University Park, PA.

Weathers, F. W., Huska, J. A., & Keane, T. M. (1991). *PCL-C for DSM-IV.* Boston: National Center for PTSD—Behavioral Science Division.

Webb, C. A., DeRubeis, R. J., Dimidjian, S., Hollon, S. D., Amsterdam, J. D., & Shelton, R. C. (2012). Predictors of patient cognitive therapy skills and symptom change in two randomized clinical trials: The role of therapist adherence and the therapeutic alliance. *Journal of Consulting and Clinical Psychology, 80*, 373–381.

Weissman, A. N., & Beck, A. T. (1978, August–September). *Development and validation of the Dysfunctional Attitude Scale: A preliminary investigation.* Paper presented at the meeting of the American Psychological Association, Toronto, Ontario, Canada.

Wells, A. (1997). *Cognitive therapy of anxiety disorders: A practice manual and conceptual guide.* Chichester, UK: Wiley.

West, R. (2005). Time for a change: Putting the transtheoretical (stages of change) model to rest. *Addiction, 100*, 1036–1039.

Westerberg, J., Edlund, B., & Ghaderi, A. (2008). A 2-year longitudinal study of eating attitudes, BMI, perfectionism, asceticism and family climate in adolescent girls and their parents. *Eating and Weight Disorders, 13*, 64–72.

Westerberg-Jacobson, J., Edlund, B., & Ghaderi, A. (2010). Risk and protective factors for disturbed eating: A 7-year longitudinal study of eating attitudes and psychological factors in adolescent girls and their parents. *Eating and Weight Disorders, 15*, e208–e218.

Westra, H. A., Arkowitz, H., & Dozois, D. J. (2009). Adding a motivational interviewing pretreatment to cognitive behavioral therapy for generalized anxiety disorder: A preliminary randomised controlled trial. *Journal of Anxiety Disorders, 23*, 1106–1117.

Wheatley, J., Brewin, C. R., Patel, T., Hackmann, A., Wells, A., Fisher, P., et al. (2007). I'll believe it when I can see it: Imagery rescripting of intrusive sensory memories in depression. *Journal of Behavior Therapy and Experimental Psychiatry, 38*, 371–385.

Wheatley, J., & Hackmann, A. (2011). Using imagery rescripting to treat major depression: Theory and practice. *Cognitive and Behavioral Practice, 18,* 444–453.

White, C., & Schweitzer, R. (2000). The role of personality in the development and perpetuation of chronic fatigue syndrome. *Journal of Psychosomatic Research, 48,* 515–524.

Whittal, M. L., Woody, S. R., McLean, P. D., Rachman, S. J., & Robichaud, M. (2010). Treatment of obsessions: A randomised controlled trial. *Behaviour Research and Therapy, 48,* 295–303.

Wild, J., Hackmann, A., & Clark, D. M. (2007). When the present visits the past: Updating traumatic memories in social phobia. *Journal of Behavior Therapy and Experimental Psychiatry, 38,* 386–401.

Wild, J., Hackmann, A., & Clark, D. M. (2008). Rescripting early memories linked to negative images in social phobia: A pilot study. *Behavior Therapy, 39,* 47–56.

Wilksch, S. M., Durbridge, M. R., & Wade, T. D. (2008). A preliminary controlled comparison of programs designed to reduce risk of eating disorders targeting perfectionism and media literacy. *Journal of the American Academy of Child and Adolescent Psychiatry, 47,* 939–947.

Williams, J. M. G., Teasdale, J. D., Segal, Z. V., & Kabat-Zinn, J. (2007). *The mindful way through depression: Freeing yourself from chronic unhappiness.* New York: Guilford Press.

Woods, D. W., & Miltenberger, R. G. (Eds.). (2001). *Tic disorders, trichotillomania, and other repetitive behavior disorders: Behavioral approaches to analysis and treatment.* New York: Springer.

Yang, H., & Stoeber, J. (2012). The Physical Appearance Perfectionism Scale: Development and preliminary validation. *Journal of Psychopathology and Behavioral Assessment, 34,* 69–83.

Yerkes, R. M., & Dodson, J. D. (1908). The relation of strength of stimulus to rapidity of habit-formation. *Journal of Comparative Neurology and Psychology, 18,* 459–482.

Zuroff, D. C., & Blatt, S. J. (2006). The therapeutic relationship in the brief treatment of depression: Contributions to clinical improvement and enhanced adaptive capacities. *Journal of Consulting and Clinical Psychology, 74,* 130–140.

Zuroff, D. C., Blatt, S. J., Sotsky, S. M., Krupnick, J. L., Martin, D. J., & Simmens, S. (2000). Relation of therapeutic alliance and perfectionism to outcome in brief outpatient treatment of depression. *Journal of Consulting and Clinical Psychology, 68,* 114–124.

Zuroff, D. C., Kelly, A. C., Leybman, M. J., Blatt, S. J., & Wampold, B. E. (2010). Between-therapist and within-therapist differences in the quality of the therapeutic relationship: Effects on maladjustment and self-critical perfectionism. *Journal of Clinical Psychology, 66,* 681–697.

Index